Clinics in Developmental Medicine No. 145
A NEURODEVELOPMENTAL APPROACH
TO SPECIFIC LEARNING DISORDERS

© 1999 Mac Keith Press
High Holborn House, 52–54 High Holborn, London WC1V 6RL

Senior Editor: Martin C.O. Bax
Editor: Hilary M. Hart
Managing Editor: Michael Pountney
Sub-editor: Suzanne Miller
Indexer: Jill Halliday

Set in Times and Avant Garde on QuarkXPress

The views and opinions expressed herein are those of the authors and do not necessarily
represent those of the publisher

Accuracy of referencing is the responsibility of the authors

First published in this edition 1999

British Library Cataloguing-in-Publication data:
A catalogue record for this book is available from the British Library

ISSN: 0069 4835
ISBN: 1 898683 11 5

Printed by The Lavenham Press Ltd, Water Street, Lavenham, Suffolk
Mac Keith Press is supported by Scope (formerly The Spastics Society)

Clinics in Developmental Medicine No. 145

A Neurodevelopmental Approach to Specific Learning Disorders

Edited by

KINGSLEY WHITMORE
Department of Child Health
Chelsea and Westminster Hospital
London

HILARY HART
Mac Keith Press
London

GUY WILLEMS
Paediatric Neurology Service
William Lennox Neurological Center and
Saint-Luc University Hospital
Brussels

1999
Mac Keith Press

Distributed by 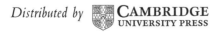 CAMBRIDGE
UNIVERSITY PRESS

CONTENTS

CONTRIBUTORS

Martin Bax, DM, FRCPCH	Senior Lecturer in Child Health, Imperial College School of Medicine, London, UK
April A Benasich, PhD	Assistant Professor of Neuroscience, Center for Molecular and Behavioral Neuroscience, Rutgers University, Newark, NJ, USA
Peter Born, MD	Research Assistant, Department of Neuropediatrics, John F Kennedy Institute, Glostrup, Denmark
J Keith Brown, MB ChB, FRCPE	Consultant Paediatric Neurologist, Edinburgh Sick Children's NHS Trust, Royal Hospital for Sick Children, Edinburgh, Scotland, UK
Philippe Evrard, MD	Professor and Chief, Pediatric Neurology Service, Xavier-Bichat Medical School (University of Paris VII Denis-Diderot), Hôpital Robert-Debré, Paris, France
Christopher Gillberg, MD	Professor, Department of Child and Adolescent Psychiatry, Annedals Clinics, Göteborg University, Göteborg, Sweden
Neil Gordon, MB ChB, MD, FRCP	*Formerly* Paediatric Neurologist, Manchester Children's Hospitals, Manchester, UK *(Retired)*
Mijna Hadders-Algra, MD, PhD	Senior Lecturer in Developmental Neurophysiology, Department of Medical Physiology, Section of Developmental Neurology, University Hospital Groningen, Groningen, The Netherlands
Elina Lindahl, MD, PhD	Department of Child Neurology, Hospital for Children and Adolescents, University of Helsinki, Helsinki, Finland
Hans C Lou, MD	Professor of Developmental Neurology, Department of Neuropediatrics, John F Kennedy Institute, Glostrup, Denmark
Robert A Minns, PhD, FRCPE	Consultant Paediatric Neurologist, Edinburgh Sick Children's NHS Trust, Royal Hospital for Sick Children, Edinburgh, Scotland, UK

Thomas G O'Connor, PhD	Lecturer in Developmental Psychology, Departments of Psychology and of Child and Adolescent Psychology, Institute of Psychiatry, London, UK
Anne O'Hare, MD, FRCP	Consultant Paediatrician, Edinburgh Sick Children's NHS Trust, Royal Hospital for Sick Children, Edinburgh, Scotland, UK
Robert C Pianta, PhD	Associate Professor, Curry School of Education, University of Virginia, Charlottesville, VA, USA
Helene J Polatajko, PhD, OT(C)	Professor and Director, School of Occupational Therapy, Faculty of Health Sciences, The University of Western Ontario, London, Ontario, Canada
Peder Rasmussen, MD	Senior Lecturer in Child Neurology, Department of Child and Adolescent Psychiatry, Göteborg University; and Child Neuropsychiatry Clinic, Sahlgren University Hospital, Göteborg, Sweden
Sonia Sharp, PhD	Chief Educational Psychologist, Educational Psychology Service, Education Department, County Hall, Aylesbury, Buckinghamshire, UK
Romy V Spitz, PhD	Postdoctoral Fellow, Child Language Program, University of Kansas, Lawrence, KS, USA
Jim Stevenson, PhD, FBPsS, CPsychol	Professor of Psychology and Health, Centre for Research into Psychological Development, Department of Psychology, University of Southampton, Southampton, UK
Kingsley Whitmore, MRCS, LRCP, DCH	Research Paediatrician in Community Paediatrics, Westminster Children's Hospital, London, UK
Guy Willems, MD	Associate Head of Department, Paediatric Neurology Service, William Lennox Neurological Center and Saint-Luc University Hospital; and Developmental Neurology Unit, Catholic University of Louvain, Medical School, Brussels, Belgium

FOREWORD

The authors of this book address the issue of specific learning disorders. By that, they mean those disorders of learning that seem to have a biological basis – the reading and spelling difficulties, clumsiness, dyscalculia and dysgraphia, the attention-deficit disorders. Together all these constitute a complex group of disorders and the difficulty of studying them is compounded by problems of definition and categorization, which are discussed in the first chapter.

There are also differences in the terminology used by experts in the various relevant fields in different parts of the developed world. For example in Europe, where it is no longer respectable to talk about 'mental retardation', people now talk, instead, of moderate or severe learning disabilities or disorders, whereas in North America the term *learning disorders* is largely reserved for the group of children with whom this book is concerned.

Equally, learning disorders clearly relate to functioning in the preschool child. For example, depending on which study you look at, something over half of children who have a speech and language problem at age 3 years go on to have a problem with reading when they reach school age. In general the editors decided not to review those data here. There are many studies on the preschool child and in the important area of preschool language; one is the recent overview *Language, Learning and Behaviour Disorders: Developmental, Biological and Clinical Perspectives,* edited by Beitchman, Cohen, Konstantareas, and Tannock (Cambridge University Press). The editors of the present book have, however, included a look at some of the other precursors of learning difficulties.

This book had its origin in a workshop organized by the Little Foundation, where the problem of specific learning disorders was discussed with a view to prevention. A concluding discussion at the workshop suggested that if our knowledge of specific learning disorders was applied, it could be used to lead to prevention, or, rather, such effective early intervention that the child would not get into difficulties. The editors were therefore asked to create a book providing the understanding that could lead to effective prevention. The task was not a simple one. They have called on an international group of authors who have created a depth and diversity of information and knowledge that should allow the reader to provide effective help for children who may either have a specific learning disorder or be at risk of developing one.

MARTIN BAX, DM
Imperial College School of Medicine

1
WHAT DO WE MEAN BY SLD? A HISTORICAL PERSPECTIVE

Kingsley Whitmore and Martin Bax

This book is about some of the problems that some children have in learning. Nowadays, when time and money are scarce and keywords in scientific publications are reduced to capital letters, such problems are commonly referred to as 'SLDs' – but we need to be aware that the letters *S, L,* and *D* do not always stand for the same words. Most readers are likely to assume that they are short for *specific learning disorder* – but some authors use them to mean *specific language disorder* and others, *specific learning disability, dysfunction, difficulty, defect,* or *disturbance* – these last five words all conveniently beginning with the letter D. No one to our knowledge has yet described the conditions in question as disadvantages, though as regards development, disadvantage is certainly what children with SLD experience, both academically and socially. It is equally certain that the two words beginning with *L, language* and *learning,* are not synonymous; nor are most of those beginning with *D,* especially *difficulties, disabilities,* and *disorders.* A further anomaly is that while readers might rightly assume that *S* stands for *specific,* meaning 'precise' or 'clearly defined,' authors seldom make it clear whether it is the *L* or the *D* that is specific and that when *D* stands for *disorder* a specific disorder is one that can*not* be clearly defined!

Those of us who struggle to find a rational, applicable concept of SLD will find complication rather than clarification from a study of various classifications of learning disorders produced during the past 45 years. The two systems most widely quoted are those of the American Psychiatric Association (*Diagnostic and Statistical Manual of Mental Disorders* – DSM) and of the World Health Organization (WHO) (*International Classification of Diseases* – ICD) (Table 1.1). These are disconcerting not only because of the extent to which they differ despite attempts to make them more compatible but particularly because of how each vacillates with ensuing versions (Rispens and van Yperen 1997).

DSM-I (American Psychiatric Association 1952) identified learning disturbances as one of several special symptom reactions, along with speech disturbance and enuresis. The next edition (DSM-II; American Psychiatric Association 1968) described the same phenomena as 'specific learning disturbances'. The word *learning* disappeared from DSM-III (American Psychiatric Association 1980), which defined disorders of reading, arithmetic, language, and articulation each separately as a 'specific developmental disorder'. The next revision, DSM-III-R (American Psychiatric Association 1987), retained 'specific developmental disorders' (SDDs), but as a subgroup of 'developmental disorders', the other two subgroups

TABLE 1.1
Changes in terminology and classification of specific learning disorders

By the American Psychiatric Association (DSM)	By the World Health Organization (ICD)

DSM-I *Special symptom reactions*
(1952) • Learning disturbance
     • Speech disturbance
      (Enuresis and sleep somnambulism)	

	ICD-7 *Other and unspecified character,*
	(1957) *behaviour, and intelligence disorders*
	     • Specific learning defects
	     • Stammering and stuttering
	     • Other speech impediments
	     • Acute situational maladjustment

DSM-II *Special symptoms*
(1968) • Speech disturbance (stuttering)
     • Specific learning disturbance
      (Tics, enuresis, and disorders of
      sleep)	

	ICD-9 *Specific delays in development*
	(1978) • Specific reading retardation
	     • Specific arithmetical retardation
	     • Other specific learning difficulties
	     • Developmental speech/language disorders
	     • Specific motor retardation

DSM-III *Specific developmental disorders*
(1980) • Developmental reading disorder
     • Developmental arithmetic disorder
     • Developmental language disorder
     • Developmental articulation disorder
      (Mixed and atypical developmental
      disorders)	

DSM-III-R *Developmental disorders*
(1987) • Mental retardation
     • Pervasive developmental disorders
     • Specific developmental disorders
     (SDDs)
      • In academic skills
        • Developmental arithmetic disorder
        • Developmental expressive writing
         disorder
        • Developmental reading disorder
      • In language and speech
        • Developmental articulation disorder
        • Developmental expressive language
         disorder
        • Developmental receptive language
         disorder
      • In motor skills
        • Developmental coordination disorder	

(Table continues on the next page)

TABLE 1.1
(Continued)

By the American Psychiatric Association (DSM)	By the World Health Organization (ICD)
	ICD-10 *Disorders of psychological development*
	(1992) • Including SDD of speech and language
	• (Including acquired aphasia with epilepsy)
	• SDD of scholastic skills
	• SDD of motor function
	• Pervasive developmental disorder
DSM-IV *Disorders usually first diagnosed in*	
(1994) *infancy, childhood, or adolescence*	
Learning disorders	
• Reading disorder	
• Mathematics disorder	
• Disorder of written expression	
Motor skills disorder	
• Developmental coordination disorder	
Communication disorders	
• Expressive language disorder	
• Mixed receptive–expressive language	
disorder	
• Phonological disorder	
• Stuttering	

(Based on findings in Rispens and van Yperen 1997.)
DSM, *Diagnostic and Statistical Manual of Mental Disorders;* ICD, *International Classification of Diseases;*
SDD, specific developmental disorder.

being 'mental retardation' and 'pervasive developmental disorders'. 'Developmental coordination disorder' was for the first time classified as an SDD in motor skills. The latest edition, DSM-IV (American Psychiatric Association 1994), has renamed developmental disorders as 'disorders usually first diagnosed in infancy, childhood, or adolescence'; the word *specific* has vanished from all levels of classification; and 'learning disorders' have been reinstated as a main subgroup, alongside 'motor skills disorder' and 'communication disorders'. Curiously the latter includes phonological disorder, which, we are repeatedly informed, is the underlying dysfunction in most children who have difficulty in learning to read (see Snowling 1996) – which is classified as a learning disorder.

In the WHO classification ICD-7 (World Health Organization 1957), specific learning defects were differentiated from speech impediments as one subgroup of other 'character, behaviour, and intelligence disorders'. In ICD-9 (World Health Organization 1978) 'other specific learning difficulties' became one of the five subgroups of 'specific delays in development', which included specific retardations in reading, arithmetic, and motor skills. In ICD-10 (World Health Organization 1992), under a heading of 'disorders of psychological development', the term *learning* disappeared from the classification (as it had from DSM-III in 1980). SDDs of speech and language, of scholastic skills, and of motor function, and pervasive developmental disorders, all became subgroups of 'disorders of psychological development'.

Such contradictions in the terminology and classification of learning disorders are exasperating, but perhaps it is not too surprising that they have arisen if we bear in mind that there is still no clear consensus as to what it is that is being classified. It is easy to be critical, but if viewed in a historical context all these changes become more tolerable and even exciting – evidence of how, as civilized society enters the information age, it is taking another step towards unravelling the mysteries of the mind.

Different professional approaches

The present contradictions appear at first to result from unresolved differences between the medical, educational, and psychological approaches to the unravelling of learning problems, sparked off more than 100 years ago by doctors' and teachers' coincidental interest in the school dunce: a child who was slow at learning, a stupid person. Stupidity (lack of intelligence) has always been the hallmark of 'mental retardation', as the first learning disorder to be studied by doctors in the middle of the 19th century was then called. Doubtless for generations there had also been teachers who had been puzzled by the paradox of otherwise intelligent children who could neither read nor write. As Gordon reminded us (1992), such children were very likely to have been described by their teachers in the 1860s as 'thoroughly stupid'. Difficulty in learning to read (so-called dyslexia, although the term actually means difficulty with language) has since been the specific learning problem that has received the most attention from a variety of disciplines. Interestingly it was a doctor who first used the term *word blindness* to describe the loss of previously normal reading skills associated with sudden aphasia in adults who were found at autopsy to have acquired lesions in their left cerebral hemisphere (Kussmaul 1877) and it was a doctor who suggested the term *dyslexia* (Berlin 1887). Furthermore it was a general practitioner (Morgan 1896) who first described a case of 'congenital word blindness' in an intelligent, 14-year-old boy. In general, doctors are primarily interested in the nature and cause of morphological changes that might account for a patient's symptoms and signs – i.e. the aetiological aspects, why a child has a neurological defect that interferes with the child's development or behaviour – since this is the key to treatment (mitigation or cure) and prevention of the disorder or disease. In contrast, teachers and, more recently, psychologists are mainly interested in fathoming how children normally learn particular academic and social skills and in determining at which stage the normal learning process has been interrupted – i.e. they are interested in the functional aspects of problems in development and behaviour, since there may be alternative methods of helping a child to learn a skill that circumvent the effect of morphological changes, whatever their cause may be. It has not been easy to reconcile these different aspects to produce a single classification that satisfies both objectives, though many have tried.

The helpfulness of an aetiological classification in understanding disorders was clearly shown when Down (1866) recognized three main groups of people with severe mental disability, or 'idiots': the congenital, the accidental, and the developmental. This classification led to the identification of another form of mental retardation, Down syndrome (previously called 'mongolism'), and to the idea that mental retardation was probably not a single entity but was due to a variety of pathologically and aetiologically different disorders capable of damaging the brain and causing abnormal behaviour. A decade later Ireland (1877) suggested that there might be at least 10 identifiable causes, one of which he astutely called 'idiocy from deprivation'.

The association between stupidity and abnormal behaviour is particularly interesting in relation to brain damage. Little (1862) was well aware in his first description of cerebral palsy that a cognitive defect was often present in addition to a motor defect but that the latter alone could result in such bizarre behavioural responses, due to lack of motor control, as to suggest that mental retardation was present when it actually was not. Still (1902) later described a group of children with hyperactive behaviour similar to that shown by children with mental retardation, though often more severe, *in the absence of demonstrable evidence of brain damage.* He postulated that this was nevertheless the result of either organic or moral factors. Thus the germ of the idea was formed that brain damage was the common factor in mental retardation, cerebral palsy, and hyperkinesis.

The introduction of IQ tests

The construction of a test of intelligence by two French physicians (Binet and Simon 1908) was a landmark in the history of learning disorders, enabling an 'intelligence quotient' (IQ) to be calculated. Eventually such tests were accepted as providing a sufficiently objective, scientific, and accurate measurement of a child's intellectual potential to warrant the use of an IQ score of approximately 70 or less (i.e. lower than 2 standard deviations below the mean) as the principal diagnostic criterion of mental retardation. This was not good news for some children whose IQ was less than 70: it could lead to standardized decisions by a doctor that they should be educated as if they were mentally retarded, regardless of the reason for their subnormal IQ scores. For instance in the UK, where education for primary school children (aged 5 to 11 years) has been compulsory since 1880, statutory regulations made school doctors responsible for ascertaining which pupils suffered from such a disability of mind or body as to require special educational treatment. Until the 1970s, in an uneasy partnership with teachers and educational psychologists and after attending special courses in the administration of an intelligence test, school doctors relied heavily on IQ scores of 70 or less to bolster their diagnosis of mental retardation. If the retardation was only mild, they formally 'ascertained' that a child was a 'handicapped' pupil (in this case 'educationally subnormal'), needing education in a special school. Children with an IQ of less than approximately 60 were very likely to be ascertained to be ineducable or unsuitable for education in school, and thus to be deprived of the help of qualified specialist teachers.

However, the use of an IQ cut-off score was good news for children who had an IQ of more than 70 but were failing in school in spite of being taught by qualified teachers, because it sparked off intensive and wide-ranging studies of child development in general and child psychology in particular, by practitioners and researchers of many disciplines interested in learning, which continue unabated today. Important classification of such pupils began to emerge in the 1930s and 1940s. Burt (1937), on the basis of his surveys in London schools, distinguished three principal groups: (1) the dull and backward, whose *mental* ratio was 70 to 85% of normal and whose disability was general and innate; (2) the educationally retarded or merely backward, whose *educational* ratio (performance) was less than 85% of normal for their age and whose disability was also general, but was acquired; and (3) children with a specific disability, whose 'defect' was not general, but limited. There are obvious inconsistencies in this psychological classification, but Burt confessed that it was chosen as a means to an end, as a practical aid rather than a scientific finality. And he explained that the term *specific disability* – 'its psychology is still in its infancy' – was used to describe a poorer result on selected tests of particular intellectual processes (such as visual or auditory perception, reasoning, and various aspects of attention and memory) than the responses of another child whose mental age was less than 85% of that particular child's *mental* age.

Schonell (1942), after summarizing the four most important types of forces or influences that contribute to the individual differences between children (intellectual, emotional, physical, and environmental factors), emphasized that many deviations from average scholastic performance were natural variations that did not need special consideration. He regarded pupils as backward only if their inability to reach a standard of scholastic performance normal for their age was sufficiently marked to warrant special remedial measures. Such backwardness might be in all or most subjects (general backwardness) or in only one or two (specific backwardness); and it might be primarily due to either innate or acquired (extrinsic) factors. So he described three types of backward children: (a) those who were generally backward because they were to some extent innately mentally dull; (b) those who were generally backward, not because they were innately dull, but because of some acquired condition; and (c) those who were specifically backward in only one or two subjects. His classification of types of backwardness, which he also used as 'categories of convenience', was therefore very similar to Burt's, save in three important respects, perhaps reflecting their different disciplines. As an educationist rather than a psychologist, Schonell suspected that both the generally and the specifically backward pupils usually owed their problems to a combination of innate and acquired factors, and he appreciated that a specific disability in only one subject was the exception rather than the rule, disability in reading frequently being associated with backwardness in spelling and written composition. He was also more discriminating in his classification than Burt, being careful not to use the terms *backward* and *retarded* as if they were interchangeable: Schonell regarded backwardness in children as poor performance relative to the average for their age group and retardation as poor performance relative to personal intellectual capacity. And, finally, he realized that this latter kind of underachievement (learning problem) could arise in dull as well as in bright pupils, though among bright pupils it was most often referred to as a specific learning disability (especially in the case of dyslexia).

The era of brain damage
In the 5 years between Burt's and Schonell's studies the association of inattentive or hyperkinetic behaviour, or both, with brain damage dominated medical interest in the field of SLD. This interest had been reawakened by reports of the emergence of such behaviour in children after recovery from encephalitis (in the 1918 pandemic). Although these children were not mentally retarded and were found to be physically and neurologically normal on

examination, some of the many new tests being devised to assess cerebral function revealed, in many cases, perceptual–motor and learning defects. These defects were similar to those being observed among soldiers who had survived head injuries during the First World War. When Werner and Strauss (1939) came to use such tests on children whose mental retardation was exogenous (associated with pre-, peri-, or postnatal brain insult), they too found a combination of problems of attention, hyperactivity, and perception not detected in children whose mental retardation was endogenous (largely familial in origin). As such problems had already been seen in association with other abnormal physical signs after seizures, measles, lead poisoning, and so on, which were known to cause brain damage sometimes, Werner and Strauss suggested that when the problems occurred, apparently spontaneously, in the absence of mental retardation or abnormal neurological signs, they were a result of *minimal* brain damage. This concept proved to be significant in the search for the causes of learning problems and in promoting interdisciplinary cooperation in their study and classification.

Since the introduction of child guidance clinics in the 1920s and the advent of psychodynamic methods of dealing with behavioural problems in intellectually normal children, the prevailing theory had been that children who were neither stupid nor socially disadvantaged but who could not read must be emotionally disturbed. The theory of minimal brain damage offered an alternative explanation, but it was some time before an influential consensus emerged. There was undoubtedly a recognizable group of what were later described as highly discrepant children (Paine et al. 1968) with a complex of symptoms, including specific learning, perceptual–motor, and general coordination deficits; hyperkinesis and short attention span or distractibility; and, in some cases, equivocal neurological signs and a borderline abnormal EEG (Clements and Peters 1962). What was not so widely accepted was the aetiological concept of brain damage as a homogeneous diagnostic entity. Not all children with recorded brain damage have such symptoms and signs, while many who do have them have no verifiable history or evidence of damage to their brains. In addition, the tests then available for differentiating between brain-damaged and non-brain-damaged children were suspect, having been based on the testing of mentally retarded children, and were not necessarily appropriate for children of normal intelligence with learning or behavioural problems. These tests were also lacking in standardization and reliability and were not based on a rational theory of brain function (Herbert 1964). Clements and Peters had already started using the term *minimal cerebral dysfunction* to describe discrepant children with the least conspicuous symptoms, such as solitary dyslexia or dyscalculia, because it allowed for the possibility that their symptoms were genetic in origin or even due to a delay in maturation rather than actual damage to the central nervous system. In the same year an international, multidisciplinary study group in England recommended that 'the convenient but possibly illogical term minimal cerebral dysfunction [should be used] rather than the anatomical term minimal brain damage', mainly because a 'disorder of brain function is the evidence used for applying a diagnostic label of minimal brain damage' (Bax and Mac Keith 1963). For similar reasons, in the USA a Task Force on Terminology and Identification (Clements 1966) opted for *minimal cerebral dysfunction syndrome* – not that minimal cerebral dysfunction was any more a diagnosis than minimal cerebral damage, but, as Paine and his colleagues pointed out, it was a less presumptuous way of describing a variety of unrelated minor dysfunctions, some neurological, some behavioural, and some cognitive, due to a variety of 'dimensions, some innate, some traumatic and psycho-social' (Rodin et al. 1964) in a group of children who they suspected 'would merge imperceptibly into the normal population at one end of the scale and at the other into more obvious ones of brain damage, such as cerebral palsies and mental retardation'. It is curious that both working parties retained the term *minimal*. Quite apart from implying that in children with this syndrome, either the symptoms or the lesions or both are minimal, which is not always the case, the use of this term was a tacit acceptance of the concept then bedevilling child neurology (Ingram 1973) that minimal signs (commonly referred to as 'equivocal' or 'soft' signs) indicate subclinical affections rather than major neurological disorders, though it was widely realized that there is no constant correlation between severity of dysfunction and severity of a causal brain lesion. Follow-up studies have since shown that lifelong disability may result from minimal cerebral damage. Ingram forthrightly declared that 'the use of the term "soft signs" was diagnostic of soft thinking'. Silver and Hagin (1990) and Spreen (1995) discussed this topic in more detail; it is one of continuing interest, for, as Touwen and Sporrel (1979) shrewdly observed, while terms like *soft, equivocal,* or *minor* should be discarded, 'a neurological sign which can be properly assessed must be called a sign, whatever its significance may be…and its significance must be looked for'.

In retrospect it can be said that Strauss and Werner's observations were a timely reminder of the primacy of the organic cerebral substrate governing children's ability to learn. Clements and Peters (1962) eloquently asserted that in the assessment and diagnosis of children with learning and/or behavioural problems 'we must search as carefully among the myriad possibilities of organic causation as we have in the past among inter-personal, deprivation and stress factors'. Their exhortation was all the more significant because they were child psychiatrists. Equally important was Strauss's conclusion that mentally retarded children with brain damage might do better if the methods used to teach and help them were more specifically geared to their particular cognitive (perceptual–motor) and behavioural (distractibility) problems than the methods that were being used at the time, indiscriminately, for all mentally retarded children. He and a colleague described some suitable methods (Strauss and Lehtinen 1947) and suggested that similar ones might also help brain-damaged children who were not mentally retarded. For the first time it seemed that an aetiological concept of learning and behavioural problems might lead to an educationally appropriate prescription. Cruickshank and his associates (1961) were among the first to show that this could be so.

Early attempts to agree terminology
Unfortunately the disagreement between those who favoured a medical/aetiological rather than an educational/functional approach to terminology and management rumbled on in the USA through the 1950s, until the inadequacies of available teaching resources and the concern of parents helped to bring about a working agreement. Responding to an invitation from the parents of 'perceptually handicapped' children to address their conference in 1963, after discussing the danger and relative uselessness of specific diagnostic labels,

Kirk (who spent his early career working with mentally retarded children but may be better remembered today for his development of the Illinois Test of Psycholinguistic Abilities [ITPA]; Kirk et al. 1968) advocated the use of the term *learning-disabled* instead of *brain-damaged, perceptually handicapped,* etc. A year earlier (1962) he had defined a learning disability as

a retardation, disorder, or delayed development in one or more of the processes of speech, language, reading, spelling, writing, or arithmetic resulting from possible cerebral dysfunction and/or emotional or behavioural disturbance and not from mental retardation, sensory deprivation, or cultural or instructional factors.

In 1966 the Task Force on Terminology and Identification (Clements 1966) adopted a similar definition for the syndrome of *minimal cerebral dysfunction:*

children of near average, average or above average general intelligence with certain learning or behavioural disabilities ranging from mild to severe, which are associated with deviations of function of the central nervous system [which] may manifest themselves by various combinations of impairment in perception, conceptualization, language, memory, and control of attention, impulse, or motor function.

Two years later the National Advisory Committee on Handicapped Children (1968) submitted to the US Congress the following definition of 'children with *specific learning disabilities*':

children who have a disorder in one or more basic psychological processes involved in understanding or in using language, spoken or written, which [may] manifest itself in imperfect ability to listen, think, speak, read, write, spell, or do mathematical calculations. Such disorders include such conditions as perceptual handicaps, brain injury, minimal brain dysfunction, dyslexia and developmental aphasia. [The term] does not include learning problems which are primarily the result of visual, hearing or motor handicaps, of mental retardation, or emotional disturbance, or even of environmental, cultural or economic disadvantage.

According to Harris (1995), citing Farnham-Diggory (1978), *specific learning disabilities* in general came to describe the same difficulties previously called 'minimal brain damage' or 'cerebral dysfunction', though outside the USA neither term was ever regarded as applying only to children of average or above-average intelligence. Of course Farnham-Diggory did not know that such disabilities would be renamed 'specific disorders' (DSM-III; American Psychiatric Association 1980) and later simply 'learning disorders' (DSM-IV; American Psychiatric Association 1994). This change in terminology no doubt disappointed Cruickshank, who, interestingly, maintained in 1970 that 'if the unfortunate term learning disabilities [was] too deeply ingrained to be soon changed', it should certainly be modified to *specific learning disabilities,* because 'irrespective of the presence or absence of diagnosed neurological dysfunction, learning disabilities are essentially and almost always the result of perceptual problems based on the neurological system'. Nor would Farnham-Diggory have known that 3 years later the National Joint Committee on Learning Disabilities, which represented six professional organizations in the USA concerned with such disabilities, would issue a revised definition of learning disabilities (Hammill et al. 1981):

Learning disabilities is a general term that refers to a heterogeneous group of disorders manifested by significant difficulties in the acquisition and use of listening, speaking, reading, writing, or mathematical abilities. These disorders are intrinsic to the individual, and are presumed to be due to central nervous system dysfunction. Even though a learning disability may occur concomitantly with other handicapping conditions...(including sensory impairment, mental retardation, emotional disturbance, psychogenic factors, and environmental influences)...it is not the direct result of those conditions or influences.

This is now the definition most often used (Hammill 1990), although it differs noticeably from that of 1967 and also from those of DSM-III-R (in 1987) and DSM-IV (in 1994) and to a lesser extent from that of ICD-10 (World Health Organization 1992). In spite of a clear preference (previously expressed by a multidisciplinary seminar of the foremost experts in special education in the USA) for educationally relevant behavioural terminology, and little concern for aetiology (Hallahan and Cruickshank 1973, Levine et al. 1980), learning disabilities continued to be described in terms of both function and cause. The list of skills to which the term was to apply also remained the same, still excluding dexterity, but problems in learning them were to be referred to as generic rather than specific. The final sentence in the definition is masterfully ambiguous. Hammill's interpretation was that problems in self-regulatory behaviour, social perception, and interaction do not by themselves constitute a learning disability. This interpretation seems correct in view of the fate of a subsequent recommendation of an Interagency Committee on Learning Disabilities (1987) that social skills should be added to those specified in the National Joint Committee's definition. There may not have been a clear mandate for this proposal; in any case, for legal and economic reasons it was not accepted by the US Department of Education (Silver and Hagin 1990).

It is curious that the National Joint Committee should have become more cautious, attributing learning disabilities to central nervous system dysfunction again (though not to minimal dysfunction this time) rather than more specifically to disorders in psychological processes, as in the 1967 report. Since that report, evidence had been accumulating that while the hyperactivity and attentional problems sometimes associated with learning disabilities, for example in children with attention-deficit/hyperactivity disorder (ADHD), might be reduced by medication, the learning problems were not (Silver and Hagin 1990). The inference was that the cortical functions involved in the learning disability must be at a higher level than those involved in the motor and/or sensory neurological abnormality. Developmental neuropsychologists have been extensively researching these higher functions during the past 20 years, groping their way towards an understanding of how the brain works and why for no apparent reason in some children it does not function efficiently in respect of a particular skill they want to perform. A theoretical framework for such knowledge that is currently attracting much interest stems from the notion that higher-order functions are domain-specific, or modular (Fodor 1983, Karmiloff-Smith 1992), or, as Gardner (1983) prefers to imagine, that they are a product of multiple intelligences. *Domain-specific* is the general term favoured to cover a number of particular kinds of functions (domains), such as language. Brain modules are seen as more specific information-processing units (microdomains) within each domain, e.g. a phonological module in the language domain; and all such functional systems are

TABLE 1.2
Modular brain functions and learning disorders

Function	Localization	Disorder
Phonological processing	Left perisylvian	Dyslexia
Executive functions	Prefrontal	Attention-deficit disorder
Spatial cognition	Posterior right hemisphere	Specific mathematics/handwriting disorder
Social cognition	Limbic, orbital, and right hemisphere	Autism spectrum disorder
Long-term memory	Hippocampus, amygdala	Amnesia

(From *Diagnosing Learning Disorders: A Neuropsychological Framework,* Pennington BF, 1991, New York: The Guilford Press, p 5, by permission. Copyright © 1991 The Guilford Press.)

assumed to be subserved by (dependent upon) normal neuroanatomical growth and maturation of different parts of the central nervous system (Harris 1995; Pennington 1991).

Pennington provides a simplified model of five domains of function that govern successful performance of children in school and are most relevant to an understanding of their learning disorders (Table 1.2). He emphasizes that his theoretical framework is explicitly neuropsychological: it assumes that disorders in all five domains are examples of specific brain dysfunction caused by genetic and environmental factors that disrupt brain development. He refers to them as specific disorders of function because the dysfunctions are specific and because the term *learning disorder,* as it does not exclude mental retardation or acquired aetiologies, is broader than *learning disability.* Obviously the human brain has many functions in addition to those shown in Table 1.2, from perception to motor control, but the five listed are the ones that Pennington identifies as accounting for 'all or nearly all the learning disorders encountered by most clinicians'. He defends the exclusion of motor problems as a specific dysfunction because they are primary only in some cases of difficulties in writing, many other cases of which have a spatial cognition dysfunction. He includes attention-deficit disorder (ADD) because there are fairly large numbers of children with learning problems whose difficulties are hard to understand unless there is a category for deficits of executive function. The inclusion of autism spectrum disorder is more controversial but is another clear indication of the importance of social cognition (interaction) as a skill that has to be learned if children are to succeed in school.

In a textbook on neuropsychiatry, under the heading 'developmental disorders, Harris (1995) also differentiates between mental retardation and learning disorders. He does not regard motor discoordination as a learning disorder, though he discusses cerebral palsy as a developmental disorder in its own right, and he refers to autism in a chapter on pervasive developmental disorders. In a textbook on developmental neuropsychology, Spreen et al. (1995) describes dysfunctions frequently encountered in children, including disorders of language, learning, attention, and motor function (sensorimotor and praxis). He describes mental retardation as a developmental handicap, and autism as a psychiatric disorder. He emphasizes that the functions involved are interdependent and pure disorders are rare. Silver and Hagin (1990), respectively a child psychiatrist and a psychologist, present a clinical classification of disorders of learning based on possible causative factors, which could be either extrinsic, intrinsic, or a combination of the two (Table 1.3). They identify

TABLE 1.3
Learning disorders: clinical classification based on possible causative factors

Group I: *Extrinsic factors*	Group II: *Intrinsic factors*	Group III: *Combinations*

Social and economic deprivation
Language differences
Inappropriate or inadequate
  prior education
Emotional barriers to
  learning
	Maturational lags
	  1) Specific language disabilities
	  2) Attention deficit hyperactivity
	    disorder
	Organic defect of CNS
	Tourette's syndrome
	Autism
	Generalized cognitive immaturity,
	  cause unknown
		Categories in Group I
		  and Group II

(From *Disorders of Learning in Childhood,* Silver AA, Hagin RA, Copyright © 1990 John Wiley & Sons, Inc. Reprinted by permission of John Wiley & Sons, Inc.)

two developmentally determined intrinsic disorders due to maturational lag: ADHD, and specific language disabilities (meaning those dysfunctions in speaking, reading, spelling, writing, and mathematics that 'subsume' the use of one major area of function, language). Other disorders that these two authors consider to be based on intrinsic factors are organic defects of the central nervous system, autism, and general cognitive immaturity. Prior (1996), a practising professor of psychology, uses the term *learning difficulty* to mean at its most general level a failure to learn basic academic skills, and *specific learning difficulty* to mean a deficit in at least one area of academic achievement (reading, spelling, mathematics) associated with specific cognitive impairments in a child whose IQ is greater than 80.

So in spite of many interdisciplinary discussions, and Cruickshank's (1970) optimistic assertion nearly 30 years ago that 'sufficient common knowledge of term utilization is available to obtain a meeting of minds', problems in terminology and definition of learning disorders are still unresolved. *SLD* continues to mean different things to different people. The introduction of yet another new term, *pervasive,* into the classification 'developmental disorders' (which sometimes includes SLD) adds to the confusion, particularly when it is applied to autism as a learning disorder but not to mental retardation. One can hardly imagine a more pervasive disability than moderate to severe forms of such cognitive dysfunction. *Pervasive* may be a better word than *global,* but will it one day go the way of *minimal?* There are signs that it might (Gillberg 1991, Happé and Frith 1991).

Do differences in terminology matter?
They do. *Terminology* means 'a set of words used in a specially understood or defined sense'. A working party set up by the British Paediatric Association (1994) to consider the appropriate services for children with mental handicap, after observing how the term *mental handicap* was being replaced by *learning difficulty* or *learning disability,* concluded that while it was possible to debate terminology endlessly, it was not profitable to do so – and promptly commended an operational description of a child with a 'learning disability' as one with

an 'intellectual handicap needing extra help to experience an ordinary life...and benefit from educational opportunities...' This misdefinition exemplifies our concern about the misuse of terms whose meaning has been widely agreed, for instance in the dictionaries or (in the present context) a WHO manual (World Health Organization 1980). That manual clearly differentiated between an *impairment* (any loss or abnormality of psychological, physiological, or anatomical structure or function), a *disability* (any restriction or lack of an ability, resulting from an impairment, to perform an activity in the manner or within the range considered normal for a human being), and a *handicap* (a disadvantage for a given individual, resulting from an impairment or a disability, that limits or prevents the fulfilment of a role that is normal for such an individual, depending on age, sex, and social or cultural factors). If those definitions are used, the British Paediatric Association working party's description is tantamount to saying that a disability is the result of a handicap, a tautological nonsense matched only by the statement that one of the 'low-prevalence high severity conditions causing disability is severe learning disability (mental handicap)' (Hall 1996). Such semantic inaccuracies are inexcusable and scientifically unsound, obscuring rather than helping to clarify central issues – in this case the nature of inexplicable learning problems, disparities in the scholastic performances of some children that simply do not make sense. It is axiomatic that the only thing that one learns from history is that one does not learn from history. In their foreword to the proceedings of the International Study Group in Oxford, Bax and Mac Keith drew attention to the lessons to be learned from the meeting: 'First and foremost, surely, is how careful we must be in our use of language. If words are used...[that] confuse us they may in fact harm the patient' (Bax and Mac Keith 1963).

Undeniably there is still terminological confusion about SLD, and that confusion can harm children. Some of the confusion stems from the careless use of language; this does need further debate, which need not be endless if the discussants operate within the limits of widely agreed semantics. Much of the confusion stems from the use of the same or similar terminology that masks different concepts or definitions of 'learning' and of 'specific learning disorders'. Debate about these is essential, even though there is no resolution in sight. Rutter was pessimistic in 1978 that learning disability could ever be defined in a 'precise and persistent manner', a pessimism that underlines the difficulty of reconciling the conflicting interests of those seeking or proposing a definition.

POINTS OF VIEW OF RESEARCHERS AND ADMINISTRATORS OF SERVICES
Whereas we had at first thought that the important differences were between medical experts studying learning disorders (impairments) and educational experts dealing with their consequences (disabilities), we now realize that the more important differences lie between, on the one hand, researchers (who are primarily interested in fathoming the causes of inexplicable learning difficulties) and service administrators (whose primary interest is ensuring there are sufficient, appropriate services – medical, educational, and social – for children who have learning difficulties) and, on the other hand, paediatricians and teachers (whose responsibility is to diagnose and educate individual children with such difficulties). The principal casualties in this conflict of interests are individual children and services, because some children suffer through not being legally eligible for certain

13

forms of special education, and the people responsible for organizing services remain unaware of the true prevalence of learning disorders and hence of the true need for the service. This situation has arisen, most often in the USA, because for reasons of expediency administrators of educational services have chosen to adopt researchers' definition of a learning disorder.

According to Rapin (1996a) it was Myklebust who, in 1954, for research purposes, started to use exclusionary criteria to sharpen the identification of children with discrete developmental language disorders, in order to elucidate their nature and cause. Understandably these criteria included diagnosed defects in vision and hearing (extrinsic factors already known to account for some children's learning difficulties) and mental retardation. The National Advisory Committee's definition (1968) of specific learning difficulties, quoted above, amplified these criteria and was incorporated in legislation in the USA [PL 94-142. Education for All Handicapped Children Act of 1975] requiring free and appropriate education for mentally retarded children of school age. Regulations were introduced defining the various handicaps that made a child eligible for special education, which education authorities had a statutory duty to provide. PL 94-142 specified that to qualify for special education as learning disordered, a child must be normally intelligent (with an IQ not lower than 2 standard deviations below the mean) and have certain skill deficiencies due to specific disorders, amounting to severe discrepancy between ability and achievement, such as 50% below the expected level.

Dissatisfaction among the practitioners who were required to quantify exclusion and discrepancy criteria in mathematical terms continues to this day. The dissatisfaction concerns the primacy still accorded to the IQ as an accurate measurement of ability, and how expected competence in any skill can be measured. These issues are not confined to the USA.

In a brief review on intelligence tests, Smith and Cowie (1993) traced the enormous influence these tests had on educational thinking. Binet, Simon, and, later, Terman in the USA constructed such tests to differentiate children who were successful in school from those who were failing: in other words the children who were from those who were not capable of learning the skills typically taught and used in schools. These test-makers were not intending to measure an abstract cognitive quality. Unfortunately the following generations of psychologists, notably Burt in the UK, too readily believed that cognitive ability was what the tests did measure and that, unlike physical growth and development, such ability was an attribute that never varied, but was innate and independent of a child's experience and environment. Although today's psychologists may not yet be able to agree on a definition of intelligence, they are well aware of the danger of relying on psychometry to determine the methods of education most suitable for children who 'fail'. A summary IQ of 70 still provides the best cut-off for an operational definition of mental retardation (see Anderson 1986), but for many years educational psychologists have been reluctant to depend on such IQs in their clinical assessments: responses to particular subtests providing, for example, verbal and non-verbal IQs may be much more helpful in identifying individual cognitive strengths and weaknesses of educational importance. Nor has it yet been proved that the psychological-process deficits judged to account for the specific learning difficulties of children with normal IQs are not also present in children with mild mental retardation, perhaps tipping the scales to put their summary IQ more than two standard deviations below the mean. No IQ-related differences in response to the teaching methods for which children with developmental learning disorder are eligible have been found (Stanovich 1988).

There are, similarly, considerable doubts about the validity and reliability of many of the tests currently used to assess any discrepancy between ability and achievement, bearing in mind that such assessment has to allow for chronological age and for age-appropriate experience of education. Furthermore, although the original guideline of a 50% discrepancy was withdrawn in 1977, there has since been considerable variation in the methods adopted by different states in the USA in arriving at their own interpretations of 'severe' (or 'substantial' – DSM-IV). In 1978 Eisenberg warned that 'the categories of exclusion' would deny services to a significant number of children with learning disabilities, 'particularly those who suffer from socio-cultural disadvantages and emotional disturbances.' Today the categories of discrepancy have the same consequence for some children whose learning disability is due to where they live (Silver and Hagin 1990). The suggestions of a working party convened in 1983 by the US Department of Education (Reynolds 1984) to identify the best measurement solutions that might be applied failed to resolve all the theoretical and practical issues – a failure that surely calls into question the strict use of mathematical definitions of clinical (behavioural) problems.

In the UK, after 60 years' experience of a system of 'special educational treatment' based on legally defined categories of handicap diagnosed by a doctor (since 1944 there have been 11 such categories, including that of educational subnormality), the use of categories has been abandoned. The decision to abandon them followed the publication of the report of the Warnock Committee (1978), whose members were adamant that children should not be pigeon-holed into categories of handicap, because their special educational needs were more complex than a single category could specify, arising from the interaction of factors within the children and factors in their environment (experience). Consequently the 1981 Education Act introduced a more flexible system based on the identification of need rather than a diagnosis of disorder. Under that act a child 'has special educational needs if he has a learning difficulty which calls for special educational provision', meaning provision which is additional to, or otherwise different from, 'that made generally for children of his age'. Not surprisingly there has been much difference of opinion as to what 'generally' means, because it depends so much upon the availability and use of resources. Resources are not the subject of this book. More relevant here is the Act's use of the term *learning difficulty* to mean 'a significantly greater difficulty in learning than the majority of children of the same age have'.

This concept was endorsed and amplified in the 1993 Education Act and Regulations, which placed duties and responsibilities on local education authorities to meet the 'special educational needs' of children with learning difficulties. In 1994 the Department of Education issued guidance to local education authorities in the form of a Code of Practice on the steps a school should initially take to determine the reasons for a child's difficulties and how to deal with them. This advice was presented separately for the following 'forms of learning difficulty or disability': learning difficulties, specific learning difficulties, emotional and behavioural difficulties, physical disabilities, sensory impairments, and other sundry medical conditions. Just as the definition of *learning difficulty* did not refer to specific causal factors, so the Code emphasized that specifying particular difficulties did not mean these were to be regarded as new statutory categories. It also accepted that children's learning difficulties might 'encompass more than one area of (special educational) need'. It may seem disingenuous that the same term, *learning difficulty,* should be used generically to cover all difficulties in learning and particularly to describe one form of difficulty (i.e. 'a general level of academic attainment significantly below that of peers'), but we should not forget the centuries-old cultural role of schools as centres promoting learning. It is enough for both clinical paediatric and special educational purposes (though not necessarily for research purposes) that the Code describes the specific learning difficulties of some children quite simply as 'significant difficulties in reading, writing, spelling, or manipulating numbers, which are not typical of their general level of performance', adding that evidence of other difficulties such as in language function, coordination, working memory, and associated emotional and behavioural difficulties, including inability to concentrate, should always be sought. Thus the Code tacitly recognizes that these are all identifiable elements in the learning of the communication skills essential for effective social interaction.

A PAEDIATRIC POINT OF VIEW
It is important at this stage that the third interested party should join the debate: the paediatricians, psychologists, and teachers who work together in schools. All of these practising professionals who deal with individual children are frequently frustrated by having to temper their recommendations for special education to accommodate an impersonal definition of learning difficulties chosen for research purposes that have been adopted for economic and administrative reasons by those who provide services. Trapped in such an unholy alliance, these practitioners become reluctant spokespersons for their patients. We cannot speak for school psychologists or teachers, but we believe that paediatricians should present an essentially pragmatic, clinical point of view. In explaining this we shall be particularly careful in our use of words.

A dictionary definition of *learning* would be along the lines of 'gaining knowledge of or skill in, by study, experience, or being taught; acquiring or developing a particular ability'. Smith and Cowie (1993), however, give a definition representative of psychologists and ethnologists who use the term as referring to 'the influence of specific environmental information on behaviour...The way an animal behaves depends upon what it learns from the environment.' In Chapter 2 Brown and Minns explain why such a simplistic concept of learning, as being an enduring internal representation of an environmental experience (Dudai 1989), is inadequate. First, it implies that the 'environment' is only the world into which a child is born, ignoring the reality that a child (person) lives also in an internal environment. This anatomical–chemical 'milieu' also generates stimuli, primarily factors of structural maturation, that initiate behaviour. New behaviours can therefore be learned as a result of either internally generated (i.e. innate, or pre-programmed) stimuli or externally generated stimuli (i.e. social experience). So there are different types of learning that result in reflex, pre-programmed, and conditioned behaviour and in motor, emotional, and cognitive learning.

Secondly, the simplistic definition of learning ignores conscious awareness of environmental stimuli, which is essential if they are to be recognized and understood – a prerequisite for normal cognitive behaviour. Theoretically a child with any degree of difficulty in learning to understand any environmental stimulus could be described as learning-disabled, but as the label would apply equally to a child who is profoundly intellectually backward and to one who is highly intelligent but has a slight difficulty in learning to read, it is a singularly uninformative oversimplification, of little use to clinicians. On the other hand it is unreasonable that in any classification of disorders of development, only those relating to the learning of reading, writing, or arithmetic (the 3 Rs) should be designated learning disorders, when problems in other activities seem just as likely to be due to difficulties in learning.

The question then arises why some children have such learning problems. It is customary to refer to the reasons for learning problems as 'disorders' – probably in part because it was doctors who were the pioneers in seeking explanations for dyslexia and because they succeeded in discovering specific biological deviations from the normal, e.g. chromosome and metabolic abnormalities, in certain children with severe, extensive learning problems (mental retardation). The WHO manual does not offer a definition of *disorder,* but a dictionary definition is 'a bodily or mental ailment or a disturbance, disease', so it makes sense medically to refer to these two causes of learning problems as disorders. However, dictionaries also define the word disorder as 'want of order, confusion, disarray'. No doubt it is in this sense that the WHO regards a disturbance in psychological function (behavioural deviation from the normal) as an impairment. The implication is that even when the structure of the brain seems to be normal, its constituent parts can fail to function effectively together, like a mechanically sound engine that is not properly tuned.

To this extent it is reasonable at present to classify all learning problems for which no environmental cause can be found as intrinsic neurodevelopmental *disorders,* provided it is not forgotten that this classification is no more than a supposition based on the precedent of known pathological aetiology in some children. In most specific neurodevelopmental disorders, difficulty in learning is a reality but its causes are not certain: the difficulty is not contingent upon its aetiology and does not in itself constitute a learning disorder. The pundits tell us, surely quite rightly, that the commonest specific learning difficulty in reading is not a disease, but a symptom. Nevertheless the condition still appears in the latest *International Classification of Diseases,* ICD-10 (World Health Organization 1992), and is increasingly referred to as specific developmental dyslexia, as if the label had been dignified as a diagnosis. The reason for calling the condition a specific disorder is either the assumption that it causes a specific disability or because it is more convenient to use one adjective to qualify both cause and effect, the assumption then being that it is common knowledge that in the medical sense *specific* means 'cause unknown'! (Rutter and Yule 1975, Silver and Hagin 1990).

Neither of these assumptions is justified. Rispens and van Yperen (1997) have also cautioned against too hasty an acceptance of the specificity of developmental disorders, just as others have been unimpressed by the evidence for a distinction between a specific developmental disorder and other types of developmental delay (Henderson and Bartlett 1995). Parents of disabled children, and individuals and organizations involved in the welfare of such children, seem to feel more comfortable with a medical diagnosis. Thirty years ago Bowley (1969), an educational psychologist, observed that once it had been made clear that the syndrome of motor, perceptual, and reading difficulties was due to minimal brain damage (as was then thought), everybody's attitude to treatment changed. Professionals need to be more realistic and to demand evidence in cases of specific learning difficulties, because we cannot yet be certain that they are due to structural defects in brain tissue.

The claim of neuropsychologists that specific learning difficulties are due to a disorder in psychological processing of information from the environment is a conjecture about computation that is also far from proven and is perhaps even less well supported by evidence than the hypothesis of minimal brain damage. Only time will tell whether it turns out to be correct, but the hypothesis has certainly stimulated exciting advances in neuroimaging and other research seeking to ascertain possible relations between postulated specific psychological processes and cerebral morphology, especially in those parts of the brain thought to be crucially involved in a particular functional skill. In the case of dyslexia Rumsey (1996) judges the results to be promising but as yet inconsistent, warning that deviations in neuronal activity shown by some functional imaging studies are not actually confined to such crucial areas. Born and Lou discuss this topic in more detail in Chapter 12. However, the answer is not as simple as that. Even if it were to be shown without doubt that certain unusual features always characterized the relevant neurological structures in children with a specific learning difficulty, the degree of deviance in structure and in function would still have to be studied extensively before such morphological differences could be described as pathologically abnormal.

That point has certainly not been reached in respect of any 'specific learning disorders'. In reporting the results of imaging and anatomical procedures, authors are often noticeably non-committal, referring for instance to 'altered' anatomy, 'deviations' in neuronal activity, 'deficits', or 'differences'. After postmortem examination of subjects known to have had dyslexia, Galabardia and his colleagues (1989) described the symmetries they found in the language-relevant and typically asymmetrical planum temporale, and the neuronal ectopias in the cerebral cortex, not as pathological, but as 'developmental anomalies'. Rapin (1996b) has drawn attention to the preponderant role of genetic factors in dyslexia, while Rumsey (1996) refers to genetic influences. There is evidently considerable uncertainty in respect of specific learning disorders about the precise point at which a natural difference in morphological features becomes a pathological abnormality. So, while accepting that the learning of skills initially depends upon organic (neurological) structure, one should not assume either that structural differences are necessarily pathologically abnormal or that functional difficulties that cannot be accounted for by extrinsic factors are necessarily the result of intrinsic neurological disorders. In paediatrics and in special education the term *abnormal* connotes defects and impaired functions. However, if, on neuroimaging, the brains of gifted children showed significant differences from the norm that might account for enhanced performance, it is inconceivable that these differences would be regarded as pathologically abnormal. Such differences may indeed exist in gifted children, since the structural organization of the central nervous system can be influenced by genetic factors and also through its stimulation, as has been shown experimentally in the visual cortex of cats (Blakemore 1974) and after the use of visual techniques to treat dyslexia (Bakker et al. 1995).

These are the main reasons why we believe paediatricians should be pragmatic and clinical in their neurodevelopmental approach to learning disorders – realistic rather than idealistic. It is surely not too much to ask that all those in this field of work should use a common language, so that each knows exactly what the others mean when they use certain words. Even today researchers and clinicians use terms such as *learning* and *attention* differently (Denckla 1996).

Specific learning disorder or neurodevelopmental dysfunction?

We have followed convention in using the term *specific learning disorder* in the title of this book, but it describes the problems of the children concerned no more satisfactorily than the labels it has replaced.

The terms *minimal brain damage* and *minimal cerebral dysfunction* were unsatisfactory because in many instances there was no evidence of minimal damage or of cerebral dysfunction. The latter term has posed conceptual problems as our knowledge of the patterns of genetic factors involved has grown. Can one describe a child who finds it particularly difficult to learn arithmetic as having a dysfunctioning cerebrum?

The label *specific learning disorder* is unsatisfactory because in the minds of many people, especially, but not only, educationists and parents, *learning* means academic learning: acquiring and applying skills in reading, writing, and arithmetic. The label has never wittingly been extended to including the learning of skills in attention, or in moderating levels of activity, or of motor skills (save in respect of traditional sports); but children have to learn these, too, and while most children learn them easily, some learn them only with difficulty.

The label *SLD* is also unsatisfactory, because it dogmatically describes the learning problems as *specific disorders,* implying that their cause is an identifiable organic defect, whereas the evidence for this is as yet inconclusive. The concept that such disorders are specific also raises the thorny issue of comorbidity. As many of our authors have pointed out, children with one specific learning problem often have other such problems, for example dysgraphia as well as dyslexia, or both with ADHD. To refer to these problems as 'morbidities' is inappropriate if one bears in mind that their aetiology is uncertain. Pennington (1991) uses the term *association,* which is safer and probably nearer the mark. Furthermore to be consistent one would then have to make multiple diagnoses to account for a variety of specific disorders, though in practice only a single diagnosis is made, e.g. dyslexia or ADHD.

No objections arise when problems in learning are described as *specific difficulties* or even *disabilities* (i.e. dysfunctions that are observable in the classroom), provided they are viewed pragmatically as relative symptoms or signs that vary with age, an amalgam of maturation and experience. Thus, difficulty or failure in learning a skill exists only when a society deems the skill to be necessary. In illiterate societies, of which there are examples today in the developing world as in medieval periods in the Western world, reading and writing were not a social requirement. Eleventh-century knights, indeed, despised the skill, leaving it to monks. (They might, of course, have qualified for a diagnosis of developmental coordination disorder if they proved poor with the sword!) Nowadays, a 3-year-old child cannot be considered dyslexic, because 3-year-olds cannot normally read; nevertheless their speech and language delay may presage a reading difficulty at 7 or 8 years of age. Nor should we too readily dismiss Stanovich's contention (1994) that the term *specific dyslexia* should be discarded, 'conceptualising reading disability as residing on a continuum of developmental language disorder'. Shaywitz et al. (1992) have gone further, maintaining that dyslexia is not an all-or-nothing phenomenon but varies along a continuum, blending imperceptibly into normal reading ability: 'there is in fact no such disorder as dyslexia' – as Rutter and Yule maintained in 1975! One has to ask how far such theories apply to other specific learning disabilities. Stevenson (in Chapter 7), in discussing genetic factors in more detail, concludes that 'ADHD is an extreme of normal variation'.

In the face of such uncertainties and possibilities it would be preferable to use the term *neurodevelopmental dysfunction (NDD)* rather than *SLD*. Substitution of *neurodevelopmental* for *learning* signals the role of the nervous system and of development in problems: the use of *dysfunction* instead of *disorder* acknowledges poor (impaired) performance, which from observations can be categorically specified, without implying a known specific defect.

This is what is meant by a neurodevelopmental approach. It is consistent with the WHO definitions of *impairment, disability,* and *handicap* (World Health Organization 1980), which recognizes that problems that children may have in learning a skill are a consequence of unusual failure (due to a variety of possible reasons) in either neuroanatomical structure or physiopsychological function.

The fact that so often specific dysfunctions are associated with one another suggests that NDD should be regarded as a syndrome rather than a series of single diagnoses, one of which is elite. This distinction is important for both research and special education. It can draw attention to the possible need for a combination of teaching methods. In 1972 Denckla maintained that while specific and definable learning disorders might not yet be diagnosable, definition of syndromes might contribute knowledge of specific and definable brain mechanisms and finding physical causes for some learning problems; 20 years later she proved her point (Denckla 1996).

Denhoff and Robinault (1960) suggested an overall grouping of syndromes as cerebral dysfunction and put these specific learning disorders in this group with motor disorders such as cerebral palsy. Disorders such as cerebral palsy are beginning to have a known impairment, such as brain lesions due to periventricular leukomalacia, and therefore the diagnosis can have both aetiological and diagnostic value. Hence the child can be excluded from the neurodevelopmental group, which we would restrict largely to the topics that are the subject of discussion of this book.

REFERENCES

American Psychiatric Association. (1952) *Diagnostic and Statistical Manual of Mental Disorders.* (DSM-I). Washington, DC: American Psychiatric Association.

— (1968) *Diagnostic and Statistical Manual of Mental Disorders.* 2nd ed (DSM-II). Washington, DC: American Psychiatric Association.

— (1980) *Diagnostic and Statistical Manual of Mental Disorders.* 3rd ed (DSM-III). Washington, DC: American Psychiatric Association.

— (1987) *Diagnostic and Statistical Manual of Mental Disorders.* 3rd ed, revised (DSM-III-R). Washington, DC: American Psychiatric Association.

— (1994) *Diagnostic and Statistical Manual of Mental Disorders.* 4th ed (DSM-IV). Washington, DC: American Psychiatric Association.

Anderson M. (1986) Understanding the cognitive deficit in mental retardation. *Journal of Child Psychology and Psychiatry* **27:** 297–306.

Bakker DJ, Licht R, Kapper EJ. (1995) Hemi-spheric stimulation techniques in children with dyslexia. In: Tramontana MG, Hooper SR, editors. *Advances in Child Neuropsychology. Volume 3.* New York: Springer-Verlag. p 144–77.

Bax M and Mac Keith R. (1963) *Minimal Cerebral Dysfunction: Papers from the International Study Group held at Oxford, September, 1962.* Clinics in Developmental Medicine No. 10. London: Spastics International Medical Publications / William Heinemann Medical Books.

Berlin R. (1887) *Eine Besondere Art Der Wortblindheit [Dyslexia].* Wiesbaden.

Binet A, Simon T (1908) Le développement de l'intelligence chez l'enfant. *Année Psychologique* **14:** 1.

Blakemore C. (1974) Development in mamalian visual systems. *British Medical Journal* **30:** 152–7.

Bowley A. (1969) Reading difficulty with minor neurological dysfunction: a study of children in junior schools. *Developmental Medicine and Child Neurology* **11:** 493–503.

British Paediatric Association. (1994) *Services for Children and Adolescents with Learning Disability (Mental Handicap).* London: British Paediatric Association.

Burt C. (1937) *The Backward Child.* London: University of London Press.

Clements S. (1966) *Minimal Brain Dysfunction in Children: Terminology and Identification.* NINDS Monograph No. 3. Public Health Service Publ. No. 1415. Washington, DC: US Government Printing Office.

— Peters JE. (1962) Minimal brain dysfunctions in the school-age child. *Archives of General Psychiatry* **6:** 185–97.

Code of Practice on the Identification and Assessment of Special Educational Needs. (1994) Department for Education, London: HMSO.

Cruickshank W. (1970) Perceptual learning disorders. *Journal of Learning Disabilities* **5** (7).

— Bentzen F, Ratzeburg F, Tannhasser M. (1961) *A Teaching Method for Brain Injured and Hyperactive Children.* New York: Syracuse University Press.

Denckla MB. (1972) Clinical syndromes in learning disabilities: the case for 'splitting' vs. 'lumping'. *Journal of Learning Disabilities* **5:** 401–6.

— (1996) Biological correlates of learning and attention: what is relevant to learning disability and attention-deficit hyperactivity disorder? *Developmental and Behavioral Pediatrics* **17:** 114–9.

Denhoff E, Robinault IP. (1960) *Cerebral Palsy and Related Disorders: A Developmental Approach to Dysfunction.* New York: McGraw-Hill Book Co

Department of Education. (1994) *Code of Practice on the Identification and Assessment of Special Educational Needs.* London: HMSO.

Down CJ.(1866) Ethnic classification of idiots. *Clinical Lecture Reports. London Hospital* **3:** 259.

Dudai Y. (1989) Some basic notions and their ontogenesis. In: *The Neurobiology of Memory: Concepts, Findings, Trends.* New York: Oxford University Press. p 3–18.

Education Act 1981. Chapter 60. London: HMSO.

Education Act 1993. London: HMSO.

Eisenberg L. (1978) Definitions of dyslexia: their consequences for research and policy. In: Benton AL, Pearl D, editors. *Dyslexia: An Appraisal of Current Knowledge.* New York: Oxford University Press. p 29–42.

Farnham-Diggory S. (1978) *Learning Disability – A Psychological Perspective.* Cambridge, MA: Harvard University Press.

Fodor JA. (1983) *The Modularity of Mind.* Cambridge, MA: MIT Press.

Gardner HG. (1983) *Frames of Mind – The Theory of Multiple Intelligences.* London: Heinemann.

Gillberg C. (1991) Debate and argument: Is autism a pervasive developmental disorder? *Journal of Child Psychology and Psychiatry* **32:** 1169–70.

Gordon N. (1992) George Eliot and specific learning difficulties. *Developmental Medicine and Child Neurology* **34:** 926–7. (Letter).

Hall DMB, editor. (1996) *Health for All Children.* Oxford: Oxford University Press.

Hallahan D, Cruickshank W. (1973) *Psychoeducational Foundations of Learning Disabilities.* Englewood Cliffs, NJ: Prentice-Hall.

Hammill D. (1990) On defining learning disabilities: an emerging consensus. *Journal of Learning Disabilities* **23:** 74–85.

— Leigh J, McNutt G, Larsen S. (1981) A new definition of learning disabilities. *Learning Disability Quarterly* **4:** 336–42.

Happé F, Frith U. (1991) Is autism a pervasive developmental disorder? Debate and argument: How useful is the 'PDD' label? *Journal of Child Psychology and Psychiatry* **32:** 1167–8.

Harris JC. (1995) *Developmental Neuropsychiatry. Volume 2. Assessment, Diagnosis and Treatment of Developmental Disorders.* New York: Oxford University Press.

Henderson SE, Bartlett AL. (1995) The classification of specific motor coordination disorders: some problems to be solved. Paper presented at the Workshop on Classification of Specific Developmental Disorders, Utrecht University.

Herbert M. (1964) The concept and testing of brain-damaged children: a review. *Journal of Child Psychology and Psychiatry* **5:** 197–216.

Ingram TTS. (1973) Soft signs. *Developmental Medicine and Child Neurology* **15:** 527–30. (Annotation).

Interagency Committee on Learning Disabilities. (1987) Report to Congress Health Research Extension. October 1985 (Public Law 99-158). Washington, DC:

Ireland WW. (1877) *On Idiocy and Imbecility.* London: Churchill.

Karmiloff-Smith A. (1992) *Beyond Modularity – A Developmental Perspective on Cognitive Science.* Cambridge, MA: MIT Press.

Kirk S. (1962) *Educating Exceptional Children.* Boston: Houghton Mifflin.

— (1963) Behaviour diagnosis and remediation of learning disabilities. In: *Proceedings of the Conference on the Exploration into the Problems of the Perceptually Handicapped Child.* Association for Children with Learning Difficulties, First Annual Meeting, Evanston, IL.

— McCarthy J, Kirk W. (1968) *Illinois Test of Psycholinguistic Abilities.* Revised edition. Urbana [IL]: University of Illinois Press.

Kussmaul A. (1877) Diseases of the nervous system and disturbances of speech. In: Von Zeimssen H, editor. *Cyclopaedia of the Practice of Medicine. Volume 14.* New York: W Wood.

Levine MD, Brooks R, Shonkoff MD (1980) *A Paediatric Approach to Learning Disorders.* New York: John Wiley and Sons.

Little WJ. (1862) On the influence of abnormal parturition, difficult labours, premature birth, and asphyxia neonatorum, on the mental and physical condition of the child, especially in relation to deformities. *Transactions of the Obstetrical Society of London* **3:** 293.

Morgan WP. (1896) A case of congenital word blindness. *British Medical Journal* **2:** 1378.

Myklebust HR. (1954) *Auditory Disorders in Children: A Manual for Differential Diagnosis.* New York: Grune and Stratton.

National Advisory Committee on Handicapped Children. (1968) *Special Education for Handicapped Children.* First Annual Report, US Department of Health, Education, and Welfare, January 31, 1968.

Paine RS, Werry JS, Quay HC. (1968) A study of 'minimal cerebral dysfunction'. *Developmental Medicine and Child Neurology* **10:** 505–20.

Pennington BF. (1991) *Diagnosing Learning Disorders: A Neuropsychological Framework.* New York: Guilford Press.

Prior M. (1996) *Understanding Specific Learning Difficulties.* Hove, Sussex, UK: Psychology Press.

Rapin I. (1996a) *Preschool Children with Inadequate Communication: Developmental Language Disorder, Autism, Low IQ.* Clinics in Developmental Medicine No. 139. London: Mac Keith Press.

— (1996b) Practitioner review – developmental language disorders: a clinical update. *Journal of Child Psychology and Psychiatry* **37:** 643–55.

Reynolds CR. (1984) Critical measurement issues in learning disabilities. *Journal of Special Education* **18:** 451–76.

Rispens J, van Yperen TA. (1997) How specific are 'specific developmental disorders'? *Journal of Child Psychology and Psychiatry* **38:** 351–63.

Rodin E, Lucas A, Simon C. (1964) A study of behaviour disorders in children by means of general purpose computers. *Proc. Conf. Data Acquis. Proc. Biol. Med.* Oxford: Pergamon.

Rumsey JM. (1996) Developmental dyslexia: anatomic and functional neuroimaging. *Mental Retardation and Developmental Disabilities Research Reviews* **2:** 28–38.

Rutter M. (1978) Prevalence and types of dyslexia. In: Benton AL, Pearl D, editors. *Dyslexia: An Appraisal of Current Knowledge.* New York: Oxford University Press.

—Yule W. (1975) The concept of specific reading retardation. *Journal of Child Psychology and Psychiatry* **16:** 181–97

Schonell FJ. (1942) *Backwardness in the Basic Subjects.* London: Oliver and Boyd.

Shaywitz SE, Escobar MD, Shaywitz BA, et al. (1992) Evidence that dyslexia may represent the lower tail of a normal distribution of reading ability. *New England Journal of Medicine* **326:** 145–50.

Silver AA, Hagin RA. (1990) *Disorders of Learning in Childhood.* New York: John Wiley and Sons.

Smith PK, Cowie H. (1993) *Understanding Children's Development.* Oxford: Blackwell Publishers.

Snowling M J. (1996) Annotation: Contemporary approaches to the teaching of reading. *Journal of Child Psychology and Psychiatry* **37:** 139–48.

Spreen C, Risser AT, Edgell D. (1995) *Developmental Neuropsychology.* Oxford: Oxford University Press.

Stanovich KE (1988) Explaining the differences between the dyslexic and garden-variety poor reader. *Journal of Learning Disabilities* **34:** 1137–52.

— (1994) Does dyslexia exist? *Journal of Child Psychology and Psychiatry* **35:** 579–95.

Still GF. (1902) The Coulstonian Lectures on some abnormal physical conditions in children. *Lancet* **1:** 1008, 1077, 1163.

Strauss A, Lehtinen L. (1947) *Psychopathology and Education of the Brain Injured Child.* New York: Grune and Stratton.

Touwen BCL, Sporrel T. (1979) Soft signs and MBD. *Developmental Medicine and Child Neurology* **21:** 528–29. (Annotation).

Warnock Committee. (1978) Report of the Warnock Committee (Chairman Mrs H M Warnock): Special Educational Needs. Cmnd 7212. London: Her Majesty's Stationery Office.

Werner H, Strauss A. (1939) Problems and methods of functional analysis in mentally deficient children. *Journal of Abnormal and Social Psychology* **34:** 37.

World Health Organization. (1957) *International Classification of Diseases.* 7th revision (ICD-7). Geneva: World Health Organization.

— (1978) *International Classification of Diseases.* 9th revision (ICD-9). Geneva: World Health Organization.

— (1980) *International Classification of Impairments, Disabilities, and Handicaps: A Manual of Classification Relating to the Consequences of Disease.* Geneva: World Health Organization.

— (1992) *The ICD-10 Classification of Mental and Behavioural Disorders. Clinical descriptions and diagnostic guidelines.* (ICD-10). Geneva: World Health Organization.

2
THE NEUROLOGICAL BASIS OF
LEARNING DISORDERS IN CHILDREN

J Keith Brown and Robert A Minns

THE NEUROLOGICAL SUBSTRATE OF LEARNING

Fifteen per cent of school-age children are thought to have some type of learning disorder. This figure not only depends upon the definition of the term *learning disorder* but also varies widely if estimates of prevalence are based upon the provision of special education, which varies greatly between cities in the same country, ranging in Scotland for example from 45 to 150 per thousand children. Even teachers' predictions at grade 2 (age 8 years) of achievement in grade 3 are good only if the problem is global; they do not accurately pick out the children with specific reading disability (Salveson and Undheim 1994).

Children who have learning disorders may be seen by professionals from many different disciplines: education, psychology, speech pathology, occupational therapy, medicine. Each professional group is inclined to use its own terminology and to have its own model. The medical model has tended to rest upon ideas current in the USA: of learning disability (LD), attention-deficit disorder (ADD), minimal brain damage (MBD), and hyperkinesis. As a result there has been a drive to search for causes of 'minimal brain damage' – birth trauma, lead poisoning, food additives, colouring agents, salicylates, or abnormalities of copper, zinc, or other trace elements – and to prescribe treatment with drugs such as Ritalin (methylphenidate hydrochloride) or special diets, e.g. salicylate-free or additive-free. In this chapter we further complicate the picture by describing a neurological model for learning disorders (Brown 1981, O'Hare and Brown 1998).

What is learning?

Learning has been defined as an experience-dependent generation of an enduring internal representation, or a lasting modification of such a representation (Dudai 1989). Although rather clumsy, this definition implies the necessity of an environmental stimulus or experience, some form of perception of that stimulus, and then some persisting, recallable internal representation (memory trace) of it. By this definition spontaneous or internally generated behaviours – innate learning such as hatching behaviour, courting, mothering, mourning, forced exploration, standing, walking – are not learned. The definition is also deficient in that it ignores conscious awareness, which is required for recognition and understanding. Neurologically there are three types of learning, which use different circuits within the brain: motor, emotional, and cognitive learning. The latter depends upon some form of language or symbol system.

Learning can also be studied at the social level of interaction between persons; at the level of an organ – the brain; at the cellular level – the neuron; and at a molecular level – protein synthesis.

The brain is the organ of learning

Alexandrian anatomists, around 300 BC, suggested that learning was sited in the brain, and Hippocrates felt that study of the mind should begin with the brain. Plato in 385 BC thought that body and mind were separate and that mind could exist in two worlds, one physical and one not. The soul was a separate entity and determined actions and thoughts. Even as late as the 1970s, however, philosophers and some psychologists thought that neuroscience was irrelevant to the study of learning and the mind (Churchill 1992). One still feels that some scholars and philosophers regard the mind as independent of the brain and that even if they accept that the brain plays a part they regard it as a black box full of amorphous jelly that soaks up learning like a sponge. Descartes thought that the mind was in the brain but that mind and soul came together in the pineal gland. This is not essentially different from Eccles's and Popper's modern idea of three worlds. One can measure light, sound, and the chemicals of smell and taste with scientific instruments and so prove that they exist without any need of a human mind. There is, however, the enigma of love, beauty, and pain, which, as Eccles stressed, have no existence outside the person and the person's nervous system.

Here we take the pragmatic view that all components and processes of mind depend upon normal brain structure and function (Table 2.1). Even consciousness, the mental process that is the most difficult to understand, indisputably depends upon a normally functioning brain. Obviously a major sensory or perceptual disorder such as partial hearing from chronic 'glue ear' (serous otitis media), severe peripheral deafness as in missed high tone deafness, central or word deafness, a severe refractive error, or partial blindness will seriously limit input and so will affect learning. Because this chapter is about the brain and learning, perceptual problems, although extremely important, are not considered further here.

The heart can be likened to a pump, the lungs, to bellows, and the kidney, to a filter, but the brain has usually been regarded as too complicated to characterize so simply. *The brain is the organ of learning,* most neurological diseases are in effect a loss of learning, and neurological abnormalities such as abnormal tone and reflexes are release phenomena at a lower level from the damaged machinery.

THE BRAIN IS COMPOSED OF LEARNING UNITS, OR MODULES

The cerebral cortex consists of some ten thousand million neurons and ten times as many glial cells. It is made up of small subunits, or modules, that are in essence a form of 'computer chip' (Table 2.2). Each module is genetically determined at the time of primitive cell division in the germinal matrix. There are many millions of modules and each can be considered to form a basic learning unit consisting of a physical means of permanent memory storage together with a switch system.

TABLE 2.1
Functions of mind and brain

Perception	Motivation	Reasoning
Attention	Arousal	Expression
Discrimination	Language	Emotional perception
Recognition	Concept formation	Emotional feelings
Consciousness	Thought	Emotional expression
Short-term memory	Intelligence	Drives
Long-term memory	Dominance	

TABLE 2.2
Make-up of the brain

5% primary areas

95% association areas

4 000 000 modules
    Each 25 μm in diameter
    Each connects with mirror image on opposite side
    2500 neurons per module
        10 000 synapses per neuron
    500 output-type pyramidal cells per module

(Based on Eccles 1979.)

Many of these modules have specified anatomical connections and are preprogrammed with a type of operational program or learning strategy committing the module to serve a preset function. These operational programs are a kind of read-only memory (ROM), which gradually evolves as the child grows, thus allowing developmental and psychological testing: indicators that can be tested include, for example, sitting, crawling, standing, walking; the order in which the child draws a cross, circle, square, diamond, etc.; the order in which consonants are learned in speech; and the development of syntax. Some developmental psychologists cannot accept this idea of innate, preprogrammed learning strategies, and they argue that all learning is environmentally determined.

The brain is a developing organ
In addition to being an organ of learning, the brain is a developing organ. The development is genetically controlled and can be thought of as happening in phases:

Phases of brain development (cerebral morphogenesis)
Prenatal
    1   Cell division and specification in subependymal germinal matrix of embryo
    2   Cell migration along the Bergmann glial fibres
    3   Cell differentiation
    4   Cell long process, axon, formation

Postnatal

    5   Myelination
            Rapid phase
            Slow phase
                of long association fibres
                of short association areas
    6   Dendritic maturation, Nissl substance formation, synaptogenesis
    7   Cell death (apoptosis) and dissolution, pruning of terminal axons, stabilization of synapses
    8   Hemispheric dominance
    9   Psychogenesis
   10   Full brain maturity
   11   Senescence

The brain does not reach full maturity developmentally until well on in the second decade of life. This means that genetic control does not cease at birth and that genetic disease may manifest itself much later, when a particular stage of brain development is reached, as in developmental dysphasia, developmental dyspraxia, and developmental dyslexia. There is a rapid phase of development in the first 4 years after birth, during which the weight of the brain increases by some 1000g from its weight at birth (Fig. 2.1). Development of dendritic connections, synaptic stabilization, myelination, formation of Nissl substance (rough endoplasmic reticulum), and maturation of association pathways are postnatal and follow an orderly, predetermined sequence (Conel 1939, Dekaban 1959, Brown 1997).

The cerebral cortex forms from primitive neuroectodermal cells, which are formed in the subependymal region of the germinal matrix. Each cell in the germinal matrix can divide only a fixed number of times, usually 12. These cells appear to be genetically destined for a particular area of cortex. They get there by migrating along 'guide wires', which are the processes of radially arranged astrocytes – Bergmann's glial fibres. The primitive cells swarm up the Bergmann's fibres by amoeboid movement. It is thought that the layer of the cerebral cortex to which the cell migrates is predetermined at the time of mitosis in the germinal matrix; if the cell is transferred to another embryo it will continue to form neurons in the same predetermined layer of cortex. Each guide wire, in all mammals, allows 130 cells to move into vertical arrays in the future cortex. The Bergmann's fibres themselves are in bundles of about eight, allowing about 1000 cells to form a unit in the cerebral cortex that is the embryological basis of the learning modules mentioned earlier (Fig. 2.2). Sir John Eccles taught that the cerebral cortex can be regarded as being made up of small cortical units or modules, each connected to its mirror on the opposite side through the 20 000 000 fibres in the corpus callosum. Mountcastle, using electrical stimulation and recordings, found that the cortex is made up of vertical units 0.5 to 1.0 mm in diameter. The cells gradually become organized into the classical six layers of the cortex and become more spread out, with a horizontal stratification replacing the primitive vertical stratification of the cell layers. Lamination starts at 25 weeks' gestation and the dendritic explosion

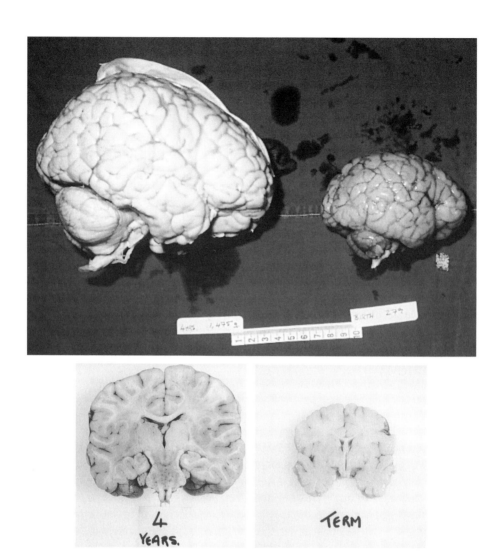

Fig. 2.1. Brain of a 4-year-old compared with that of a newborn infant, demonstrating the enormous amount of growth in size of the brain in the first 4 years of life.

is at 32 weeks. The six layers of cerebral cortex develop in an odd sequence of 5 – 6 – 3 – 4 – 2 – 1. The layers, outer to inner, are as follows:

1   molecular or plexiform layer: has few cell bodies and a lot of parallel fibres
2   outer granular layer: short cortico/cortical fibres
3   pyramidal cell layer: long cortico/cortical and transcallosal fibres extending to layer 3 on opposite side

28

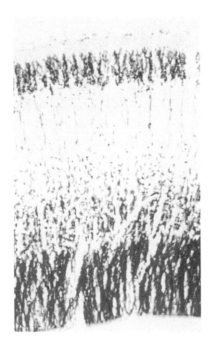

Fig. 2.2. A section of fetal brain to show that the migration of cells from the subependymal matrix to form the future cerebral cortex is in columns that determine the modular (learning-unit) structure of the cerebral cortex.

4 inner granular layer: no pyramidal cells but has cell bodies; layer is thick in somatosensory cortex and thin in motor cortex
5 inner pyramidal layer: large Betz cells; layer is thick in motor cortex and thin in somato-sensory cortex. Connections with colliculi and spinal cord come only from layer 5
6 multiform cell layer: corticothalamic fibres

Brodmann described histological variations from area to area within the mature cortex; he gave these areas numbers, thus producing a map of the cortical cellular organization. In the motor cortex, layer 5 is thick with the large pyramidal cells and layer 4 (which contains no pyramidal cells) is thin, whereas in the sensory cortex, layer 4 is thick and 5 is thin. Pyramidal cells in layer 5 tend to connect with the periphery, whereas those in layer 3 are cortico/cortical and extend across the corpus callosum to the same layer in a mirror module on the opposite side as well as extending long intracortical connections within their own hemisphere. These connections between and within hemispheres gradually develop over the first 16 years of life.

Neurons sprout an axon first, then dendrites. In any region of the brain, the dendrites of neurons with a short axon differentiate later than the dendrites of principal neurons, which have a long axon. The young neuron has relatively short, thick dendritic processes, but these develop a complex system of branches. Such branching greatly increases the

29

surface area of the dendrites, which form more than 90% of the postsynaptic surface of the neuron. Each type of neuron has a characteristic size, shape, and pattern of dendritic branching. The axons make contact with the dendrites at projections from the dendritic surface – the dendritic spines. An excess of these spines is formed, and those not making synaptic connections elongate and drop off while those making connections thicken and shorten. The spines, about 2000 per cortical neuron, are all formed by 6 months after birth and are the same then as at age 7 years. The spine connections are more easily damaged than actual dendritic branching. Paldine and Purpura (1981) postulated that failure of normal dendritic spine formation is the basis of many learning disorders, as in Down syndrome, hypothyroidism, ventilated preterm infants, and West syndrome. Use of a system modifies the pattern of dendritic branching and synapse formation: for example visual stimulation of the retina defines the retinotopic maturation of the calcarine visual cortex.

Establishment of specific synaptic interactions between neurons is essential for neuronal functional activity. Establishment of dendritic synaptic connections as a result of use of a pathway is the rationale for programmes of early infant stimulation, and lack of such stimulation could explain any permanent effects of early psychosocial deprivation. In experiments stimulation of one eye and occlusion of the other causes the optic nerve on the stimulated side to myelinate more quickly. Animals deprived of light have a thinner visual cortex. Experiments in cats have even more interesting results, in that during the phase of rapid brain growth, especially of the visual cortex, visual stimulation affects the actual structural organization of the cortex and the synaptic connections that form (Blakemore 1974). Blind infants have high metabolic activity in the visual cortex as it tries to establish some connection. All this evidence suggests that an ability developing within the brain can go only so far driven by biology alone and then requires stimulation for completion of the maturation process. It is interesting, therefore, that there is a built-in, preprogrammed behaviour that ensures that a new ability is used before it has any meaning or cognitive drive, as in forced visual pursuit, forced grasping, forced utterances, and forced exploration.

Many more neurons are formed in embryonic life than are present in the mature nervous system. Many neurons are eliminated as their axons are establishing synaptic contacts. This is called the phase of selective cell death or apoptosis. As many as 50% of anterior horn cells and retinal ganglion cells may be eliminated by such 'naturally programmed cell death' (Oppenheim and Chu-Wang 1983).

Myelination is the most obvious postnatal aspect of brain development (though it actually begins before birth) and takes place in a definite order, in the so-called myelinogenetic cycles of Yakolev and Lecours (1967) (Fig. 2.3). Although somatically the fetus develops in a cephalocaudal direction, i.e. arms before legs, in the cerebral cortex the leg area and visual (calcarine cortex) area myelinate first. At birth a baby has a little myelin in the internal capsule, the leg area of the cortex, and the median longitudinal bundle in the brainstem. Myelination is then very rapid from about the 38th week of development to 6 weeks after birth, when the whole of the cerebellar white matter, olives, brainstem, and leg area of the cortex myelinate very quickly. The corpus callosum starts to myelinate at 8 weeks after birth. The pyramidal tract is 50% myelinated by age 1 year, and myelination continues rapidly to age 4 years. It then continues, but much more slowly, in the association areas

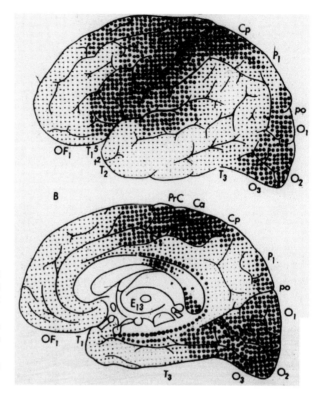

Fig. 2.3. A myelinogenetic chart showing areas that myelinate early (dark dots) and those that myelinate late (smaller dots).

Note that the angular gyrus and the frontal poles both mature late.

(See also Yakolev and Lecours 1967.)

and finally the subcortical frontal region, until age 16 years. The myelination of association fibres connecting one part of the cerebral cortex with another has been given as the reason why puberty comes about when frontohypothalamic pathways mature or why the ability to reason from a scientific experiment may not occur before the age of 13 years.

MRI has made the study of myelination a clinically useful possibility (Fig. 2.4). The following order of myelinogenesis is seen: posterior limb of the internal capsule, genu of the corpus callosum, occipital U fibres, frontal U fibres, periventricular frontal white matter, and peritrigonal white matter.

As long ago as 1906 Flechsig showed that there are three stages in the postnatal maturation of the cerebral cortex: (i) The earliest areas to develop are the primary areas, such as the primary motor cortex (Brodmann's area 4), the somatosensory cortex (Brodmann's area 41), and Heschl's gyrus, that is, all the areas of cerebral cortex that receive information through the senses from the environment. All these areas either have rich connections to the thalamus, and *no* long intracortical connections, or else have long efferent projections to the periphery, that is, the muscles. Included among these early-developing primary areas is the limbic system. These primary areas make up only 5% of the brain's surface. (ii) The second areas to develop are the association areas, which usually lie adjacent to the primary motor or sensory area and include for example the visual association area (Brodmann's area

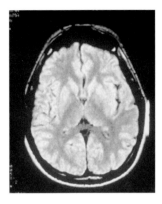

Fig. 2.4. An MRI to demonstrate the pattern of myelination ('dark' areas) in normal brain.

18) or the auditory association area (Wernicke's area). These areas all have long intracortical association pathways and are connected via the corpus callosum to their equivalent region in the opposite hemisphere. (iii) Flechsig called the third and last part of the cerebral cortex to mature during childhood 'terminal zones': the anterior pole of the frontal lobe and the angular gyrus, areas that have no thalamic connections. These are the areas that have to do with future planning, seeing the consequences of one's actions, impulse control, and the amalgamation of visual material (letters) with sounds (phonemes) as well as right/left orientation – all areas of function that have been found to be abnormal in children with learning disabilities.

It can be seen that if there if there is delay in brain maturation from any cause, then parts of the brain that are important in motivation and cognitive learning will be delayed in particular. Since the brain grows more slowly in boys and the left hemisphere grows more slowly than the right, it is not surprising that learning difficulties will arise more often in language skills in boys, no matter what the cause of slowing down of brain growth.

Learning is localized in the brain

Much as a computer disk must be formatted to arrange the memories in a retrievable form at specified addresses, the cerebral cortex is formatted with learning at specific predetermined addresses, and this learning is classified and retrieved by a language.

Descartes, in 1649, thought that the pineal gland, the seat of the soul, moved to and fro between the right and left cerebral hemispheres searching for memories. It was Auburtin (1825–1893) whose gruesome experiment started the search for localization. He had a patient who in attempting suicide blew off the front of his skull. Auburtin showed that by pressing on the patient's exposed frontal lobes with a spatula he could arrest the patient's speech. Broca (1861) later showed that it was expression, not comprehension of speech, that was situated in the frontal region on the left side. Wernicke showed that aphasia with loss of comprehension was due to left-sided lesions, and Dejerine completed the elucidation of language dominance by showing that reading and writing skills were also dependent upon an intact left cerebral hemisphere (Brain 1961).

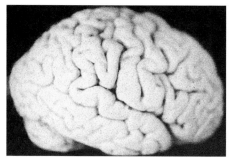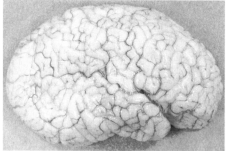

Fig. 2.5. Brains showing (left) normal gyral topography and (right) how this can be distorted by stretching, causing polymicrogyria, which allows normal function but interferes with any attempt at anatomical localization.

Paul Broca's work suggested that motor speech is localized in the inferior motor strip, i.e. Broca's area. The localizations of various other functions – of vision in the occipital area (Brodmann's area 17); of motor skills, as visualized in Penfield's familiar homunculus, in the precentral gyrus (Brodmann's area 4); of somatic sensation in the posterior central gyrus (Brodmann's area 1); and of hearing in the superior temporal Heschl's gyrus (Brodmann's area 41) – are all primary motor and perceptual areas (Fig. 2.5). The areas of the cortex representing lips and hands, which are very important for speech and learned manipulative skills, have an input of particularly high neuron density and are disproportionately large for the size of the organs they represent. All these primary 'hard-wired' areas, constituting only 5% of the area of the cerebral cortex, are not plastic, but rather their functions are dictated by the anatomy and cannot be replaced if the area is damaged. These are the areas damaged in cortical blindness, cerebral palsy, and cortical deafness from neuronal necrosis. The premotor area is hard-wired to the pyramidal tract; the calcarine cortex, to the optic tract; Heschl's gyrus, to the auditory system; and sensory fibres from the thalamus, to the postcentral gyrus. These various areas are either the primary reception areas for perception or the final organization areas for muscle movement patterns. 'Learned' abilities are stored not in the primary areas but in the adjacent association areas. A path can be traced from the retina by way of the optic nerve to the lateral geniculate nucleus and then by the optic radiation to the calcarine cortex (Brodmann's area 17) and then onward to the visual association area (Brodmann's area 18), which is connected across the splenium of the corpus callosum to area 18 on the opposite side. Area 18 is connected to the motor system (affecting visuomotor skills), to the limbic system (affecting emotion, e.g. in response to beauty), and via the angular gyrus to the auditory system (affecting reading).

Localization of function was further elucidated by seeing the clinical deficits associated with focal pathology, such as the tumours and infarcts of classical neurology, and then by gunshot wounds, and finally by studies using direct stimulation of the exposed human brain (Penfield and Roberts 1959).

In the Wada test for cerebral hemispheric dominance (Wada and Rasmussen 1960), injecting 150 to 200mg of 10% sodium amytal solution into the carotid artery on one side causes anaesthesia of that hemisphere and a transient contralateral hemiparesis. In 119 people tested in this way (Milner 1971), 90% of right-handers were found to have their speech centre in the left hemisphere and 10% in the right. Among the left-handers the speech centre was on the left in 64%, on the right in 20%, and bilateral in 16%.

A less invasive (and less discriminating) way of testing cerebral dominance for language is dichotic listening: i.e. listening to different sounds, such as two different words, presented simultaneously through headphones to the two ears. The word discriminated is usually the one that is presented to the ear (usually the right) contralateral to the hemisphere dominant for speech.

The study of cortical localization has been revolutionized, however, by the advent of local blood flow studies using radioactive xenon, of positron emission tomography (PET scans), of studies of regional cerebral metabolism for glucose and oxygen, and now by SPECT and functional MRI. These methods have the big advantage that they can be used to study normal rather than diseased brains. Before their advent one would always wonder if any complicating hypoxia, ischaemia, or effects of raised intracranial pressure was diffuse, rather than being confined to the immediate area of disease, even when there was a circumscribed contusion, tumour, or infarct.

Using these modern techniques one can show the motor planning occurring in the motor association area, execution by the precentral gyrus, and sequencing by the supplementary motor area (Fig. 2.6). Speaking or writing can be shown to be associated with the association area for lips, tongue, and palate (Broca's area) or the hand (graphomotor centre). The visual areas can be shown to 'light up' differentially when a person is looking at scenes or faces compared with the response to language-based materials. As definition improves one can show separate visual processing areas for faces, geometric forms, central colour vision, speed of movement, and written words. The motor eye field and the visual area are both involved in tracking a moving object.

Neuroimaging by CT and MRI is now possible in people with dyslexia, whose images are usually normal. One of the most dramatic new findings from functional MRI, which may account for the predominance of males among children with speech, language, reading, and spelling problems, is that speech is very definitely localized in the left Broca's area in males, whereas females use both hemispheres, with bilateral representation (Reid and Rumsey 1996). The visual association area can also be shown to be involved in the recognition of written letters and words; the left temporal lobe, in phonological and auditory word recognition; and the left posterior temporal cortex, in reading aloud. Activation of the left posterior temporal cortex in word recognition gives credence to previously postulated localization (Howard et al. 1992, Price et al. 1994, Rumsey et al. 1995). Blood flow and metabolism increase in the planum temporale on the right in response to music and on the left in response to the spoken word. Language and visual areas are both involved in reading. Language areas also light up when a person is lip-reading. The limbic and postulated emotional areas of the brain are highly metabolic in panic attacks, and in depression there is abnormal activity in the anterior cingulate cortex, particularly on the right. Attention is thought to depend upon normal function of the anterior cingulate and prefrontal cortex.

Fig. 2.6. Single-photon emission tomograms showing how function can be demonstrated non-invasively.

In the normal, awake, vigilant person there should always be frontal flow and metabolism (shown here by bright areas). Use or loss of function shows as a rise or fall in flow in the corresponding area.

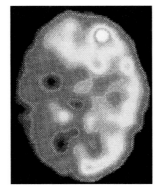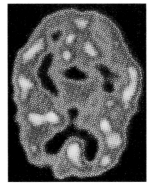

All these investigative methods have shown that learning of specific modalities is indeed localized within the brain, in line with the teachings of classical neurology. Paul Broca showed that expressive speech came from the left hemisphere in an area adjacent to the motor strip for the lips, tongue, and palate, and this phenomenon has been verified with most of the techniques just mentioned. Writing appears to be localized in the graphomotor area, again on the left (in right-handers) and adjacent to the area for motor control of the right hand. Reading depends upon the visual association area on the left, i.e. that area is involved in the recognition of visual symbols with a linguistic meaning. The integration of phonological aspects of heard speech with the graphemes of written speech requires the angular gyrus.

The right hemisphere controls the recognition of musical tones and memory of tunes. We sing as we speak, and the difference between an American and a German accent is as much one of intonation pattern as of the actual pronunciation of words. The intonation pattern accompanying speech can be likened to a continuous Gregorian chant. We express ideas in words from the left hemisphere but feelings in non-verbal communication from the right hemisphere, so we normally communicate using both hemispheres. The pyramidal system is used to produce the words, while the extrapyramidal system contributes emotional intonation, expression, and stress. Prosodic recognition of expression in speech, facial expression, and reception of non-verbal or emotional communication is lost in autism. It is thought that expression of emotion through intonation and gesture (i.e. expressive prosodia) also depends upon the right hemisphere: this may be lost in extrapyramidal diseases such as parkinsonism. The right frontal lobe, which is bigger than the left, integrates emotional with cognitive processes and has strong limbic connections. Visual recognition of objects and discrimination of faces, forms, geometric shapes, colour, and direction sense (i.e. cognitive maps) depend upon the visual association area of the right hemisphere. There is a specific visual area for the recognition of human faces, an ability that can be specifically lost in prosopagnosia (face agnosia), probably because of a lesion in the medial occipitotemporal cortex (Damasio et al. 1982). It is thought that non-language-dependent hand skills such as constructional praxis and drawing of shapes may also be more represented

TABLE 2.3
Usual hemispheric localization of function

Right cerebral hemisphere	Left cerebral hemisphere
Visual recognition of faces, shapes colour, objects, pictographs	Word recognition
Space, shape, direction (visuospatial) skill	Understanding – concepts
	Reading
Drawing	Writing
	Spelling
Constructional praxis	Speech
Facial expression	
Gesture recognition	
Manipulative and spatial (visuomotor) skill	Verbal reasoning
Musical appreciation	
Intonational pattern imposed on speech; singing	Arithmetic, number
Flight	Fight
Gestalt function	

on the right, just as writing is on the left. The usual localization of function in the two hemispheres is as shown in Table 2.3.

Modalities of learning

We have explained that the cerebral cortex is made up of many millions of modules, each with a built-in program allowing learning to proceed in a set way at a predetermined rate, and that the cerebral cortex is formatted like a computer disk, with preset addresses learning specific tasks. These learning modules have a preset hard-wiring and software system enabling them to function in a specific modality, i.e. to collect and store a defined data set.

There is a tendency to think that specific learning disorders affect only reading and writing, but in fact any of the modalities shown in Table 2.4 can be lost in isolation. Many such disabilities are signalled by the prefix *dys-*, which should be interpreted as meaning merely 'difficulty with'. The prefix *a-*, as in *alexia, agraphia,* or *aphasia,* means a total absence of the ability in question. The meanings of some common terms for specific learning disabilities are listed here:

dysphasia – word-deafness
dyslexia – word-blindness
dysgraphia – writing paralysis
dyscalculia – number-blindness or -deafness
dysmusia – tune-deafness
articulatory dyspraxia – word-dumbness
constructional dyspraxia – constructional paralysis
visuospatial agnosia – shape-blindness

36

TABLE 2.4
Types of specific loss of learning, seen in acquired brain disease

Dyspraxias/Apraxias
  Writing
  Constructional
  Oculomotor
  Articulatory
  Dressing
  Walking

Agnosias
  Visual
      For faces (prosopagnosia)
      Spatial (space, shape, and direction)
      For objects
      For colour (also, colour anomia)
      For reading (written symbols)
      For geometrical, chemical, and other symbols
  Tactile
      Astereognosis
      Asomatognosia (body image)
  Auditory
      Word-deafness
      Tune-deafness (receptive dysmusia)
      Expressive dysmusia

Dysphasias
      Central word-deafness
      Receptive dysphasia (Wernicke's area affected)
      Expressive dysphasia (Broca's area affected)
      Conductive dysphasia
      Transcortical dysphasia (word-deafness)
      Nominal dysphasia
      Specific dyslalia
      Dyslexia
      Spelling dysgraphia

Dyscalculia

Dysprosodias
      Receptive
      Expressive

---

astereognosis – shape-numbness
proprioceptive loss – position-numbness
anaesthesia – pain-numbness

Cerebral hemispheric dominance (the fixation of learning)

LATERALIZATION AND BRAIN ASYMMETRY

The brain is anatomically asymmetrical, and so is behaviour, even before birth. After birth, 80% of infants continue to show a strong preference for the direction of head-turning, and grasp reflexes disappear asymmetrically. By the age of 10 months most infants show a definite

37

preference for the right hand. Older children also show asymmetry on standing and walking. There is an obvious foot preference in kicking a football. Eye preference is often affected by refractive error, but tachistoscopic presentation of material in each visual field will confirm that there are asymmetries of visual perception. Equally, studies using dichotic listening will reveal a preference of the right ear for speech and the left ear for music in normal right-handed individuals. People clasp their hands or fold their arms in what appears to be a genetically determined way. Ninety per cent of people are right-handed and in most cases the speech centres will be on the left side. Unilateral electroconvulsive therapy also showed that in over 95% of right-handers speech was in the left hemisphere (though 10% of right-handers also have a speech centre in the right hemisphere): one may therefore lose speech in association with a left hemiplegia. More rarely Broca's area and Wernicke's area may be on opposite sides to each other – Broca's on the right and Wernicke's in its usual place on the left. There are many ambidextrous or non-right-handed people who cannot be strictly classified as right- or left-handed – for example 60% of children labelled left-handers are definitely left-handed, about 20% are ambidextrous, and 20% use their left hand to write but their right hand for most other tasks.

About 9% of the population are left-handed and about 60% of these people nevertheless have their speech centres on the left side of the brain; on Wada testing 7 of 44 left-handed people were found to have bilateral representation of speech. Most left-handed children have no learning disability, but there does seem to be a preponderance of left-handedness in reports of children with specific learning disabilities. Boys are more strongly left-handed than are girls of a corresponding age, an observation in agreement with recent studies suggesting that language skills are more firmly unilateral in the male than the female. Studies have, on the whole, tended to suggest that it is not left-handedness but ambilaterality and left-ear dominance for speech that are significantly associated with reading difficulty. Steenhuis et al. (1993) showed that in 1829 adult males and 3631 females the factors most likely to be associated with reading difficulty were being male, being non-right-handed, and being right-eyed.

Both sides of the brain can process speech and language, but there is normally a genetic bias towards left hemispheric dominance and right-handedness. If this gene is absent, handedness and the location of the speech centre will both be randomly allocated, so that 50% may be right-handed and 50% left-handed: this theory explains why a few people who are right-handed have their speech centre on the left side, why monozygotic twins may be one right-handed and the other left-handed, and why, of the children of two left-handed parents, 70% are right-handed.

ESTABLISHMENT OF HEMISPHERIC DOMINANCE
It is thought that the very young infant uses both sides of the brain, with a mirror pattern of learning for each modality such as speech, reading, shape-copying, drawing, writing, and movement. The more learning is required for a skill (speech, reading, typing, facial recognition), the more it needs to be lateralized in the brain. The more distal and lateralized to one hand a skill is, again the more it is lateralized in the brain. And the more midline a motor activity is, such as biting, chewing, swallowing, or bladder and bowel control, the

less lateralized it is in the brain. In the absence of a corpus callosum the cerebral hemispheres act as two separate brains, with the memories from one hemisphere entering consciousness without reference to the other. If the posterior corpus callosum of an adult is cut through, tactile and visual stimuli presented to the non-dominant hemisphere cannot be identified verbally. Callosotomy before puberty, however, does not cause a disconnection syndrome (Sauerwein and Lassond 1997).

If bilateral learning were to persist into school years, mirror interference would be a constant problem, especially when direction is important, as in speaking, reading, writing, and drawing. Mirror interferences show up clinically in various ways:

• reversal when copying shapes
• reversal of patterns, e.g. in block design, Raven's matrices
• poor crossed commands
• right/left confusion on self or mannikin
• difficulty with imitation of gestures
• finger agnosia
• dysgraphaesthesia
• mirror movements to opposite side and mouth
• mirror posture (seen on the Fog test)
• speech reversals in sound, word, or phrase
• reading reversals: *was/saw, god/dog*
• writing reversals: *b/d, m/n;* or in words: *no/on*
• suppression of one eye with squint: no diplopia or amblyopia

Many of these developmental signs have been confused in the past with abnormal, 'soft' neurological signs and attributed to minimal brain damage. In an adult many of the signs would be regarded by a neurologist as signs of parietal lobe dysfunction or of a lesion of the angular gyrus. Normal children less than 7 years of age manage quite well without being able to identify which fingers are touched, without necessarily being able to recognize shapes traced on their hands or to discriminate weights or textures, and this inability does not produce proprioceptive ataxia or clumsiness. Finger agnosia, for example, is thought to be due to the fact that normally we identify which side of the middle finger is touched, and if there is a mirror confusion the wrong side can be identified, causing inaccuracy. Similarly, a shape traced on the hand may be reversed in exactly the same way as *god* and *dog* or *was* and *saw* in reading and writing. Many children have been classified as clumsy because they had the motor symptoms of associated movements and mirror movements with a degree of dysdiadochokinesia and had difficulty with alternating movements such as opening one hand and closing the other, as well as an immature Fog test and choreiform movements (Walton et al. 1962, Gordon and McKinlay 1980).

If such interference and confusion are to be prevented from continuing, one directional pattern must be suppressed in favour of the other, by a mechanism called 'reciprocal cerebral inhibition': learning becomes localized to one side of the brain, in one place, with inhibition of the opposite side through the corpus callosum. This is what we mean by 'aquisition of hemispheric dominance', which tends to occur between 3 and 7 years of age. Acquisition of dominance is genetically controlled and its variability has a normal distribution. There are also some families in which dominance is acquired more slowly, and again this will be more obvious in the boys than in the girls. Some children do not achieve hemispheric dominance until well into the school years and so have difficulties in school; the occasional child never achieves it completely.

Although we generally speak of the left hemisphere as the dominant one, this is technically wrong, as the right hemisphere is dominant for vision and spatial skills. It seems that mirror-image learning appears to be suppressed at the same time as the brain's alpha rhythm appears, and the suppression could consist in inhibition or switching off of the mirror modules.

THE FRONTAL LOBE DIARY

The frontal lobe constitutes 30% of the cerebral hemisphere in man and only 10% in the monkey. It is the anterior pole that is peculiar to man and forms the tertiary developmental area (Walsh 1994). Being one of the last areas, along with the angular gyrus, to reach full maturity, it therefore is one of the areas likely to be retarded in development in any disorder that slows down the rate of whole brain development. The frontal lobe contains posteriorly the motor cortex, containing both Broca's speech area (Brodmann's area 44) and the graphomotor, i.e. writing, area. The motor eye field and the higher control of micturition are thought to be in the middle frontal gyrus. The medial part of the frontal lobe, along with the cingulate gyrus, has a strong limbic connection, regulating mood and the feeling of emotion, and an autonomic component to do with peristalsis, respiration, and blood pressure, which are often also involved with strong emotion.

Studies of cerebral blood flow show that in the normal awake, alert state the anterior pole of the frontal lobe is continuously perfused. Death, anaesthesia, or dementia is associated with a loss of this perfusion. Arousal, attention, current thought, and consciousness appear therefore to be associated with frontal lobe activity. Bilateral frontal lobectomy or infarction does not, however, cause coma or sleep (and so we know that the frontal lobe is not necessary for consciousness) nor does it affect scores on intelligence tests (and so we know that this lobe is not the site for intelligence). Frontal lobe function has become a topical subject for psychologists studying 'executive function'.

The four basic functions of the frontal lobe are (1) to plan the future (the frontal lobe diary), (2) to check for the presence of danger, (3) to inhibit basic drives, and (4) to focus attention. This lobe is thought to be important in planning for the future; it contains current working memory, and it allows us to 'say to ourselves'. It provides a 'devil's advocate', seeing the danger or worst consequences of the planned actions, and so provides the higher (moral) control of basic drives of thirst, hunger, sex, and so forth to prevent unwarranted aggression, gluttony, alcoholism, and sexual excess. It has to do with producing a plan of action in problem-solving. It also has to do with sustaining attention, with the initiation of activity, and with drive through curiosity; without this lobe the adult patient tends to be inactive, without initiative, apathetic, and unmotivated. Children with frontal lobe dysfunction cannot concentrate on one task for long and are easily distracted.

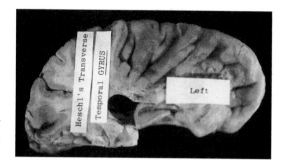

Fig. 2.7. Brain with lateral part cut away to reveal the concealed superior surface of the temporal lobe with Heschl's gyrus for hearing, and the planum temporale.

THE TEMPORAL LOBE

Diseases of the temporal lobes are particularly likely to be associated with learning disability. The temporal lobe is a vital junction of cognitive, emotional, and autonomic functions as well as being vital for memory function. The fact that speech reception in Heschl's gyrus and the storage of the lexicon basic to language function are dependent upon the planum temporale makes this part of the brain particularly important in considering the brain and learning. The medial temporal cortex belongs to the phylogenetically old cortex, or archicortex, with no thalamic connections but rich limbic and hypothalamic ones, whereas most of the cerebral hemispheres, including the lateral part of the temporal lobe, are neocortex and have structured thalamic connections.

The hard-wiring of the auditory system takes impulses from the cochlea via the eighth nerve to the cochlear nucleus and then decussates and passes via the lateral lemniscus to the inferior colliculus and then via the medial geniculate nucelus of the thalamus to Heschl's gyrus in the temporal lobe. This pathway can be verified using electrocochleography, brainstem evoked responses, and cortical auditory evoked responses. Heschl's gyrus is not visible from the surface of the brain but is very prominent if the superior surface of the temporal lobe is exposed (Fig. 2.7), where it can be seen to consist of two or three transverse gyri. It is thought that there are at least six cochleotopic maps in each area of Heschl's gyrus. The transverse gyri of Heschl are thought to be responsible for auditory discrimination, e.g. distinguishing sounds with a linguistic meaning (for example differentiating between *colour* and *collar)* from those with an emotional connotation such as tenderness, anger, sarcasm. The system is very accurate and discriminates between sounds with only a few hertz' difference in frequency or milliseconds' difference in time, e.g. *ta* and *da*. This system is thought to be abnormal in children with speech delay and some therapies are based on stretching out the times over which sounds are presented. Localization of sound direction, stereophonic sound, loudness, pitch, rhythm, stress, and tune (intonation), as well as word differentiation, are all part of normal learning.

Planum temporale

Behind the mountains of Heschl's gyrus is the flatter plane, the planum temporale, of the auditory association area, which is identical with Wernicke's area. This is the area of the brain that differs most between the higher apes and humans. It is the most asymmetrical area of the brain and is thought to be the anatomical basis of speech; in particular is the site of the word store – the lexicon – of language. Heschl's gyrus is longer and often fatter on the left, and the left planum temporale is the bigger. Wada has shown that these asymmetries are present in utero and are not the effects of language acquisition. The left occipital lobe is the wider, the left sylvian fissure is 6.0 mm longer than the right, and the left angular gyrus is the more prominent. The left planum temporale tends to be larger than the right and contains about 17 times more cells (Geschwind and Levitsky 1968). In a study of 100 brains the planum temporale was larger on the left in 65, larger on the right in 11, and equal on right and left in 24.

The importance of the planum temporale in the genesis of learning disabilities has become clear from the Boston studies (Livingstone et al. 1991). Using celloidin sections stained by the Nissl method, these researchers studied the brains of five males and three females with dyslexia. In the males they found (1) right/left symmetry of the planum temporale, rather than asymmetry; (2) defects in the auditory and visual systems; and (3) focal neocortical areas of dysplasia – from 30 to hundreds of areas of ectopic tissue, in contrast with the very few found in 10 normal control brains from the Yakolev collection.

Such ectopias are in layer 1 of the neocortex, which normally contains very few neurons. They are mainly on the left and along the sylvian fissure and are occasionally overlaid by polymicrogyria, indicating perturbation before 26 weeks of gestation. Similar abnormalities have been described in the hippocampus, septal nuclei, mamillary bodies, amygdala, cerebellum, and olives in autism (Bauman and Kemper 1985).

Memory

Memory is absolutely basic to learning: if we cannot store any new memories we cannot learn anything new. Loss of memory is one of the first and most important symptoms of dementia. Memories once laid down are difficult to erase; they may last 70 years and resist sleep, coma, anaesthesia, drugs, or concussion.

Complex strategies such as the classification and storage of related memories into *concepts,* thus making it possible to understand and to reason (see below). Memory systems are seen in the genetic memory coded in DNA, lymphocyte memory, and neuronal memory. Clinically it may be very difficult to decide if a patient's main difficulty is aphasia, dementia, or a primary memory disorder.

EXPLICIT AND IMPLICIT MEMORY

Explicit memory encodes information about autobiographical knowledge as well as factual knowledge. Another name for this type of memory is *declarative memory* (memories that can be reported verbally). The stored information of explicit memory is the result of processing by our perceptual apparatus. Once stored, it can be recalled deliberately. However, later recall is not merely a faithful reproduction of the original stored information but rather a modified representation of past experience in which the sensory information is used as clues to reconstruct the past event in a newly formed later recall.

Implicit memory has an automatic, or *reflex,* quality and in this chapter the term is applied mainly to motor learning. The formation and recall of an implicit memory are not dependent on cognition, but rather are automatic, without deliberate effort. Repetition, i.e. practice over several trials, is responsible for its formation. It can be expressed primarily by improved performance rather than in words.

SHORT-TERM AND LONG-TERM MEMORY

Short-term, or *labile, memory* endures for seconds or minutes; it is working memory – the equivalent of RAM (random-access memory) in computer terms. It is the memory necessary for acquiring new data by perception from the environment. It is the memory into which we also bring previously stored memories from the cerebral cortex. Material must be brought into short-term memory before it can be processed by recognition or reasoning. It enters consciousness only when held in short-term memory. Thought is what we are currently thinking about and therefore is the current content of short-term memory. Short-term memory is closely related to consciousness; it is the capacity – i.e. how much information can be held in consciousness at any one time – for thinking. It probably relies on oscillating circuits in the reticular formation, or possibly – according to Hebb's less appealing suggestion – modification of synapses. Just as the memory in a pocket calculator or RAM in a computer is lost when it is switched off, so short-term memory is lost with sleep, electroconvulsive therapy, anaesthesia, or distraction.

Loss of attention, as when we are distracted, clears the short-term memory. This is why, when changing the subject of thought, as when writing a paper, we walk around to clear our minds, have a cup of coffee, listen to music. Paying attention holds the current content of consciousness, while distraction allows the loss of current thoughts. Interest holds the attention and so maintains the content of consciousness, which can then be processed by reasoning. The content of short-term memory lasts only a few minutes, even with rehearsal, after which it is forgotten if it is not transferred to long-term stores. Digit span and repeating sentences of varyious lengths test the capacity of short-term memory.

Long-term, or stable, memory endures for days, years, or even decades and can be compared to hard-disk memory in computer terms. It is the memory required to demonstrate a learned behaviour over longer periods of time. It holds all significant data of our lives and, very importantly, holds it in sequence, so giving us our concept of time. Unlike short-term memory, it is hard to change or displace.

The long-term memory is a permanent store, not destroyed by sleep, anaesthesia, or electroconvulsive therapy but only by destruction of that particular area of cortex. Penfield, in his original studies on electrical stimulation of the cerebral cortex in the awake human, conducted during operations for epilepsy, confirmed that past memories and experiences could be brought back by low-voltage stimulation of the cerebral cortex and that different memories were awakened by stimulating different parts of the cortex, suggesting that some form of 'hard-copy' storage occurred in the cortex. This idea is also supported by certain disorders – in which, for instance, one language, English, may be lost but another, e.g. Gaelic, may be preserved. Equally specific agnosias, such as the inability to recognize faces or the central loss of colour vision, mean that memories underlying specific skills must be localized. Loss of selective memory, such as the loss of one's own autobiography, can occur in pathological conditions and is strong evidence for the localization of specific aspects of memory

43

(Mimura et al. 1997). Specifically grammatical aspects, such as small-word aphasia (loss of *it, in, on, at*) or even the specific loss of collective nouns, suggest that even the rules of grammar may be localized (Semenza et al. 1997). As outlined we feel that the site of this hard-copy store is in the specific learning modules that make up the cerebral cortex.

Storage of memories must also be sequential, since sequence gives us a concept of time, of past and present. In aquired brain damage, memories of a few days or a few years preceding the damage may be lost (retrograde amnesia) while all others remain intact, or no new memories may be added to existing stores (anterograde amnesia). How this continuous and sequential tape-recording of memories is achieved is not known. It explains why time distortion is part of amnesic syndromes. The time sequence can be entered through hypnosis, and a current anxiety is whether 'false memories' can be placed in a past time sequence, as by suggesting that a parent sexually abused the patient as a child. The patient may then remember the suggestion in the time frame of memory from the past, even though the suggestion was only recent, and this may convince the person that the memory is true. Distortion of the time frame also causes the phenomena *déjà vu* and *déjà fait.*

'SEARCH' AND 'SAVE'
Search – recalling old memories
Material is drawn from long-term memory stores into short-term memory by a 'search' command via the frontal lobe and the reticular formation, and if this process is faulty the result is difficulty in recall – in *RE-MEMBERING.* This process must be different from the activation of the medial temporal lobe structures required to memorize, i.e. save new memories, since recall of past stored memories is normal after bilateral medial temporal lobectomy. Faulty searching is also seen when as we get older we have difficulty in remembering names but not concepts and yet a few minutes later recall is perfect. This phenomenon shows that the store is still there: it is the recall that is faulty. In searching the cerebral cortex for stored memories that form part of a concept, the brain is *associative,* not *logical.* That is, all parts of the cortex are searched for a recognizable component of the concept, and the brain does not go through every step of a mathematical, logical program as occurs in a computer. We understand less about the neurology of recall than about that involved in saving memories. How does one search such vast memory stores in all parts of the cerebral cortex so rapidly? Eccles has shown that the apical dendrite of a neuron contains a structure known as a cartridge, which can switch the neuron on or off, so that if all the neurons in a module are switched on then any pattern of surface stimulation that they have previously met and for which they have a memory trace or protein would be signalled by the neuron firing.

Saving new memories
Placing new material from short-term memory and conscious perception or reasoning into long-term memory stores requires the anterior temporal lobe to be intact, and specifically the hippocampus: the brain's equivalent of the 'save' command on a computer. Lesions of the lateral surface of the temporal lobe – i.e. of the neocortex – do not prevent the laying down of new memories. The memory system within the temporal lobe is quite extensive.

The hippocampal formation includes the hippocampus, the dentate gyrus, the subiculum, to which the hippocampus projects, and the parahippocampal cortices. The subiculum and the entorhinal area are really a continuation in neocortex of the hippocampus. The dentate gyrus consists of small, dense granule cells and the hippocampus consists of large pyramidal cells. There are also GABAergic basket cells, which inhibit the hippocampal pyramidal cells. The hippocampus is divided into three parts, CA1, CA2, and CA3. Bilateral loss of pyramidal cells in CA1 appears to be specifically involved in memory loss. Afferents to the hippocampus come mainly from the entorhinal cortex, which in turn is connected with nearly every association area in the neocortex (permanent memory stores) and septal nuclei (attention and consciousness). The acetylcholinergic fibres of these nuclei produce a long-lasting excitation of hippocampal pyramidal cells. One of these nuclei is the basal nucleus of Meynert, which is always affected in Alzheimer's disease. Efferent fibres project back to the parahippocampal cortex, hypothalamus, mamillary bodies, and cingulate cortex. The complete circuit required from the temporal lobe involves the fornix, which arises in the subiculum, the indusium griseum along with the mamillary bodies, and the medial dorsal nucleus of the thalamus. Lesions of the mamillary bodies were originally thought to be the basis of memory loss in alcoholism and post-traumatic Wernicke's encephalopathy, but the damage is now thought to be more extensive, also involving the medial thalamus.

Uncal or amygdaloid lesions, i.e. of the archicortex (archipallium) alone, do not disrupt memory if they do not go deep enough to involve the hippocampus. Dott, in Edinburgh, found that cutting the fornix on both sides in the human did not disrupt memory. The amygdala is thought to be needed for emotional rather than cognitive memory. It is still not definite whether the seat of memory is the hippocampus itself or the adjacent bundle of white matter, the temporal stem. Studies of the neurotransmitter choline acetyltransferase, which is essential for memory function and is deficient in Alzheimer's disease, including that seen in Down syndrome, suggests that the basis of memory is a primary gray matter processing unit in the hippocampal formation. It is thought that normally the amygdala/hippocampal complex on the left has to do with verbal memory and that on the right, with spatial memory. If one side is damaged or removed the opposite side can take over; if both sides are damaged the long-term storage of any new memories is severely disrupted. This was starkly demonstrated in the people studied by Brenda Milner (Milner 1971), the most famous being HM, who had bilateral anterior temporal lobectomies for epilepsy. After such bilateral damage to the amygdala/hippocampal complex, one can still hold information – numbers, names, telephone numbers, short messages, lines of poetry – for seconds or minutes in short-term memory, but the information disappears on distraction and is not permanently stored. One cannot recognize any new faces that are seen after surgery but has no difficulty with faces learned before surgery. HM took one year to find his way around a new house. Motor learning is preserved and new motor skills, e.g. playing ping-pong or pool, can be learned. This case study proved most vividly the difference between motor and cognitive memory and between short- and long-term memory. CW, the chorus master of the London Sinfonietta, similarly lost the ability to store new memories after temporal lobe destruction from herpes simplex encephalitis. After this damage he could still play the organ and read music, but life was a constant brief new snapshot.

PHYSICAL STORAGE OF LONG-TERM MEMORY IN THE CEREBRAL CORTEX

The cell and memory

Memory could be stored by oscillating circuits, as in a pocket calculator or the RAM in a computer, whose contents are erased when the computer is switched off, when there is a power failure, or when the person is asleep or distracted. Memory could be due to temporary changes in synapses, to changes in protein molecules, or, since there are so many billion nerve cells, even to one memory per cell. Whatever the explanation, long-term memory must reside in some permanent, physical, molecular change.

Synapses

Some change in a synapse as a result of stimulation is thought to act as the memory trace underlying and responsible for memory. The reason such changes are thought to take place in the synapse is that its size, the amount and type of the neurotransmitter it releases on arrival of the action potential, and the type and number of receptors in the subsynaptic membrane all affect the magnitude, duration, and type of the postsynaptic event: such changes could be thought of as an analogue gradation of a digital signal.

Post-tetanic potentiation means that there is a significant increase in the excitability of subsynaptic membrane after a train of several impulses; that is, use of the system increases its excitability. It persists for a few hours and then the subsynaptic membrane returns to normal. This short-term synpatic enhancement may be related to the temporary accumulation of calcium ions within the terminal.

Long-term potentiation differs from post-tetanic potentiation in that it can persist for days, weeks, or even months. Stimulation is greater with larger numbers of impulses and the involvement of several brain areas. Repeated or persistent firing of a synapse may cause some subtle changes that increase the efficiency with which it thereafter excites the postsynaptic cell; in order to induce this change, simultaneous presynaptic and postsynaptic activities are required. There is strong evidence that the NMDA (*N*-methyl D-aspartate) receptor is involved in the induction of long-term potentiation.

Memory and patterns of cell-surface stimulation

The surface membrane of the neuron and its dendrites is covered with some 10 000 synapses by dendrites from other cells ending at boutons terminaux. This arrangement can be regarded as potentially etching a picture on the surface of the cell, with each bouton terminal being the equivalent of a pixel on a computer screen. The area of cell membrane is vastly increased by the dendrites – the total membrane area of the Purkinje cell, for example, is enormous. Nissl substance abounds in cells that have a large input from which they have to select and compute, such as pyramidal cells in the motor cortex, Purkinje cells in the cerebellum, and anterior horn cells in the spinal cord (Fig. 2.8). The boutons terminaux can impose a specific pattern over an area of membrane, drawn as if in pixels on the cell surface. If there were a biochemical system whereby the RNA of Nissl substance could synthesize a protein (type of neuronal antibody) that would allow memory of that pattern of surface stimulation, this learned pattern would be recognized (remembered) if it were subsequently experienced again, and the neuron could fire: that is, the neuron would function as a memory and a switch.

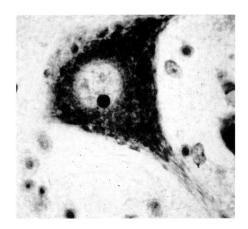

Fig. 2.8. A normal neuron (dark area), whose denseness is due to the presence of large amounts of RNA in polyribosomes of the Nissl substance.

Molecular memory

The synthesis of specific 'memory molecules', as occurs in immunological memory, is an attractive hypothesis of the method of memory storage proposed by Holger Hyden and coworkers (Hyden and Lange 1967; Nicholls 1994). Drugs (e.g. cytostatics or high-dose phenytoin) that block protein synthesis are thought to interfere with the learning of new material. Drugs (e.g. benzodiazepines) that affect neurotransmitters may also affect memory. Repetition of a memory reinforces it in the same way as repeated immunizations reinforce an antibody response in a lymphocyte.

De novo protein synthesis depends on the neuronal genome, that is, nuclear DNA, and requires communication between the cell surface and the nucleus (Agranoff 1980, Montorolo et al. 1986). A neurotransmitter released from a nerve ending crosses the synapse and binds to the postsynaptic membrane on the cell surface. Here it may have one of two actions: (a) ionotropic, when it binds to a channel across the cell membrane – an ionophore – which will then allow sodium, potassium, calcium, or chloride ions to flow into the cell and so set up an electric current; or (b) metabotropic, when the neurotransmitter attaches to a receptor on the cell membrane and causes a change in the cell's metabolism. Acetylcholine, serotonin, noradrenaline (norepinephrine), dopamine, insulin, nerve growth factor, steroid hormones, and neuropeptides all have their effect on the cell by means of metabotropic receptors, of which there may be as many as 100 types. It is thought that acetylcholine and glutamate are particularly involved in memory function. These neurotransmitters are the *primary messengers.* They cause the release of regulatory G proteins, which are activated if they combine with GTP (guanosine triphosphate) and are in an inactive form if combined with GDP (guanosine diphosphate). There are at least 20 G proteins, and a single receptor can activate several of them, not only causing an amplifier effect but also making that receptor biochemically specific. If many receptors are stimulated, a pool of G proteins is produced that will obviously reflect the pattern of stimulation. The G protein also activates *second messengers,* such as cyclic AMP, inositol phosphates, arachidonic acid, carbon monoxide, or nitric oxide, and these form an intracellular messenger or communication system.

Nitric oxide seems vital to the memory function of neurons, allowing them to remember previously experienced signals. These second messengers in turn activate protein kinases that phosphorylate certain amino acids such as serine, tyrosine, and threonine; this phosphorylation changes the shape of protein molecules and so their function. In this way genomic read-out and protein synthesis can all be affected by a pattern of cell-surface stimulation. Specific proteins such as alpha cam K2 appear to be needed for animals to learn. Long-term neuronal memory associated with protein synthesis may cause the development of new spines on the dendritic trees, which is another way in which cell stimulation would affect developmental anatomy (Smith 1989, Kandel et al. 1995).

Second messengers can also be activated by the binding of intracellular calcium to calmodulin, which is present in the hippocampus at a high concentration (2% of the total protein content). Each calmodulin molecule binds four calcium ions. The calcium enters the cell via the NMDA receptor, and hence glutamate (the neurotransmitter at the NMDA receptor) is also a regulator of cell memory. More exciting has been the study of a second type of glutamate receptor, the AMPA (alpha-amino-3-hydroxy-5-methylisoxazolepropionic acid) receptor, especially as a group of compounds, called ampikines, that enhance the sensitivity of this receptor to glutamate have been shown to enhance learning markedly in experimental animals and are an exciting area of research in Alzheimer's disease. Benzodiazepines work on the GABA receptor in the same way that ampikines facilitate the AMPA receptor and have the opposite effect, impairing memory and learning. Oestrogen is also thought to inhibit learning, and women often complain of memory problems during pregnancy and the puerperium. It has been suggested that the phase of the menstrual cycle affects grades in secondary school girls (Boyle 1997).

Causes of failure of long-term memory storage
Disruption of the architecture of the whole cerebral cortex, as in cortical dysplasias of tuberous sclerosis, lissencephaly, Miller–Dieker syndrome, familial micrencephaly, fetal alcohol syndrome, and maternal cocaine addiction, will result in severe learning failure with a global cognitive learning disorder, also called mental retardation. Destruction of the cortex by neuronal necrosis due to hypoxia/ischaemia, to severe trauma, or to a storage disease produces severe global learning defects. Focal dysplasias may cause more localized or specific learning disorders, but the highly selective loss of certain memories is more likely due to tumours or focal infarcts.

Unilateral surgical ablation of the anterior temporal lobe or more specifically the medial temporal lobe results in failure to store verbal material if ablation is on the left, or spatial material if on the right. There are many diseases of this area, which has a high glutamate concentration and is therefore particularly sensitive to hypoxia; for example memory may appear to be poorer after a myocardial infarct or cardiac surgery. It is not surprising that carbon monoxide poisoning can cause a severe Korsakoff syndrome. Korsakoff syndrome is also seen in alcoholism, thiamine deficiency, head injury, tumour infiltration, and raised pressure with uncal herniation. This syndrome also involves the failure of transfer or saving of new material from short- to long-term memory stores. The patient is aware of the memory defect and so makes up material to cover the defect – i.e. confabulates.

Sixty per cent of children with epilepsy have a learning defect: memory defects are common and so of course is hippocampal or mesial temporal sclerosis. In psychomotor fugue states the person may perform very complex behaviours but have no stored memory of the events. In non-convulsive status epilepticus all learning may come to a halt for days, weeks, or months.

Herpes simplex encephalitis, posterior hypothalamic tumours, and basal tuberculous exudate of the mamillary area are also associated with amnesic syndromes. Hypothalamic tumours going into the mamillary area can produce failure to store new memories.

In transient global amnesia the person fails to store any memories for, on average, 4 hours and yet is fully conscious, with no effects on the IQ and no epilepsy seen on EEG. Recovery is complete. This phenomenon appears to occur in temporal lobe ischaemia with migraine.

Consciousness (arousal)

We can try to explain many brain functions in a mechanical way, as with our computer simile, but as in all science eventually one comes upon a brick wall – What is space? What is energy? What initiated the big bang? and, in the case of the biological sciences, What is consciousness? This is the enigma that remains, allowing philosophy to reign over neuroscience. Nevertheless consciousness as we know it cannot exist without a brain and in some brain diseases is lost forever. Even our deepest emotions, such as love, hate, happiness, or deep depression, can exist only in the conscious brain. Consciousness is difficult to define. Descartes' dictum 'I think, therefore I am' (*Cogito, ergo sum*) falls short as a definition of consciousness, since the converse is not true: if I cannot think I may be demented, deluded, or hallucinating, but I am not unconscious. We do not know what is going on in the conscious mind of another person if they do not communicate with us. A non-anaesthetized person given curare remains fully conscious, but how does an outsider determine that there is a personal inner awareness?

Is consciousness, if only microconsciousness, a feature of all living cells and does a huge protoplasmic conglomerate such as the brain merely amplify it into macroconsciousness? The brain could amass a large amount of consciousness by joining billions of cells in the form of what Graham Cannon in Manchester used to call 'organismal control', and death could then be simply the permanent loss of this organismal control centred in the brainstem reticular formation and a return to a mass cellular microconsciousness.

Do we simply need a nerve net such as the reticular formation linking millions of cells as one unit to give us consciousness? Does the size of the cerebral cortex merely store more information for the content of consciousness? Some experts in artificial intelligence have claimed that a computer if made powerful enough would automatically become conscious. The most telling argument against this idea is that loss of intelligence in people with global learning disorder or severe dementia does not mean a loss of consciousness, but only a diminution in its content.

Consciousness depends upon intactness of the reticular activating system and septal nuclei. A child may have a gross lesion of the lower brainstem (i.e. lower pons and medulla), as with a pontine glioma, so that all body movement, speech, and swallowing are paralysed, and yet be fully conscious and able to think normally. This is also true in akinetic mutism resulting from a bilateral upper brainstem lesion. Similarly a whole cerebral hemisphere may be removed, thus limiting the subsequent content of consciousness (thought processes), and yet the child will be fully conscious. Extensive disease of both cerebral hemispheres may cause severe mental defect or dementia and so limit or even abolish all cognitive learning (as in post-traumatic persistent vegetative state), thus grossly restricting the content of consciousness, and yet the child may still be conscious. There is a relatively small area of the upper brainstem, thalamus, and septum that appears to be necessary to sustain consciousness, and a small lesion here – as in tentorial herniation secondary to raised intracranial pressure, primary midbrain injury in trauma, localized encephalitis, or tumour – may cause prolonged coma. An irreversible lesion in the brainstem, e.g. central ischaemic neuronal necrosis, can result in permanent failure of cortical arousal and of consciousness: this is why the concept of brain death depends upon brainstem function rather than the cortex.

Most comas are due to (a) tentorial herniation from raised intracranial pressure, (b) hypoxia, or (c) drugs affecting the reticular formation. Primary upper brainstem tumours and infarcts are uncommon; upper brainstem infarcts and haemorrhages are usually secondary to raised intracranial pressure.

Hypnotic drugs have specific actions on the reticular activating system. There may be natural endogenous hypnotics such as natural benzodiazepines in the same way that there are natural endogenous opioids. The brain comprises about 2% of the body weight (1.5/70 kg) but accounts for 20% of the body's oxygen consumption. The most effective way to reduce consciousness and flatten the EEG is to reduce cell metabolism by hypoxia. This suggests that consciousness requires a constant energy supply and is an active process in the cell. The reticular formation, hippocampus, and basal ganglia have the highest oxygen uptake.

It is lesser degrees of loss of cortical arousal that are important to the teacher. The teacher is likely to notice if a child is overtly sleepy and lethargic, but may not always find it easy to spot more subtly impaired arousal. A child who is taking certain anticonvulsant medications, who is using other drugs or alcohol or sniffing solvents, who is bored, or who was watching television till late at night may be drowsy, with impaired speed and accuracy of thought.

Attention
Attention is the willed or voluntary selection of a topic to hold within consciousness, utilizing short-term memory in order to allow mental processing (thinking). Attention is the focusing of conscious awareness upon (i) a particular motor activity – especially while it is being learned; (ii) a specific sensory input or perception; or (iii) memories and concepts retrieved from long-term memory stores into short-term memory. Sustained attention requires a high level of arousal, and a drowsy or bored child will have a short attention span. Distraction is the opposite of 'paying attention': the child loses attention, short-term memory is cleared, and the train of thought is lost. Attention is accompanied by the rejection of simultaneous unwanted sensory stimuli, which are said to be 'gated out' – e.g. environmental noise as distinct from speech sounds, sensation from muscles or skin (due to seating and

clothing), and visual stimuli other than those relevant to the task at hand. If such irrelevant stimuli are not gated out they enter conscious awareness and interfere with thought processes, so that one may 'lose the stream of thought' – i.e. one is distracted and this clears short-term memory. Attention is also lost (a secondary attention deficit arises) when the material is boring, irrelevant, or anxiety-provoking, and likewise attention is sustained when the material is interesting and excites curiosity.

It is thought that the intralaminar thalamic nuclei and the prefrontal lobes are important in the maintenance of attention. It is a well-documented clinical observation that certain drugs such as phenobarbitone and benzodiazepines can disrupt attention, causing the child to be more distractible. Frontal lobe damage after head injury can often be demonstrated by SPECT scans and is associated with a major attention deficit. Functional scans suggest that in attention-deficit disorder (ADD) there is abnormal frontal lobe perfusion, which can be improved with methylphenidate. True ADD coexists with specific learning disability in about 30% of cases, but treatment of one cannot be guaranteed to improve the other.

True lead poisoning with clinical signs can cause severe overactive behaviour, but there is no conclusive evidence that the lower concentrations that often cause such concern result in any behavioural abnormality. Also unconvincing is the evidence that colouring agents, salicylates, or food additives (in Europe, often identified with so-called E numbers) cause a true toxic encephalopathy with selective damage to the prefrontal lobes and intralaminar thalamic nuclei. Children with coeliac disease certainly are overactive in the true sense, with a measurable increase in motor activity and restlessness, and are also very irritable; these signs are possibly due to a true toxic encephalopathy from absorption of larger peptides, which is ameliorated by a gluten-free diet.

Primary attention deficit is an unlikely diagnosis if a child's loss of attention is situational – for instance if the child does not pay attention when trying to read and yet will perform the most boring tasks when succeeding, or will watch television or videos or play computer games for long periods, or will sit patiently for several hours during assessment or computer-based psychometrics. Anxiety can certainly disrupt attention: the child will concentrate if succeeding, but loses concentration, fidgets, and becomes restless as soon as an area of difficulty arises and failure is imminent. In a great many children with learning disorder the attention defect is a secondary situational problem due to induced anxiety, not a primary biological defect.

For many years a primary disorder of attention has been postulated as a major cause of learning disability. Attention-deficit/hyperactivity disorder (ADHD), which is considered in more detail in Chapter 6 of this book, is not a primary reason for speech and language failure or for dyslexia and dysgraphia. There may be a primary attention deficit, hyperactivity alone, or a combination of the two. Attention disorder on its own is usually situational – due to anxiety from chronic failure – and the solution is a good remedial teacher who makes the child feel secure and not a failure and who motivates the child rather than prescribing large doses of sympathomimetic amines. This is not to deny the existence of a hyperkinetic syndrome, thought to affect 5 to 10% of school-age children, or its presence in 30% of children with specific learning disability. Poor concentration and distractibility show concordance in twin studies, suggesting a true genetic basis for these conditions.

Since the prefrontal area and the angular gyrus are the two last areas of cerebral cortex to develop, the combination of behavioural and learning symptoms is not unexpected (BA Shaywitz et al. 1995).

For a sustainable diagnosis of ADHD the condition must be diagnosed before the age of 7 years, and at least six symptoms must be attributable to attention deficit and six to hyperactivity or poor impulse control, i.e. 'rages'. It is five times more common in boys than girls. The condition must also not be situational: it must occur both at school and at home. Anxiety about parental marriage breakdown and inconsistent discipline, particularly during the 'terrible twos' stage, may cause hyperactivity at home, and anxiety from an undiagnosed learning disability may be manifest mainly at school.

Children with epilepsy, especially complex partial seizures arising in the temporal lobe, or children with brain damage due to asphyxia at birth, encephalopathy of low birthweight, hydrocephalus, or head injury may certainly show attention deficit and learning disability. However, most children with specific learning disability do not have brain damage.

In the case of children with global delay in cognitive learning, the deficit in cognitive learning means that they cannot sustain thought on a particular subject. For example they may not be able to sustain play through imagination and 'saying to themselves' in order to know what to do with a toy car or airplane. Such children cannnot sustain play, but flit from toy to toy or activity to activity, so appearing to have a defect of attention that is actually secondary to the cognitive difficulty.

TYPES OF LEARNING

In the first part of this chapter we discussed, in terms of brain structure and function, the neurological substrate that underpins how a child learns. There are three separate neuroanatomical circuits, subserving motor, emotional, and cognitive learning, and a new behaviour can arise purely as a result of neuroanatomical maturation or as an effect of environmental experience. Learning can be divided into several categories:

- Reflex behaviour
- Preprogrammed behaviour
- Conditioned behaviour
- True learned behaviour
  - Motor learning
  - Emotional learning
  - Cognitive learning

REFLEX BEHAVIOUR
In a classic reflex such as a tendon, pupillary, or protective reflex (e.g. a flexor withdrawal reflex), the same stimulus always produces the same stereotyped response. This response is a function of the wiring of the nervous system and its appearance does not require environmental experience or repetition. It varies only in its presence, absence, or intensity. Reflexes can be exteroceptive, such as the examples just given, or interoceptive. Interoceptive reflexes

control the vegetative or autonomic functions of the body: secretion of saliva and gastric acid, control of blood sugar, and emptying of the bladder and bowel are basic reflexes. Nevertheless in the normal person they can be conditioned, as the classic Pavlovian experiments showed. Even blood pressure, cardiac output, heart rate, and urine flow can be modified by emotion or forced relaxation. Reflexes are dependent upon the maturity of the nervous system and may appear at one stage and disappear at another, e.g. the asymmetrical tonic neck reflex, the Moro reflex, and feeding reflexes. A reflex in its simplest form is obligatory and unchanging, but its presence in this form is nearly always an indication of release of control in a disease state: purely reflex bladder emptying is seen in paraplegia, the tendon reflex is less state-dependent when isolated from higher centres, blood pressure may rise in response to posture, respiration may be purely automatic, and so on.

There is often a positive and a corresponding negative reflex – extensor versus flexor, ingesting versus egesting – and one of these may be facilitated over the other. Several reflexes may be facilitated together, reinforcing one another. This is seen best in feeding behaviour as opposed to feeding reflexes. A group of reflexes – rooting, cardinal points, tongue furling, sucking, stripping, and swallowing – are facilitated together for ingestion, as opposed to lip avoidance, lip pursing, tongue rolling and unfurling against roof of mouth, gagging, vomiting, choking, and coughing as egesting reflexes. Hunger, thirst, taste, and smell, as well as hyperosmolality or hypoglycaemia, will facilitate these feeding reflexes as a group into a behaviour pattern. In the young preterm infant these ingesting reflexes develop separately, becoming integrated only after the 32nd week of development, when an emerging behaviour is often referred to as the infant 'having learned to bottle-feed'.

Reflex emotional behaviours also exist: the newborn infant switches on a set cry, the feeding siren – an inspiratory stridulous noise and a long, loud expiratory vocalization – when the blood sugar falls, and this persists until the infant's hunger is satiated. If feeding is stopped the infant has a rage reaction – legs extended, face suffused, fisting and fighting of the upper limbs, arching of the back – which dramatically disappears with the first suck. When the infant is satiated the siren is replaced by a satiation grunt on expiration.

PREPROGRAMMED LEARNING

Philosophers have thought for centuries that people had 'free will' and could determine their own actions. We can now recognize many behaviours that are a stereotyped response in all humans to a particular environmental event – a kind of reflex behaviour. Such behaviours appear to be preprogrammed within the brain, in a type of preprogrammed memory. Examples are hatching behaviour, bonding, maternal behaviour (mothering), feeding behaviour, nesting behaviour (home-making), courting, sexual behaviour, mourning behaviour, forced usage (visual, oral, manipulative, and postural), punishment behaviour, fight and flight responses (to threat to security, or to frustration of a planned action or desire), and nonverbal communicative behaviours appearing in the first year of life (including, cuddling, consoling, greeting, smiling, submitting, desire to please).

Individual reflexes such as the walking, stepping, crossed extensor, and Bauer reflexes are in essence all part of the intrauterine swimming pattern required for the infant to swim into the vertex position, turn its head to the right, and so present in the typical left

53

occipitoanterior position – i.e. human hatching behaviour. The infant will swim in a coordinated fashion if submersed in water after birth, as Myrtle McGraw has shown dramatically in her films. The statoacoustic system is thought to develop at about 32 weeks gestational age, and at about this time the infant swims into the vertex position. This must be a preprogrammed learning response, because if the infant is born prematurely, if anything impedes its swimming (such as oligohydramnios, maternal fibroids, or fetal weakness from neuromuscular disease), then transverse lie or breech presentation may occur. Infants are also much more frequently born in the left occipitoanterior position, so asymmetrical head-turning is necessary for the head to engage.

As any new ability appears, such as vision, hearing, hand manipulation, and walking, a built-in program ensures that the infant uses and practises the skill – that usage is forced, and is prior to learning by volition or intent. Thus forced visual pursuit at 3 weeks of age, forced grasping and hand regard at 3 months, forced utterances (repetitive babble at 4 months), and forced exploration at 1 year are all seen (McGraw 1935). Deaf children may babble even though they will never develop speech. This shows that babbling is innate, and not a result of environmental natural selection.

CONDITIONED LEARNING

Conditioned learning requires environmental experience and the ability to lay down a memory trace. The behaviour always occurs in response to the same stimulus but is not innate and does not simply require hard-wiring of the nervous system for its production. It is often reinforced by the giving of approval and pleasure or disapproval and discomfort. It does not require understanding or meaning or cognition and can be achieved in the presence of severe learning disability. Meaning may come later, as in waving bye-bye, toilet training, repeating nursery rhymes, or singing tunes.

Conditioned memory sequence

Some degree of rote learning is a prerequisite for cognitive learning and is the basis of, or lingua franca that is a prerequisite for, concept formation and understanding. Anatomy is often learned by rote using rude mnemonics which are remembered years after, say, the branches of artery in question have long been forgotten. I can still remember, 30 years on, the mnemonic for the branches of the brachial artery – *p*rostitutes *n*ever *u*se *m*ethylated *s*pirits – and an even ruder one about Oscar for the branches of the carotid artery.

Repeating nursey rhymes and singing 'baa baa black sheep', 'twinkle, twinkle, little star', and 'pop goes the weasel' are simply the rote learning of memory sequences. Children do not know that 'ring a ring of roses' commemorates death from bubonic plague or that goosey goosey gander commemorates intolerance of Roman Catholicism.

Children can have speech without language, as in the cocktail party personality, mynah bird syndrome, or parroting, when they may learn and repeat, sometimes ad nauseam, long conversations that they have heard, e.g. about Pay-As-You-Earn or the effect of the French market on the price of Scottish beef, without understanding the meaning of what they are saying. This is really an exaggerated form of echolalia and is sometimes seen to an advanced degree in children with the fragile X syndrome, hydrocephalus, and Williams syndrome.

Similarly children may 'learn to read' by remembering the page and word shape as an object and will 'bark at print': they recognize the print upside down or with the page half covered but they will not recognize the identical words in a different context. With practice one may learn to play 'from memory' the first page of Beethoven's 'Moonlight' Sonata and yet not be able to play anything else or read music – i.e. be musically illiterate.

TRUE LEARNED BEHAVIOUR

Motor learning

Learning new motor skills is dependent upon the frontal cortex – including motor association areas, the motor strip, and the supplementary motor area – and also the basal ganglia and the cerebellum. Motor memory (kinaesthetic memory) is not only for postural or manipulative motor skills but also for speech and writing. New motor skills can be learned in the presence of a severe cognitive defect, for example in global learning disability or in the failure of all new cognitive memory stores after anterior temporal lobectomy.

A motor skill is learned in several stages:

(1) Perform a single movement in isolation – hit a note on a piano or a typewriter keyboard, push down a clutch, copy a letter of the alphabet.
(2) Sequence several movements into a skill – sing a simple tune; write, type, or speak a word; change gears in a car; dance; ride a bicycle; swim.
(3) Practise the skill to increase speed and fluency until after several hundred practices the action does not occupy conscious effort – i.e. it becomes automatic.
(4) Then one can add prosodic or emotional overtones, i.e. intonation in speech, phrasing in poetry, rhythm and stress in music or dance, and punctuation to one's writing.

Motor learning requires concentration (attention), consciousness (arousal), motivation (application), and practice (repetition). Motor skills are not cognitive and so depend not upon a symbol system or language but upon repetition of a sequenced memory of a movement pattern, i.e. kinaesthetic memory.

Motor planning is in the premotor area, so that for speech it is in Broca's area and for writing it is in the graphomotor area. The actual execution is in the precentral motor strip but also requires the cerebellum, to adjust force, speed, and direction, and the basal ganglia for starting and stopping and for cadence. Sequencing requires the supplementary motor area. This pattern can be seen on PET scans or in functional MRI, as there is a 5% increase in cerebral blood flow when a part of the brain is active.

Motor learning of speech

Speech and language, although closely related, are not synonymous. Language, which is the basis of cognitive development, is a systematic symbol system used to develop concepts and so allow understanding (see later). Inner language is usually expressed through speech, but it can just as readily be conveyed through other means such as writing, manual signing, or musical notation. It is possible for a child to have normal 'inner language' in the absence of speech, as in akinetic mutism and Broca's aphasia. It is also possible for a child to develop speech without a commensurate level of inner language, as in the 'cocktail party

TABLE 2.5
Parts of the body that need to receive signals (+) from Broca's area
in order to say the word *spoon*

	Lips	Tongue	Palate	Voice	Breathing apparatus
S	–	+	–	–	+
P	+	–	–	–	–
O	+	–	–	+	+
O	+	–	–	+	+
N	–	+	+	+	+

–, no signal.

chatter' referred to earlier. These children recall by rote whole pieces of conversation, which they do not understand but which they produce in social situations, giving rise to a false impression of language competency (pragmatics as opposed to cognition).

Speech is based upon a phonological system. *Phonology* refers to the rules governing the way sounds are combined in speech. *Syntax,* which is closely related developmentally, refers to the grammatical structure of speech, and *semantics* refers to the underlying meaning. We discussed in the first part of this chapter how the components of grammar such as little connecting words (*at, it, as, to*), collective nouns, or proper names may be lost in isolation and so are learned as separate components of speech. The development of speech is the most sophisticated motor skill demanded of the preschool child. Its normal progress depends on the integrity of the bulbar musculature, brainstem motor pathways, basal ganglia, cerebellum, and cortical motor pathways: abnormality in these areas causes a dysarthria. Although the development of speech may be impaired independently of cognitive development, if there is a primary language disorder (dysphasia) or a global delay in cognition (learning disability) the child will be slow to speak because of a secondary speech disorder (Ingram et al. 1970).

Table 2.5 shows the sequence of signals that must be sent from Broca's area to the Rolandic motor strip, and so to the muscles of lips, tongue, palate, vocal apparatus, and breathing apparatus, in order to say the simple word *spoon:* the tune to be played by Broca on the Rolandic piano. In order to write the same word, a different series of signals is required, from the graphomotor area to the small muscles of the hand and wrist.

Development of the primary motor area of the cortex and corresponding association area of Broca along with the supplementary motor area is essential for the learning of this sequenced motor skill of speech, i.e. moving the lips, tongue, and palate in the correct sequence. The rate at which these areas develop is affected by the sex of the child, other genetic factors, and any brain damage, as described later. Simple, genetically caused slowing of development is usually referred to as *dyslalia,* while more severe disruption of phonological motor learning is really a developmental disease, *articulatory dyspraxia.* Lou et al. (1984) demonstrated decreased blood flow in the lower part of the premotor cortex (Broca's area) in three children with articulatory dyspraxia.

By the time children produce their first word with meaning (50th centile age 12 months, 90th centile 18 months), they have already developed complex preverbal communication and have all the sounds required for speech. During the first 6 months infants learn to distinguish between speech and non-speech sounds and can differentiate intonation (auditory discrimination). They can produce consonant/vowel single-syllable babble – *ma ma ma, ga ga ga.* During the second 6 months, they start to distinguish their name and the names of other family members, and babbling becomes increasingly complex. By the end of the first year they use many consistent sound sequences to represent meaning 'protowords' and combine these increasingly with non-verbal features such as eye-pointing and gesture to increase their ability to communicate.

Between 12 and 18 months, children can sequence only a limited range of consonants, i.e. *p, b, t, d, m, n,* with vowels, as in *mama, papa, dada, tata, bye-bye, pee-pee, poo, baba,* etc. Sound production gradually increases in sophistication, with acquisition of an increasing number of consonants, so that by the age of 2 to 3 years children can sequence a wider range, i.e. *k, g, s, f, h, w, j,* which at first they can put only in certain parts of a word and before or after certain consonants or blends. They will therefore omit the sound or substitute a sound that they can make (*l* for *r, t* for *k, d* for *g, d* for *j, t* for *th, s* for *i*) for the so-called later-acquired consonant, i.e. *r, sh, th, l, k, ch, dge, g, f.*

Phonology normally develops in a predictable manner. Most of the later-acquired speech sounds, at least in connective speech, are either fricative sounds or sounds that can be prolonged. There is therefore a pattern to children's speech that is consistent if one is aware of the omissions, insertions, reversals, and substitutions being used – the so-called developmental pattern. The paediatrician can recognize these characteristic alterations: omissions (*poon* for *spoon*), substitutions (*lolly* for *lorry*), insertions (*plegs* for *pegs*), and reversals (*aminals* for *animals*). Some other typical alterations are listed here:

ephelan	for	*elephant*
tolocat	for	*chocolate*
suss	for	*fluff*
odilay	for	*holiday*
teese	for	*cheese*
ottlies	for	*sausages*
Asilan	for	*Alison*

The mirror-image learning in the two hemispheres means that reversals of sounds in words and reversals of words in phrases are added to the immature motor performance. Other young children will often be able to understand the child with developmental speech problems better than adults can, and a sibling may translate, with the result that the parents may attribute the child's difficulty to laziness, arising from lack of a need to speak. Laziness is usually not the problem. A child who may be able to pronounce *s* in isolation may be unable to say, for instance, *s-s-s-s-poon* and so will say *poon.* This inability reflects how a child acquires motor skills. Phonology matures between the ages of 3 and 4 years, but some normal children continue to have difficulties with consonant clusters, especially those that can be prolonged, e.g. *ch, sh.* By the age of 5, the phonological development is largely complete and speech is entirely intelligible, though there may still be problems with *r, l,* and *th* (O'Hare and Brown 1998).

The mature adult will speak at a rate of 165 words or 250 syllables per minute. A student may hear up to 100 000 words per day and a highly educated person will have a total vocabulary of 100 000 words. In contrast, it is also suggested that any non-technical idea can be communicated successfully with a basic vocabulary of only 850 words.

Grammar, however, also has to be learned and at first children will learn simple rules that they will apply in all situations, e.g. to make a plural one adds an *s* at the end of the word (*foots, sheeps, mouses*); the past tense is indicated by adding *-ed* at the end of the word (*comed, goed, wented*). There is difficulty with the concept of time, such as today, tomorrow, yesterday, and with pronouns, such as *I* for *me*. For example a 2^1/$_2$-year-old might say:

> *It's comed off*
> *That's what me dood*
> *I amn't a menace*
> *I go get me cars*
> *I come me too as well*
> *Them cars is mine – them cars called –*
> *Off shoes on ladies wall*
> *Let's going now*
> *Going down one now he is*

Syntax develops from single words meaning a whole utterance (holophrastic speech) to a strictly structured two-term system using what are described as open and pivot words. For instance the open words could be *mummy, moon, dog, juice, place,* and the pivot words, *all gone, big, more, pretty, bye bye,* and when the child combines the two we would get, for example, *'all gone mummy', 'all gone moon', 'all gone juice', 'all gone dog',* etc. This two-term system is then gradually replaced by a simple phrase structure. At 2^1/$_2$ years of age children use an average of 3 words per utterance with a maximum of 8 words, and 95% of words are in the simple present tense. By 3 years of age children use an average of 6 words per utterance and a maximum of 15, and at this age there are 3 times more verbs in the past tense (McNeill 1970; TTS Ingram 1978, personal communication).

By the end of the second year children can understand simple questions of the type beginning with *what, where,* or *when.* By the end of the third year they understand concepts such as quantity, colour, size, and the use of prepositions. The vocabulary is small during the second year, and children may use 'overextensions', e.g. call all animals *cat.* The vocabulary rapidly increases during the third year to an average of 1000 words.

Between 3 and 5 years of age, comprehension becomes increasingly complex, e.g. adjectives and other descriptive words are recognized (*large/small, beside/inside*), and the function of objects is understood. At school entry, normal children can understand three-part instructions, are less dependent on context, and are developing abstract understanding, e.g. of time.

Cognitive learning

Cognition (from *con*, with, + *cognitio*, knowledge or understanding) is the opposite of *agnosia* (from *a-*, without + *gnosis*, feeling and understanding). With the development of understanding we are able to say 'I know', i.e. I have *know*ledge, that is, I possess a collection of acquired data on that subject that I can group and bring together into short-term memory and consciousness to form a concept, so that I can say that I understand. The basis of understanding is the formation of concepts, that is, a set of linked memories on the same topic stored at different addresses in the cerebral cortex; this allows holistic function of the whole brain. This formation of concepts requires some form of language. One does not therefore need to take sides as either a localized-language or a whole-brain-function theorist. Words (the lexicon) are localized, but inner language as implied by, for example, understanding or comprehension, requires all parts of the brain. The individual memories that form a concept are not stored at the same place. Take as an example the concept of an orange: the phonetic sound sequence, smell, taste, colour, size, texture, written spelling (i.e. graphemic sequence), and facts – that it is a citrus fruit, that it contains vitamin C, that there are Jaffas and blood oranges, that they come from Israel – are all memories stored in different parts of the brain. The time when a particular memory component of a concept was initially laid down from first perception may also differ by 50 or more years: it would take a long time if a whole lifetime of individual memories had to be gone through to extract one fact. A memory in isolation may only be retrieved by chance. It has been pointed out that in the Library of Congress in the USA, with its millions of books, if one takes a book off one shelf and places it on the shelf below it is the same as stealing the book, as it would be unretrievable at the wrong coded address. The same is true in the brain: excellent hardware with abundant but unclassified data is of little use without a language and an operations strategy to say what to do with the data – without such a strategy we would have to return to the cerebral sponge concept of 'store everything and let it sort itself out'. This is not to say that when we have developed a concept and understanding we do not 'self-program' and generate our own software systems for further development of the data through reasoning and imagination. The human brain is not 'logical' like an ordinary computer, which runs through all its information in a pre-set mathematical routine dictated by the software, but is associative, i.e. the brain scans a wide field looking for relevant data to light up (see our earlier discussion of cellular and molecular memory of modules). This image triggers the corresponding concept so that the other components of the concept are retrieved, from all the different addresses in the cerebral cortex, into short-term memory. One *RE-COGNIZES* the object and can say 'I understand what that is; I have previous knowledge'. If the orange were square, blue, or tasted like a peach, the incongruity with the previously existing concept would cause us to recognize a discordance and make us unsure whether we understood what the object was. One can enter the concept once established through any modality: vision, touch, the spoken word, the written word, smell, or taste.

Thought is the current content of consciousness, so if I am thinking about an orange, then, using our analogy with a computer, this corresponds to that section of RAM which we are currently processing (thinking about). I can process or compute these thoughts by verbal reasoning. This computation occurs in the central processing unit of my reticular formation while these thoughts are held in short-term memory, making them 'conscious'. I can compare an apple with an orange (an easy process) or socialism with communism (a narrow concept), or the substantia nigra with the locus coeruleus (a barely existing concept, so my understanding is limited). One must have multiple stored facts, i.e. knowledge about a subject, in order to form a concept. The more individual memories there are – the more components to the concept – the greater the understanding. In the mature adult these may not be solely dependent upon perception but can be abstract concepts, e.g. feminism, the Holy Spirit.

Verbal reasoning consists in comparing each individual component of the two concepts – e.g. size, shape, colour, taste, smell – to see if they are similar or different. Simple! As a result of this reasoning I can come to a decision: the two concepts are similar or very different. These mental abilites or processes of perception, recognition, understanding, verbal reasoning, and decision-making are the basis of the *mind* (mental processes) and are what we attempt to test in intelligence tests.

The way in which memories acquired at different times in our lives and stored in different parts of the brain are classified into concepts depends upon a structured symbol system that we call a language. Although this language is usually based upon words, other systematized symbol systems – such as those for chemistry, electronic circuitry, music, algebra, and arithmetic – are also languages allowing memories to be grouped into concepts and allowing the person to understand and reason. It is interesting that deaf children will say things to themselves in sign language, and that children who are both blind and deaf and who have been taught a digital language are seen to translate Braille felt with one hand into digital language with the other hand: one must not be restrictive and think of language as consisting only of words.

One cannot reason until one has formed concepts and one cannot form concepts without some basic factual knowledge. This is often forgotten in medical education, when teachers may try to teach clinical reasoning before the basic lingua franca of anatomy, physiology, and pathology has been remembered.

The inability to use a symbol system in order to create concepts and so create understanding and verbal reasoning is the basic defect in learning disability, i.e. global delay in cognitive learning, and in receptive dysphasia – i.e. specific delay in cognitive learning.

The language or lexicon (in the case of verbal language) needs to be stored in some concrete place, just as a computer language is stored. The vocabulary of an educated person is about 60 000 words and that of an expert in a very technical subject may exceed 100 000. We can speak in English using only about 46 individual sounds or phonemes and can represent the entire English language with combinations of 26 letters. Just as the hardware of many computers can operate on any language for which it is programmed, so the human brain can learn any of the world's languages. As Noam Chomsky (1972) pointed out, all languages have certain common features and there must be an operational program to allow the language to be learned and stored. We think that this is in the planum temporale and Wernicke's area of the left temporal lobe. At the same time if one loses the lexicon or cannot learn a lexicon because of congenital deafness, some other means is needed of organizing memories into concepts: pictograph, finger spelling, signing, or through vision, touch, smell, or taste.

It is thought that humans have a spatial vocabulary or lexicon of simple outline shapes or pictographs, which allow us to recognize all faces, all chairs, all houses as having certain basic common features upon which the concept can then be built up. Chinese who speak Cantonese and read Mandarin have no alphabet and hence have no spelling of the word; this shows that spoken words and their spatial representation need not be the same. It is a vital but unknown point as to whether such Chinese children ever suffer from dyslexia, or if in children with dyslexia, divorcing the spoken word from its written form (spelling) by use of pictographs that call upon the opposite hemisphere will help overcome their difficulties.

CLINICAL NEUROLOGY OF LEARNING DISORDERS

Delayed learning of speech

The whole of the left cerebral hemisphere is thought to mature more slowly in boys and speech is more firmly lateralized to the left hemisphere in boys, so that not only will motor aspects of speech be retarded but also syntax and semantics will be affected, severely in a few cases. If a child has difficulty in pronouncing words, it is not unexpected that that child's sentences will be shorter and telegrammatic and will lack propositions and conjunctions. All the causes of slowing down of normal brain development are illustrated by slowing of speech development. Environmental factors are obviously of immense importance, as children can only learn the speech that they have heard. Deafness must be considered in every case, particularly high-tone deafness due to genetics, toxicity (bilirubin, aminoglycoside antibiotics), or infection (e.g. pneumococcal meningitis). This is also why glue ear, causing temporary deafness that may affect up to 33% of all children at some time, is incriminated as a cause of slowed speech development.

Among children with delayed language learning, boys outnumber girls by 3 to 1. Signs of delayed dominance, environmental deprivation, and genetic factors have all been stressed (Rutter 1969). In Scotland certain families relating to the old clan system are known to have a higher incidence of developmental speech delay; and among the 75 affected individuals in Ingram's original study (1971), 18 had a similarly affected parent and 24 had a similarly affected sibling.

Brain damage also slows up the rate of speech acquisition, so that in about 25% of premature infants or infants asphyxiated at birth, speech development will be delayed sufficiently to require speech therapy. Many children with ataxia, e.g. after hydrocephalus or associated with hypothyroidism, have slowing up of motor learning and thus of the development of expressive speech. Forty per cent of children with congenital hemiplegia will have a delay in maturation of speech and not dysarthria or dysphasia.

Ten per cent of the population will have significantly slow speech development. Four per cent of children will have very slow speech development – 3% who are in effect normal children who are below the third centile mark (usually considered as the lower limit of normality) because they have a developmental articulatory dyspraxia, which tends to get better, and the remaining 1% who have a genetically determined severe delay that does not respond to speech therapy. The commonest and probably most important such delay is the dominantly inherited condition described 50 years ago as 'word-blind aphasia syndrome' (see Table 2.6, below) (MacMeeken 1939).

DEVELOPMENTAL RECEPTIVE DYSPHASIA (SEMANTIC DYSPHASIA)
Semantic receptive dysphasia of childhood, including central deafness, is a profound disorder of central language, i.e. the ability to use words to form concepts in order to understand, think, and reason (see above). The dominant auditory cortex has a predilection for speech as opposed to non-verbal sounds, but if this is damaged in a young child the opposite side is capable of taking over. Therefore, in congenital word deafness there must be bilateral interference with temporal lobe function. Children with this condition may be very musical and obviously able to hear, discriminate, and remember tones and pitch but not sound sequences with a linguistic meaning. In clinical practice it may be impossible to distinguish between central word deafness (the ability to discriminate between similar sounds with linguistic meanings in Heschl's gyrus) and auditory agnosia (in which the association area storing the lexicon is affected). Children with receptive dysphasia show gross auditory inattention to speech, and clearly great care must be taken to exclude a peripheral high-tone hearing loss. The congenitally deaf child is aphasic, but the child with acquired deafness already has acquired inner language (Ewing 1967). Children with receptive dysphasia are typically mute or severely dysfluent. If they do speak, their articulation is grossly defective. It is also difficult to differentiate these conditions from global learning disorder and autism.

As discussed already, the child with global learning disorder will have marked delay in the semantic aspects of language as well as all other areas of learning. Children with an isolated specific receptive dysphasia have most disruption of thought and reasoning, due to the failure of development of inner language, and this may result in a misdiagnosis of (global) learning disorder; but such children should show normal learning of other symbol systems, especially in relation to spatial abilities. They may be able to recognize and name objects but be unable to carry out more complex language tasks such as classifying or categorizing. They cannot cope with abstract notions such as time: today, yesterday, now, later.

A further complication in young children with developmental semantic dysphasias is that there may also be failure in development of non-verbal communication through gesture, eye contact, intonation, facial movements, etc., so that there is in addition a total loss of social communication. The child does not differentiate people (whom you look in the eye) from objects and does not recognize self as a person, i.e. the child shows autistic features.

ACQUIRED RECEPTIVE DYSPHASIA
Damage to the dominant temporal lobe produces a receptive dysphasia. The aetiologies include head injury with extradural haematoma, direct contusional injury, contrecoup injury, epileptic dysphasia, temporal lobe abscess due to middle ear infection, emboli, cortical thrombophlebitis, herpes simplex encephalitis, meningitis, or temporal lobe tumour. In the adult (Wernicke's aphasia) the result is a fluent aphasia with jargon speech and neologisms, but in children the clinical picture is dominated by mutism. As the mutism resolves, the comprehension difficulties persist and include the child's understanding of his own speech. Reading skills are also usually lost.

DEVELOPMENTAL PHONOLOGICAL DELAY

In some children with delayed developmnt of articulation, maturation of the motor circuit sometimes appears to be delayed, as shown by persisting extensor plantar responses. In cases of pure delay in motor learning of articulation the children's hearing, comprehension, vocabulary, and intelligence will be normal but they will be slow to say their first words after a normal period of babbling. They will have fewer words in their spoken vocabulary and these words will be pronounced in an immature way. These children may have little recognizable speech before 3 years of age and may be 7 years old before they acquire all the later-acquired consonants.

Very severe cases, usually labelled *articulatory dyspraxia,* may represent disease rather than maturational delay. This interpretation is supported by modern genetic research showing a gene associated with benign rolandic epilepsy, and a separate gene for familial articulatory dyspraxia has now been identified. The speech is very slow and motor learning may be so disrupted that the child may never develop normal articulation and may need an alternative communication system. The pattern of speech is often deviant and does not follow the classic omission/substitution pattern seen on the Edinburgh Articulation Test when normal speech development is simply slowed, but may be characterized by bizarre omissions and inconsistent substitutions, sometimes of vowels as well as consonants. By school age such children may be able to make most of the 46 speech sounds in isolation but not be able to sequence them into words. When the children reach an age when developmentally they should be able to make all the speech sounds, the specific difficulty of sound sequencing or 'word synthesis' becomes increasingly apparent. In trying to repeat a sentence after the examiner they may be able to produce the correct parsed pattern of words and syllables, thus showing that they have an inner representation of the correct syntactical pattern. There will be some words that they learn and articulate well, i.e. they may overlearn a few words or phrases. When they are anxious their speech will disintegrate further and when they speak quickly it will become even less understandable. A specific speech sound may be used in one word and not in another. In very severe cases they may not even be able to imitate certain individual sounds. They may learn to say a simple word such as *cat* and yet when trying to say *catapult* be unable to pronounce the *cat* part of the word distinctly. In severe cases the children may circumvent their severe articulation problem by contracting their sentences so that speech becomes telegrammatic, often consisting of one or two word utterances. Some children may have oromotor dyspraxia, e.g. they cannot imitate rapid repetitive lateral movements of the tongue. In a minority of cases there may be some nasal escape in speech: though the palate will move well when the children say 'ah' and the gag reflex is normal, the soft palate does not close off the nasopharynx during connected speech. This condition may be misdiagnosed as mild pseudobulbar palsy.

Reading disorders

DYSLEXIA WITH DEVELOPMENTAL SPEECH DELAY

SE Shaywitz et al. (1992) emphasized the continuum of reading difficulty, from that in normal children whose development is below the 3rd centile, to socially disadvantaged children, to children with true genetic dyslexia. The latter do not show a simple developmental lag,

TABLE 2.6
Word-blind aphasia syndrome

Information about syndrome	Reference
8% Edinburgh Children	MacMeeken 1942
Genetic to certain Scottish clans	Ingram 1960
Strong family history in children with subsequent spelling dysgraphia	O'Hare and Brown 1989
Poor auditory discrimination as infant	
Poor developmental phonemic maturation to 7 years	
Dyslexia to 12 years	
Spelling dysgraphia into adult life	

but have lifelong difficulties that are often resistant to remedial help. Population studies suggest that 3 to 7% of children have selective difficulty in learning to read (SE Shaywitz et al. 1990).

There is a strong genetic predisposition of autosomal dominant type with variable penetrance. Twin studies have confirmed the genetic concordance: 27 to 49% of parents and 40% of siblings have been found to be similarly affected. In some families the disorder has been mapped through generations, in association with chromosome 15 (Pennington 1995). Another gene locus at 6p21 has also been incriminated. Thirty-three per cent to 70% of affected individuals have a positive family history of reading retardation (Rutter 1969). Nearly half of first-degree relatives can be shown to have residual difficulties on testing (Finucci et al. 1976). It is the phonological type of dyslexia rather than the look-and-say 'visuospatial' type that shows the strongest genetic predisposition.

Males with dyslexia due to developmental speech and language delay exceed females by 4 to 1. This is hardly surprising, since the brain matures more slowly in the male, the left hemisphere matures more slowly than the right, and the angular gyrus is a tertiary area and so is the last area to develop. A dominantly inherited slowing of linguistic development will be more obvious in boys than girls. Dichotic listening studies show an excess of left ear dominance. A third of children with developmental language delay will be slow to read (Silva et al. 1983). Fifty per cent of slow readers have had slow speech development (Ingram 1963) and the syndrome of developmental speech delay is probably the single most important cause of later reading retardation (Table 2.6).

Children show a developmental progression through understanding of speech, expression of speech, reading, writing, and spelling. The infant is thought first of all to show auditory discrimination problems: the discrimination of *da* as in *dada* from *ta* as in *tata* requires extremely rapid temporal processing and hence one means of therapy is by stretching the sound (see section headed Temporal lobe). This is followed by slow phonological development but not slow comprehension. The slow phonological development may or may not be associated with more severe expressive language problems affecting the learning of grammatical rules such as the use of pronouns, tenses, and plurals. The normal phonological development has already been described in the section on motor learning of speech. Most articulation is mature by age 7 years even in children with significant delay, by which time any reading difficulty has become apparent. Children who have severe expressive phonological impairments when they start school are at high risk for reading and spelling problems. However, their speech does not become completely normal even in adulthood: on repetition of long sentences, words are omitted and tenses are changed, and there is difficulty repeating nonsense words such as *surke* and *pyte* (Welsh et al. 1987).

Reading, like speech, slowly improves, so that by the time they reach secondary school at age 12 most children who have dyslexia with developmental speech delay are competent to read and acquire information from written text. The spelling dysgraphia (discussed in a later section), however, persists into secondary school, is obvious in final examinations at university, and probably never resolves completely.

SPECIFIC DEVELOPMENTAL DYSLEXIA WITH DELAYED HEMISPHERIC DOMINANCE
Features attributable to delayed cerebral hemispheric dominance occur in 33% of dyslexic children with or without a prior history of speech delay. Such features, termed interference phenomena, are normal in younger children; it is their persistence that is abnormal. An example of such a phenomenon is *b/d* confusion (strephosymbolia), which is present in the writing of 1% of 7-year-olds (Temple et al. 1995). If the establishment of hemispheric dominance is delayed, the resulting interference phenomena may be misdiagnosed as soft neurological signs of so-called minimal brain damage, mentioned above.

PURE DOMINANTLY INHERITED DYSLEXIA
A third type of reading and spelling disorder is seen in people with true genetic word-blindness, or true dyslexia. This condition, like true articulatory dyspraxia, is a true dyslexic disease and has a poor prognosis. The term *word-blindness* is apt, as children with this condition can recognize the letters and can put a sound to each letter but cannot make a word out of the components: i.e. they cannot achieve the step of word synthesis. The condition is often inherited in a pure form, unaccompanied by slowing down of initial speech development. Such children will show reversals, insertions, omissions, *b/d* confusion, mixing of long and short vowels and of hard and soft consonants, difficulties with complex graphemes, and guessing at words with similar shapes. Table 2.7 illustrates the difficulties experienced by a boy who eventually reached university standard. They vividly illustrate the need for a scribe during examinations if a person with such a condition is not to be severely undermarked.

BRAIN DAMAGE AND DYSLEXIA
Fourthly, brain damage that slows up the rate of brain maturation, as in preterm infants and asphyxiated term infants, will slow up the rate of learning and reading skills. Children from socially disadvantaged families are poorer readers and make slower progress than other children, and although they may catch up to some degree there is still clear separation at 8 years of age. The debate continues as to how much of the difference between social groups represents genetic limitation and how much is based on preschool language experience (Ritchie 1950). We prefer not to use the term *minimal brain damage* as this suggests that so-called soft signs are the main diagnostic criteria. In mild brain damage there must be some more concrete evidence of a diagnosable syndrome based upon aetiology, such as perinatal asphyxia

TABLE 2.7

Examples of writing and spelling difficulties in a bright 15-year-old boy with dominantly inherited dyslexia and without developmental speech problems, after 8 years of remedial teaching

	Actual word	Desired word	Actual word	Desired word
Writing difficulties	active	attractive	champion	campaign
	adence	audience	gome	gnome
	bin	bun	goome	gnome
	plauside	plausible	concession	conscience
	festinate	fascinate	shoulder	smoulder
	chore	choir		
Spelling difficulties	hear	here	Britch	British
	fount	front	Britick	British
	th	the	elethant	elephant
	sodeam	sodium	dimonds	diamonds
	sodaiium	sodium	unisellar	unicellular
	matilic	metallic	commnity	community
	dus	bus	to	too
	talk	tail	bibleorgafy	bibliography
	angle	angel	kanarry	canary

(in which case behaviour must always have been abnormal in the neonatal period), and there must be a neurological diagnosis, e.g. minimal hemiparesis or ataxia. Various investigations, particularly MRI and EEG, may help. Neuropsychological tests such as a verbal–performance discrepancy of more than 2 standard deviations (i.e. 30 points) is suggestive of brain damage, but abnormalities on tests such as the Bender–Gestalt test can be produced by emotional disturbance and in themselves are not to be taken as diagnostic of brain damage. In the future, developments such as regional cerebral blood flow studies, PET, magnetron tomography, computerized EEG techniques, oxygen-15 regional cerebral metabolism studies, and particularly functional MRI offer exciting prospects of more accurate study in vivo of brain function in these children.

There is no doubt that mild brain damage due to abnormal perinatal events is seen. In our own department, we followed 32 term infants, all of whom had had abnormal behaviour (fits, impaired consciousness, tube feeding, apnoea, etc.) in the newborn period after asphyxiation at birth, usually associated with definite abnormalities on neurological examination. These 32 infants were compared with 16 control infants, all of whom were normal in behaviour and whose neurology and EEG were normal at birth. The asphyxiated infants were clumsier (50%), were slower to learn to speak (27% needed speech therapy), and showed more behavioural disturbance (70% of the parents had difficulty compared with 10% of the parents of normal controls). The motor disability can usually be classified in conventional terms as a mild hemiparesis, mild diplegia, or mild ataxia. In addition to being slow in speech development, such children are frequently slow at learning to read, and some have difficulties in concepts of space and direction, or in copying shapes. These children therefore have true mild brain damage: they have clumsiness, speech delay, behaviour disturbance, and learning difficulties. However, such children represent only 1.5 per 1000 of the population and therefore do not constitute a large fraction of the 150 per 1000 children with learning disorder.

The newborn preterm infant can show similar abnormalities in maturation, the so-called dystonic syndrome of low birthweight, and many of these children, too, show clumsiness, behaviour disturbances, and subsequent speech and reading difficulties (Drillien et al. 1980).

Difficulty with short-term memory and storing of new memories (anterograde amnesia) may occur in children who have apparently otherwise completely recovered from severe head injuries, cardiorespiratory arrest, a severe bout of status epilepticus, or tentorial herniation due to hydrocephalus.

Less well recognized as a cause of reading and writing problems, and particularly of specific number difficulty, is epilepsy arising in the left hemisphere in a male. This interferes with acquisition of language skills and in severe cases may cause epileptic aphasia (Landau–Kleffner syndrome). Less obvious degrees of interference with language skills show as naming problems, and difficulties in reading and writing may be seen in the so-called benign rolandic seizures arising in the left hemisphere. There are certain families in whom benign rolandic epilepsy coexists with articulatory dyspraxia. We believe that there is a spectrum with benign rolandic epilepsy at one end and Landau–Kleffner syndrome (malignant rolandic epilepsy) at the other. There may be interference with verbal memory even in the interictal period in people with left-sided temporal lobe epilepsy (Mayeux et al. 1980). This is nearly always associated with an epileptic discharge of the left inferior temporo-occipital region; there is a statistically very significant difference between discharges from the left and right sides, and the memory disturbance does not depend upon seizure frequency or medication. In the severe form of epileptic aphasia, good control of the discharging focus may occasionally cause dramatic improvement in speech (Racy et al. 1980). Even hemispherectomy may improve learning, which suggests that it is the epileptic discharge that is preventing the brain from learning normally. SPECT scans in such patients often show a switched-off hypometabolic brain, and it is possible that the brain's attempts to limit the discharge results in the switching off of learning in that part of the brain. An epileptic focus arising on the right side is associated, as might be expected, with lower performance scores than verbal scores (Annett et al. 1961). Some form of learning problem is thought to be present in 60% of children with epilepsy (Holdsworth and Whitmore 1974).

An acquired lesion in the left area 18 and the splenium of the corpus callosum results in a pure alexia, i.e. reading and word agnosia, or word-blindness. If the angular gyrus, which links the visual association area with the auditory association area, is damaged or matures slowly, we see the syndrome of alexia with agraphia. And if Wernicke's area, i.e. the main speech association area, is damaged, we get an alexia with agraphia and dysphasia together (Benson 1978). Children with acquired dyslexia will probably also have dysgraphia, which will look just like a primary neurodevelopmental dysgraphia (Fig. 2.9).

Acquired brain damage with neuronal necrosis or neuronal disconnections may produce alexia. Often the alexia is overshadowed by the accompanying dysphasia, as in the sensory impairment of reading that follows damage to the superior temporal gyrus. Dyslexia may

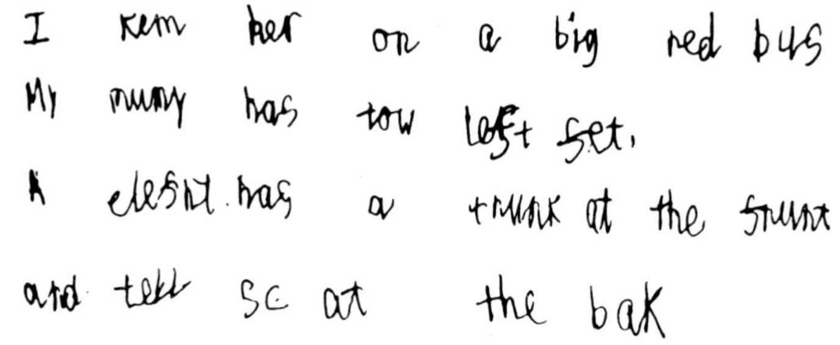

I kem her on a big red bus
My mumy has tow left fet,
A elefnt has a trunk at the frunt
and tell sc at the bak

Fig. 2.9. Dysgraphia after an acquired left frontal lesion, showing that the difficulties are similar to genetic developmental disorders.

occur with dysphasia and dysgraphia, when damage extends from the angular gyrus down to the underlying white matter. After damage to the dominant temporal lobe a child may be unable to learn to read.

Pure alexia without dysgraphia follows a lesion of the paraventricular white matter of the left occipital lobe. This may follow interference with the blood supply in the territory of the posterior cerebral artery and there may be an accompanying right hemianopia.

A rare form of reflex 'reading' epilepsy occurs in which epileptic discharges, either generalized or focal to the dominant hemisphere, are triggered by the complex cerebral activity that accompanies the language function of reading. There is often a family history, with onset of the disorder in the teens.

The vast majority of children with selective (or specific) difficulty in reading seen by a school teacher will not, however, have any brain damage at all, but will have one of the first two types of reading disorder described above.

Writing and spelling disorders (dysgraphia)
Dysgraphia is due to retarded development or to an acquired loss in the skill of writing. In speech, syntax is learned after the phonetic system develops, and in writing, syntax is learned after graphemic skills develop, so that sentence construction is related more to motor than to cognitive learning. The child may have an IQ over 130, i.e. excellent cognitive development, and yet have very severe syntactic dysgraphic difficulty (Fig. 2.10). Acquired brain damage that causes a Broca's aphasia will usually also cause a dysgraphia, since the motor association area of Broca, controlling motor learning in lips, tongue, and palate, is adjacent to the graphomotor area on the left controlling the motor learning of the right hand that is required for writing. Writing can be regarded as speech written down, and disorders of writing follow a similar classification to disorders of speech. Writing dysgraphia falls into three groups: (1) abnormalities in motor learning and execution, i.e. penmanship; (2) difficulties with the syntactic aspects of written language, i.e. spelling, sentence construction (grammar), and punctuation; and (3) abnormal content of what is written, i.e. semantic aspects of dysgraphia.

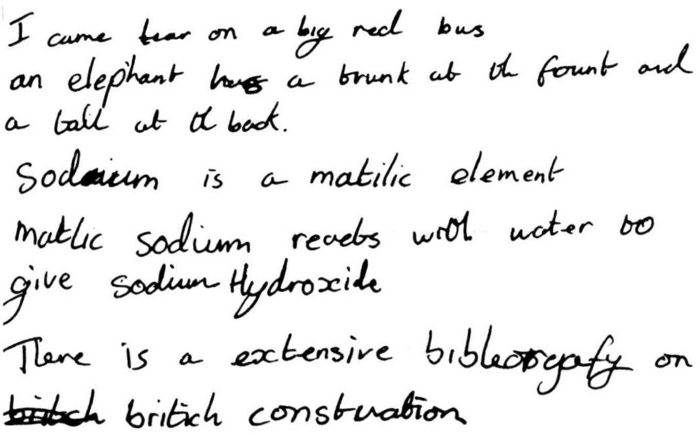

I came tear on a big red bus
an elephant has a brunk at th fount and
a ball at th bad.
Sodaium is a matilic element
matlic sodium reaebs wrth water to
give sodium Hydroxide
Thre is a extensive bibleography on
britch britch construation

Fig. 2.10. Spelling dysgraphia in a 15-year-old boy with an IQ of 130.

Thus the time-honoured division of writing skills into penmanship, spelling, and composition still holds good. Because writing is the last language skill to develop in the child, it is the abnormality that is likely to persist the longest in disorders of language development, or to be lost most easily in acquired brain disease. The child who has brain damage, for example due to a head injury, acquired after the development of speech, reading, and writing may show a persisting disorder of writing even after there has been an otherwise good recovery of speech and reading. The disability most likely to persist into secondary school in the child with slow development of speech is also dysgraphia.

INCOORDINATION DYSGRAPHIA
A movement is planned by the cerebral cortex relying upon motor memories (engrams) from past experience and practice. The smooth, coordinated execution of this planned movement is dependent upon the precentral motor cortex, the pyramidal tract, and the extrapyramidal and cerebellar systems. When pyramidal lesions are present, the child can plan but not execute the movement. The degree of distal weakness correlates well with the loss of function. Movements are slowed and this loss of speed also correlates well with the loss of skill (Brown et al. 1987, 1997). The extrapyramidal system regulates the natural speed of a movement and so the cadence of speech, gait, and writing. In cases of hypokinetic dyskinesia (e.g. Parkinsonian complex), writing is small (micrographia) and slow (bradygraphia), while the converse is the case in hyperkinetic dyskinesias. Involuntary movements may cause sudden unexpected jerks, sudden angulation of letters, blotching, or drawing of the pen across existing script. The child with executive motor difficulty has an immature grasp of the pen and in severe cases may retain the primitive grasp reflex. Fine independent movements of the fingers, without associated or mirror movement and with speedy opposition of fingers to thumb, represents the peak of neurological maturation

in the upper limb and is a useful clinical test of pyramidal maturation. Not surprisingly, children with incoordination dysgraphia often perform poorly on these tests. Analysis of their writing reveals a wide range of abnormalities that equally severely affect copying, writing to dictation, and spontaneous composition. The pen is held insecurely, with a dagger or abnormal tripod grip, and it may slip through the fingers. Writing is untidy, shaky, and blotched and there is varying pen pressure. There may be angulations and different-sized letters in a word, the words do not lie on the lines on the paper, margins are irregular, and the text slopes across the page. There may be macrographia or micrographia, with a very slow speed or a rapid, 'careless' speed. The child with this type of motor dysgraphia may be able to spell aloud correctly. A typewriter keyboard will overcome the purely executive difficulties in a child with an uncomplicated incoordination dysgraphia.

DYSPRAXIC DYSGRAPHIA
Visual copying of letters on a horizontal line moving from left to right is a primary skill in learning to write, but as the motor engram becomes established it becomes less important, i.e. one can write and spell with the eyes closed, albeit with poor spatial arrangement on the page. Alternatively one can execute the motor skill with a toe in the sand, a pen in the mouth or the opposite limb (in mirror fashion). As the motor skill is learned it becomes subconscious (see above), and it becomes more strongly associated with visual and auditory imagery and the developing knowledge of language.

Dyspraxic dysgraphia may occur in any child with brain damage and can complicate any type of cerebral palsy, so that for example a child with spastic diplegia but little or no increase in upper limb muscle tone may have quite gross dyspraxic difficulties with the hands. As with so many developmental disorders, there is a condition of pure dyspraxic dysgraphia that appears to be genetic in origin and not to be based on any neurological damage (O'Hare and Brown 1989).

If hemispheric dominance is not established, there may be interference from the opposite side, so *p* may be written for *q, b* for *d, was* for *saw, god* for *dog* (Fig. 2.11). This may occur in a pure form without any difficulty in actually writing the letters down, but if the child has additional spatial problems there will be irregularities: words may run into each other and the script may slant across the page.

Dyspraxic dysgraphia is a disorder of motor learning involving the graphomotor centre, which has the same relations to hand movements as Broca's area has to movements of lips, tongue, and palate. Affected children write slowly and cannot remember which way to move their hands to make the letters: they will make a stroke, see how it looks, half make the letter, then correct it when it looks wrong, so that they are constantly correcting by visual means on a trial-and-error basis, and crossing out, with the result that their writing looks very untidy. They can make a letter in isolation but may have enormous difficulty in putting several letters together in order to make even the simplest word. There is difficulty in distinguishing between capital and small letters and in knowing where one word ends and another begins; words often run into one another.

Some children have additional difficulties in that they not only have a genetic dyspraxia for writing but may also have difficulties with other hand skills, such as fastening buttons

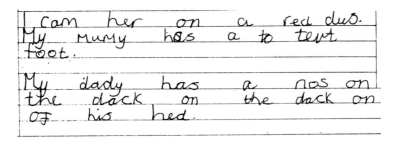

Fig. 2.11. Reversal of *b* for *d* in addition to spelling dysgraphia.

or laces, dressing, using a knife and fork, or wiring an electric plug; they have manipulative or constructional dyspraxia, which shows up as particular difficulty in sequencing (Dewey 1991). Manipulative dyspraxia and writing dyspraxia are not interdependent but may be seen together in the clumsy child with schooling difficulties.

SPELLING DYSGRAPHIA

Spelling can be defined as the production of a correct sequence of graphemes to correspond to a word of spoken speech as dictated by the rules of the particular language. Speech is the same, substituting phoneme for grapheme. It should not, therefore, surprise us that syntactical and spelling dysgraphia should so often follow a developmental speech retardation syndrome (Fig. 2.12). Mastery of spelling requires a high degree of linguistic competence and is the last language skill to develop. There are cases of isolated familial spelling dysgraphia without any preceding abnormality in speech development, again suggesting that there must be genes acting during childhood governing the maturation of individual systems within the brain.

People with spelling dysgraphia write slowly and have difficulty retrieving words from the spelling vocabulary. They tend to write words in a slavishly phonetic way: (*sodeam* for *sodium, matilic* for *metallic, dimonds* for *diamonds, pepol* for *people*) or according to dialect (*reet doun* for *right down*), and very occasionally as the child speaks them with immature speech (*led lolly* for *red lorry, doddy* for *doggy*). Complex graphemes such as *ph, ch, sh, th,* and *ough* cause particular difficulties. Spelling age is retarded on standardized tests, and mirror writing – *god* for *dog, was* for *saw, b* for *d* – adds confusion to what at first may appear an unintelligible muddle. Children with this condition have no idea of punctuation, phrase, or sentence, and spacing may be absent between words. They cannot read what they have written, even though they can read the same passage from a book. They can copy well and neatly, but writing to dictation and spontaneous composition are very poor, with short, poorly constructed, simple sentences. The children will deliberately search out words they can spell in order to try to get their ideas down on paper. This is slow and very frustrating.

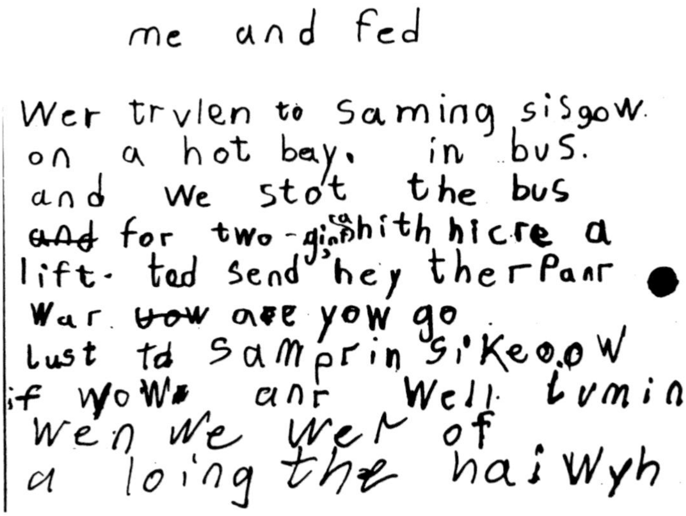

Fig. 2.12. Severe spelling dysgraphia in an intelligent boy with the genetic syndrome of slow speech, then slow reading, followed by slow spelling.

SUMMARY

The brain is the organ of learning and continues to develop throughout childhood and adolescence. Learning is localized within the brain both anatomically and for the siting of learned material. This localization can now be confirmed by modern imaging methods and is not confined to the study of gross pathological states. There are built-in strategies for the handling of data by the brain. The gradual evolution of the brain circuits, development of the localized modules, and maturation of these strategies is under genetic control. The existence of such patterns of maturation explains why children learn certain skills and behaviours in a set sequence, which allows psychometric tests to be devised which get more difficult with age. It also explains the variation in the rates of learning in different children and why some families are slow to learn in specific areas. Slowing down of brain development either globally or locally will cause delay in learning. One may see a global delay in learning, as in children with global cognitive learning disorder, or a specific delay, as in children with dyslexia, dysgraphia, dyscalculia, dysphasia, dysmusia, dysprosodia, etc. Brain growth may be slowed by insults such as perinatal asphyxia, prematurity, or head injury, but these account for only a small percentage of the total number of children with learning disability. In most children with a specific learning disability, the condition is secondary to genetic factors that slow the development of particular parts of the brain. The study of children and their families with such disorders is beginning to lead to the identification of specific genes that appear to be responsible. It is hoped that finding the organic basis of many of these disorders can bring several benefits: it can mitigate the feelings of failure or frustration on the part of child and teacher, and it can lead to an increase in the study of how the brain learns and so to an understanding of how we should teach.

REFERENCES

Agranoff BW. (1980) Biochemical events mediating the formation of short and long term memory. In: Tsukada Y, Agranoff BW, editors *Neurobiological Basis of Learning and Memory*. New York: John Wiley and Sons. p 135–47.

Annett M, Lee DL, Ounstedt C. (1961) Intellectual disabilities in relation to lateralised features in the EEG. In: *Hemiplegic Cerebral Palsy in Children and Adults. A Report of an International Study Group, Wills Hall, Bristol, 1961*. Little Club Clinics in Developmental Medicine No. 4. London: Medical Advisory Committee of the National Spastics Society. p 86–112.

Bauman M, Kemper TL. (1985) Histoanatomic observations of the brain in early infantile autism. *Neurology* **35:** 866–74.

Benson DF. (1978) Neurological correlates of aphasia and apraxia. In: Matthews WB, Glaser GH, editors. *Recent Advances in Clinical Neurology*. No. 2. Edinburgh, London, New York: Churchill Livingstone. p 163–75.

Blakemore C. (1974) Development of mammalia visual systems. *British Medical Journal* **30:** 152–57.

Boyle GJ. (1997) Effects of menstrual cycle moods and symptoms on academic performance: a study of senior school students. *British Journal of Educational Psychology* **67:** 37–49.

Brain WR. (1961) The history of thought about aphasia. In: *Speech Disorders, Aphasia, Apraxia, and Agnosia*. London: Butterworths. Chapter 4, p 30–53.

Broca P. (1861) Perte de la parole. Ramollissement chronique et destruction partielle du lobe antérieur gauche du cerveau. *Bulletin de la Société Anthropologique de Paris* **2:** 219.

Brown JK. (1981) Learning disorders: a paediatric neurologist's view. *Transactions of the College of Medicine of South Africa*. p 49–104.

— van Rensburg F, Walsh G, et al. (1987) A neurological study of hand function of hemiplegic children. *Developmental Medicine and Child Neurology* **29:** 287–304.

— Omar T, O'Regan M. (1997) Brain development and the development of tone and movement. In: Connolly KJ, Forssberg H, editors. *Neurophysiology and Neuropsychology of Motor Development*. Clinics in Developmental Medicine No. 143/144. London: Mac Keith Press. Chapter 1, p 1–41.

Chomsky N. (1972) *Language and Mind*. New York: Harcourt Brace Jovanvich Inc.

Conel J. (1939) *The Postnatal Development of the Human Cerebral Cortex*. Cambridge [MA]: Harvard University Press.

Damasio AR, Damasio H, Van Hoesen GW. (1982) Prosopagnosia: anatomical basis and neurobehavioral mechanism. *Neurology* **32:** 331–41.

Dekaban A. (1959) *Neurology of Infancy*. London: Baillière Tindall and Cox.

Dewey D. (1991) Praxis and sequency skills in children with sensorimotor dysfunction. *Developmental Neuropsychology* **7:** 197–206.

Drillien CM, Thomson AJM, Burgoyne K. (1980) Low-birthweight children at early school-age: a longitudinal study. *Developmental Medicine and Child Neurology* **22:** 26–47.

Dudai Y (1989) Some basic notions and their ontogenesis. In: *The Neurobiology of Memory: Concepts, Findings, Trends*. New York: Oxford University Press. Chapter 1, p 3–18.

Eccles J. (1979) *Gifford Lectures*. Edinburgh: University of Edinburgh.

Ewing AWG. (1967) *Aphasia in Children*. New York: Hafner Publishing Co.

Finucci JM, Guthrie JT, Child AL, et al. (1976) Genetics of specific reading disability. *Annals of Human Genetics* **40:** 1–23.

Flechsig P. (1906) Developmental localisation in the cerebral cortex in the human subject. *Lancet* **ii:** 1027–9.

Geschwind N, Levitsky W. (1968) Human brain: left right asymmetries in temporal speech region. *Science* **161:** 186–7.

Gordon N, McKinlay I. (1980) *Helping Clumsy Children*. Edinburgh: Churchill Livingstone.

Holdsworth L, Whitmore K. (1974) A study of children with epilepsy attending ordinary schools. I: Their seizure patterns, progress and behaviour in school. *Developmental Medicine and Child Neurology* **16:** 746–58.

Howard D, Patterson K, Wise R, et al. (1992) The cortical localization of the lexicons. *Brain* **115:** 1769–82.

Hyden H, Lange PW. (1967) A differentiation in R.N.A. response in neurons, early and late during learning. *Molecular Approaches in Psychology* **3:** 32–40.

Ingram TTS. (1960) Paediatric aspects of specific developmental dysphasia, dyslexia, and dysgraphia. *Cerebral Palsy Bulletin* **21:** 254–77.

73

— (1963) The association of speech retardation and educational difficulties. *Proceedings of the Royal Society of Medicine* **56**: 199–212.

— (1971) Specific learning difficulties in childhood. *British Journal of Educational Psychology* **41**: Part 1.

— Mason AW, Blackburn I. (1970) A retrospective study of 82 children with reading disability. *Developmental Medicine and Child Neurology* **12**: 271–81.

Kandel ER, Schwartz JH, Jessel TM. (1995) *Essentials of Neural Science and Behaviour*. New York: Appleton and Lange.

Livingstone MS, Rosen GD, Drislane FW, Galaburda AM. (1991) Physiological and anatomical evidence for a magnocellular defect in developmental dyslexia. *Proceedings of the National Academy of Science of the United States of America* **88**: 7943–7.

Lou HC, Henricksen L, Bruhn P. (1984) Focal cerebral hypoperfusion in children with dysphasia and/or attention deficit disorder. *Archives of Neurology* **41**: 825–9.

MacMeeken M. (1939) *Ocular Dominance in Relation to Developmental Aphasia*. London: University of London Press. p 27.

— (1942) *Developmental Aphasia in Educationally Retarded Children.*. London: University of London Press / WH Ross Foundation.

Mayeux R, Brandt J, Rosen J, Benson DF. (1980) Interictal memory and language impairment in temporal lobe epilepsy. *Neurology* **30**: 120–5.

McGraw MB. (1935) *Growth: A Study of Johnny and Jimmy*. New York: Appleton.

McNeill D. (1970) *The Acquisition of Language*. London and New York: Harper and Row.

Milner B. (1971) Interhemispheric differences and psychological processes. *British Medical Bulletin* **27**: 272–7.

Mimura M, Kato M, Watanabe R, et al. (1997) Autobiographical memory loss following herpes encephalitis. *No To Shinkei* **49**: 759–64.

Montorolo PG, Goelet P, Vastelluci VF, et al. (1986) Critical period for macromolecular synthesis in long-term heterosynaptic facilitation in aplysia. *Science* **234**: 1249–54.

Nicholls DG. (1994) *Proteins, Transmitters and Synapses*. Oxford: Blackwell Scientific Publications. p 234–44.

O'Hare AE, Brown JK. (1989) Childhood dysgraphia. Part 2: a study of hand function. *Child: Care, Health and Development* **15**: 151–66.

— — (1998) Speech and language disorders. [Section of chapter 14, Disorders of the central nervous system.] In: Campbell AGM, McIntosh N, editors. *Forfar and Arneil's Textbook of Paediatrics*. Edinburgh: Churchill Livingstone. p 833–47.

Oppenheim RW, Chu-Wang IW. (1983) Aspects of naturally occurring motorneuron death in the chick spinal cord during embryonic development. In: Burnstock G, Vrobova G, editors. *Somatic and Autonomic Nerve–Muscle Interactions*. New York: Elsevier. p 57–107.

Paldine AM, Purpura DP. (1981) Influence of extrauterine survival on branching characteristics of hippocampal neurones in preterm infants. *Experimental Neurology* **71**: 235–50.

Penfield W, Roberts L. (1959) *Speech and Brain Mechanisms*. Princeton [NJ]: Princeton University Press.

Pennington BF. (1995) Genetics of learning disabilities. *Journal of Child Neurology* **10**: 569–77.

Price CJ, Wise RJS, Watson JDG, et al. (1994) Brain activity during reading: the effects of exposure, duration and task. *Brain* **117**: 1255–69.

Racy A, Anis MA, Osborn BA, Molinari GF. (1980) Epileptic aphasia: first onset of prolonged monosymptomatic status epilepticus in adults. *Archives of Neurology* **37**: 419–22.

Reid L, Rumsey JM. (1996) *Neuroimaging: A Window to the Neurological Foundations of Learning and Behaviour in Children*. Baltimore [MD]: Paul H Brookes.

Ritchie WD. (1950) In: McLaren VM, Taylor CD, Dunlop DC, editors. *Studies in Reading*. London: University of London Press.

Rumsey JM, Nace K, Andreason P. (1995) Phonologic and orthographic components of reading imaged with PET. *Journal of the International Neuropsychological Society* **1**: 180.

Rutter M. (1969) The concept of dyslexia. In: Wolff PH, Mac Keith R, editors. *Planning for Better Learning*. Clinics in Developmental Medicine No. 33. London: Spastics International Medical Publications. p129–39.

Salvesen KA, Undheim JO. (1994) Screening for learning disabilities with teacher rating scales. *Journal of Learning Disabilities* **27**: 61–6.

Sauerwein HC, Lassonde M. (1997) Neuropsychological alterations after split brain surgery. *Journal of Neurosurgical Science* **41**: 59–66.

Semenza C, Mondini S, Cappelletti M. (1997) The grammatical properties of mass nouns : an aphasia case study. *Neuropsychologia* **35**: 669–75.

Shaywitz BA, Fletcher JM, Shaywitz SE. (1995) Defining and classifying learning disabilities and attention-deficit/hyperactivity disorder. *Journal of Child Neurology* **10** Suppl. 1: S50–S57.

Shaywitz SE, Shaywitz BA, Fletcher JM, Escobar MD. (1990) Prevalence of reading disability in boys and girls. Results of the Connecticut longitudinal study. *Journal of the American Medical Association* **264**: 998–1002.

— Escobar MD, Shaywitz BA, et al. (1992) Evidence that dyslexia may represent the lower tail of a normal distribution of reading ability. *New England Journal of Medicine* **326**: 145–50.

Silva PA, McGee R, Williams SM. (1983) Developmental language delay from three to seven years and its significance for low intelligence and reading difficulties at age seven. *Developmental Medicine and Child Neurology* **25**: 783–93.

Smith CUM. (1989) *Elements of Molecular Neurobiology.* New York: John Wiley and Sons.

Steenhuis RE, Bryden MP, Schroeder DH. (1993) Gender, laterality, learning difficulties and health problems. *Neuropsychologia* **31**: 1243–54.

Temple CM, Dennis J, Carney R, Sharich J. (1995) Neonatal seizures: long-term outcome and cognitive development among 'normal' survivors. *Developmental Medicine and Child Neurology* **37**: 109–18.

Wada J, Rasmussen T. (1960) Intracarotid injection of sodium amytal for the lateralisation of cerebral speech dominance. *Journal of Neurosurgery* **17**: 266–82.

Walsh K. (1994) The frontal lobes. In: *Neuropsychology, A Clinical Approach.* 3rd ed. Edinburgh: Churchill Livingstone. Chapter 4, p133–96.

Walton JN, Ellis E, Court SDM. (1962) Clumsy children. *Brain* **85**: 603–12.

Welsh MC, Pennington BF, Rogers S. (1987) Word recognition and comprehension skills in hyperlexic children. *Brain and Language* **32**: 76–96.

Yakolev PI, Lecours AR. (1967) The myelinogenetic cycles of regional maturation of the brain. In: Minkowstki A, editor. *Regional Development of the Brain in Early Life.* Philadelphia: Davis. p 3–70.

3
DYSLEXIA – WHY CAN'T I LEARN TO READ?

Neil Gordon

Although the term *dyslexia* has raised some controversy, it is a good label with which to identify a number of children with reading difficulties, who are indeed in need of help. As with many other labels, to say that a child has dyslexia is not to make a diagnosis, but only to identify a complex problem and, one hopes, to start a process of analysing and treating it. Stanovich (1994) considered that the term *dyslexia* should be abandoned, because even if distinct causes exist there is no evidence that they correlate with a discrepancy between reading level and IQ (see also Chapter 7). However, there is some support for the idea that at least some examples of reading disability have a distinct aetiology (Nicolson 1996). This does not exclude the possibility that other children who are slow to read are merely at the lower end of a normal distribution of reading ability. SE Shaywitz et al. (1992) found that reading–IQ discrepancy scores follow a univariate normal distribution, and that the interrelation of two different discrepancy scores, obtained for the same child in different school grades, follows a bivariate normal distribution. In their study only 9 of 108 discrepancy scores and 171 of 3402 pairs of discrepancy scores differed significantly from the expected scores – proportions well within the expected values for data with, respectively, univariate and bivariate normal distributions. It is important to differentiate between reading backwardness (which implies that with appropriate help affected children will eventually catch up with their peers) and a specific learning disorder, called dyslexia, that leads to reading retardation (Yule and Rutter 1976). For the purposes of this chapter it can be taken that *reading backwardness* denotes a difficulty in learning to read from a variety of causes, resulting in poor achievement for age, and *dyslexia* indicates a difficulty in learning to read because of a particular neurologically based disorder, resulting in unexpected underachievement for the person's general level of ability.

Causes of reading difficulties are likely to be complex, and they vary widely. School may be missed at a critical period of learning, often because of illness; teaching may be inappropriate; depression and other emotional disorders can interfere with learning; illness or injury, especially due to adverse influences during pregnancy and birth, can cause brain damage (Rickards et al. 1993); the child may have below-average intelligence; lack of opportunity and experience (for example if parents are unsupportive) can directly influence the acquisition of a learning skill; and another disorder such as deafness, impaired vision, or physical disability may play a critical role.

Loss of reading ability from disease (acquired dyslexia) is different from failure to learn to read in the first place (congenital dyslexia), but there is no reason to believe that the underlying neurological mechanisms are basically different. However, specific learning disorders frequently occur in the absence of any contributory factors, although secondary emotional complications are common enough.

About 3 to 10% of school children are thought to have dyslexia, and the ratio of males to females is between 2:1 and 4:1 (Rutter and Yule 1976), although the higher ratio may be an overestimate (Keys 1993). The term *dyslexia* is sometimes used to include dysgraphia and orthographic or spelling disorders, but these conditions do not necessarily coincide with dyslexia.

Kussmaul described word blindness in 1877, and Dejerine in 1891 described the two main types of acquired reading difficulty – alexia with agraphia, and alexia without agraphia (Critchley 1961, 1970). *Dyslexia* is generally used when reading retardation is thought to be due to a learning problem in the child rather than to absences from school, emotional disturbance, or poor teaching (Ingram 1971). The term also tends to denote slower than expected progress with remedial help: only 1 of 14 children studied in Edinburgh by Mason (1967) showed any definite improvement over a 2-year period of observation. In 1968 the World Federation of Neurology defined dyslexia as 'a disorder in children who despite conventional classroom experience fail to attain the language skills of reading, writing and spelling commensurate with their intellectual abilities'. It is accepted by convention that a delay of 2 years in the acquisition of these skills is significant. The common working definition is reading ability below the 10th centile in a child in primary grade 2 (i.e. age 7 years in the United Kingdom) who has normal overall intelligence. The determination of overall normal intelligence may be difficult, as a child who was slow in learning to speak may show retardation on oral vocabulary tests: for accurate assessment, reliance often has to be placed upon non-linguistic skills, as in drawing shapes, block design, and Raven's Matrices.

Normal development of reading
To be able to learn to read, a child obviously must have vision that is good enough to let the child see something the size of the print and discriminate letter shapes; and normal eye movements are required so the child can scan the words and the page from left to right (Luria 1973, Shapira et al. 1980). However, reading retardation in a child who has a normal IQ and has had 2 years of consecutive normal schooling is only rarely due to undiagnosed severe refractive errors or to an inability to see or discriminate letters as shapes. Even children with a total ocular dyspraxia, as in ataxia–telangectasia, can nevertheless read.

The child also has to appreciate that the spoken word is made up of a series of sounds, through a process often called phonic segmentation, and through phonemic or phonological awareness. Problems with reading can arise if the child cannot do this. This ability depends upon auditory processing in the left temporal lobe. Having learned to hear a series of sounds, the child then has to learn that, for example, each of the 46 sounds found in the English language can be represented by one or more of the 26 letters in the English alphabet, sometimes in combinations that appear to defy common sense, as with the *f* sound in *fish, phlegm, cough*. Each sound has a pictorial representation that is recognized in the visual association area in the left hemisphere. The difficulty of realizing that a word is made up of sounds is nothing compared with the task of putting a sound to a written letter, and then getting a word out of it. This is often the area of maximum difficulty, accounting for the aptness of the term *word blindness*. The written word must be heard in 'inner language' before it can be spoken as in reading aloud and before meaning can be extracted from it, i.e. before the child understands the written word.

Words, whether spoken or written, that are recognized in the language area of the temporal lobe as being in the lexicon need to be held in short-term memory and so reach consciousness while meaning is searched for. This process means that memory stores in all parts of the brain, and not just the language area, are used. Disorders of short-term memory or difficulties in holding the material in short-term memory (for example due to lack of concentration and to distractibility) will interfere with this aspect of learning. The words being read have to be held in short-term memory until enough of the phrase has been decoded to permit meaning to be extracted. Slobin (1971) gives the example of the sentence: 'Rapid righting with his uninjured hand saved from loss the contents of the capsized canoe' – i.e. only at the end of the sentence does the reader learn that it was a canoe that was being righted, and only then can the meaning be extracted. If reading is slow, distractions are more likely to occur before meaning is extracted. The same thing will happen if the material being read is badly constructed, because short, grammatically simple constructions are the easiest to read.

Reading skill, therefore, consists of a combination of learning word shapes ('look and say') and phonetic analysis of words. The phonetic approach is now thought to be the more important in the English language. Speed gradually increases, so that a good reader takes only a tenth of a second to scan a word and can read up to 400 words a minute and still extract meaning.

Types of dyslexia
A number of authors have classified dyslexias into visuospatial, audiophonic, and mixed types (Ingram 1969, Boder 1973). In most instances dyslexia is a basic defect of language development. Indeed all children who have suffered from a specific delay of language development are at risk of having difficulties in learning to read, so that there is a continuum of language disorders (Snowling et al. 1994). Also, if reading is to be taught adequately, due attention must be given to boosting phonological skills (Hatcher et al. 1994). However, a few children have difficulties in gaining reading skill because of visual-perceptual disorders (Boder 1973). If a child cannot easily recognize shapes and has difficulties with sequencing, problems in recognizing letters and their order in a word are likely to follow. Some children appear to be affected in both the visual and the language-processing spheres and are consequently the most severely disabled. The presence of deficits in both of these areas among children with dyslexia is supported by the studies of Slaghuis et al. (1993), who found that a visual-processing score and a phonological-coding test both discriminated between normal children and children with dyslexia, whereas a test of language comprehension did not. Boder (1973) based a means of assessing and remediating disorders of reading and spelling on these concepts, which perhaps have a particular attraction for doctors. The theory seems to be compatible with the physiology of the brain, and the Boder test can be used by individuals not trained in psychology (for a further description of the Boder test, see the section Examination, on page 87). Other workers (Bryant and Bradley 1985) have stressed that there is no guarantee that the different types of deficit are unique to children

with dyslexia, and it can be argued that children without reading problems might also be divided into similar groups. Olsen et al. (1989) found no suppport for the presence of a perceptual deficit to explain an orthographic, or spelling, coding disorder among the children with reading disabilities whom they studied. Nevertheless it does seem most likely that reading disabilities are, to varying degrees, a result of a complex interaction between perceptual and phonological representations (Goulandris 1994).

Causes of dyslexia
GENETIC FACTORS

Although genetic influences may certainly play a part in causing dyslexia, there must be considerable heterogeneity, with no single mode of transmission (Childs and Finucci 1983), and there is always likely to be an interaction between genetic endowment and environmental influences. There is undoubtedly aggregation of children with reading difficulties within certain families (Wolff and Melngailis 1994): in one study concordance was found in all uniovular twins but in only a third of binovular twins (Hermann 1959; and see Stevenson in Chapter 7 of this book). Evidence has been found for quantitative trait loci for dyslexia on chromosomes 6 and 15 (Cardon et al. 1994), but how these two genes affect development is not known. Maybe they affect the establishment of intracerebral tracts (Njiokiktjien et al. 1994), or cause defects of cell migration leading to faulty cortical architecture (Flowers 1993).

A history of similar learning disorders among the parents and relatives of children with dyslexia is not uncommon and can provide important clues, not only to the nature of the particular disability but to the possibility of genetic factors in aetiology. Stevenson (Chapter 7) gives more information, and references, on the genetics of dyslexia, in particular stressing that learning disorders are produced not by the effects of a single gene but rather by the action of a number of genes and environmental influences. Annett et al. (1996) claimed that dyslexia is commoner in left-handers, but the relation, if any, is probably small. In the first place genetically determined left-handers must be differentiated from left-handers who prefer to use their left hand only because of damage to the left cerebral hemisphere, as only the latter group will be more liable to learning disorders (Gordon 1986). Annett et al. (1996) found that subjects with dyslexia who also had poor phonological processing were less likely to be right-handed than controls, whereas the contrary was true of subjects with dyslexia whose phonological processing was normal. If the theory of a genetically based right shift is correct, this would suggest that there is a gene that adds to the random asymmetry by handicapping certain regions of the developing right hemisphere. This gene would be associated with benefits for speech learning but at costs to the right hemisphere, so that there might be two types of risk to learning to read: those children who inherited no copy of the gene, and might be ambidextrous, would have a weakness in the cognitive representation of speech; while those who inherited two copies, and are strongly right-handed, would have other difficulties, probably in the representation of words in visual memory. In one representative sample of individuals with dyslexia, 29% of those with poor phonological processing were left-handed, whereas none who had normal phonological processing were left-handed (Annett et al. 1996). This finding would be expected if left hemisphere function was impaired in the group with poor phonological processing. Individuals who are heterozygous, inheriting only one copy of this hypothetical gene, have been claimed to be intellectually at an advantage. This hypothetical advantage was not supported by the findings of others, who concluded that the differences were due to factors such as motivation (McManus et al. 1993). Psychosocial stress in early childhood has a particularly strong influence on the ability to read, no doubt often interacting with a genetic predisposition, and it has been shown that this acts to a much greater degree than in individuals with poor spelling (Olsen et al. 1989). This offers an opportunity for effective intervention.

ENDOCRINE FACTORS
There have been a number of non-genetic hypotheses to explain dyslexia. It has been suggested that prenatal exposure to increased levels of testosterone slows neuronal development in the left cerebral hemisphere, leading to an increased rate of left-handedness and developmental learning disorders in males; testosterone also affects the development of the thymus, increasing the risk of immune disorders at a later age (Geschwind and Behan 1982, Galaburda et al. 1985). This possibility has been supported by some researchers (Tonnessen et al. 1993) but not others. Nevertheless it cannot be entirely ruled out (Jariabkova et al. 1995).

BRAIN DAMAGE
Any pre-, peri-, or postnatal damage to the brain can interfere with normal development, and one possible result would be difficulties in learning to read. Such damage is a recurrent theme in this chapter, especially when considering non-connection and disconnection syndromes, and the role of the doctor.

The anatomy of dyslexia
Accepting that dyslexia may be due, in varying proportions, to auditory and visual defects, and that this specific learning disorder is neurologically based, what are the foundations for this claim? There may be several explanations, and it is all too easy to oversimplify the issues, but the following evidence is offered.

ANATOMICAL DEVELOPMENT – NORMAL AND ABNORMAL
The primary visual area 17 in the striate or calcarine cortex of the occipital lobe is linked to the visual association area 18 and these are both linked across the corpus callosum. A lesion in the striate cortex causes cortical blindness. Patients with right-sided lesions of the visual cortex will have visual agnosia for faces, music, shapes, colour, or objects but will not develop dyslexia. Conversely most children with dyslexia are very competent at matching, copying, and drawing shapes and do not have 'visuospatial difficulties'. The visual association area 18 on the left is needed in order to pick out shapes with a linguistic significance, i.e. graphemes and words, in the same way that the auditory association area on the left picks out sounds, i.e. phonemes and words, with a linguistic meaning. Children with dyslexia rarely have difficulty discriminating or matching letters or even copying them as geometric shapes, but they have great difficulty in matching them with the sound, i.e. making grapheme–phoneme correlations.

From studies of brain lesions causing reading and writing problems in adults, it would appear that the visual areas on both sides are linked together into the visual association area on the left, and the material is then transferred by the left angular gyrus to Wernicke's area. Audio-to-visual correlation or grapheme-to-phoneme transformation depends on an intact angular gyrus. Reading is a linguistic skill: once a word has been read it must be 'heard' in inner language, a process dependent upon the planum temporale on the left, and only then can its meaning be extracted and the word be spoken aloud if that is necessary. Even sign language has to be 'heard' in the dominant temporal lobe of a deaf person in order for meaning to be extracted. Dysplasia of the planum temporale in some individuals with dyslexia would account for the greater frequency of the audiophonic than of the visuospatial type of dyslexia. The functional MRI studies by Shaywitz's group at Yale (1992, 1995) have vividly demonstrated the neurobiological basis for specific reading disorder. The inferior frontal gyrus is activated in phonological tasks and the extrastriate cortex is activated for letter recognition; and when subjects are asked if a string of letters rhymes, the superior and middle temporal gyri are also activated – i.e. all the brain areas expected to contribute to reading do so. Using magnetic resonance spectroscopy, Rae et al. (1998) have found that among men with dyslexia, compared with controls, there are biochemical differences in the left temporoparietal lobe and in the right cerebellum. These differences may be due to changes in cell density, and their presence supports the hypothesis that cellular development or intracellular connections or both are abnormal in this condition. The findings regarding the temporoparietal lobe may correlate with defects in the magnocellular system, and those in the cerebellum may explain the frequent association of dyslexia with incoordination.

VISUAL INPUT

Information on which the acquisition of reading skill depends is conveyed to the relevant centres in the brain by visual and auditory pathways, which must function reasonably normally. A number of disorders of vision have been suggested as possible causes of dyslexia, all examples of defective integration or input. Pavlidis (1979) found that the eye movements of many affected children were defective: they were erratic in a random, scattered fashion, and regressive eye movements were more frequent than in controls and were also irregular and often bigger than the forward saccades. These children's eyes moved farther back to fixate on words than did the eyes of normal and slow readers. However, it may be that the malfunctioning of the eye-movement control system and the dyslexia have a common cause, such as a disability of central, non-modality-specific, sequential activities.

Some children with dyslexia show evidence of abnormal cerebral lateralization, resulting in impaired ocular dominance that may confuse the ocular motor system and make it harder to tell where letters and words are positioned on a page (Stein and Fowler 1982). Stein and Fowler (1985) found that a third of children with dyslexia had unstable control of vergence and tended to make visual rather than phonic errors. They claimed that monocular occlusion improved reading performance. Another interesting finding is the use of tinted yellow spectacles: it has been claimed that these can improve reading by compensating for blue light being brought into focus in front of the retina, causing blurring and glare (Fowler et al. 1991).

It has been suggested (Bakker et al. 1987) that initially reading requires mainly visuoperceptual analysis of script, relying mainly on the right cerebral hemisphere, and that at this stage reading is relatively slow; whereas advanced reading is characterized by fluency and rapidity and is a semantic–syntactic text processing mediated mainly by the left hemisphere. During normal development the functions serving this skill switch from the right to the left hemisphere at some point after 1 to 2 years of reading experience. Some children fail to make this shift and continue to rely on right hemisphere strategies and are slow readers, whereas others skip the initial process and are fast readers, and the two types of children make different errors.

Admittedly these visuoperceptual disabilities may only be a prelude to other, predominantly phonic, disorders, and their possible effects have been questioned (Metzger and Werner 1984). Nevertheless even if these findings apply to only relatively few children, there are implications for remedial teaching. If the cause of the dyslexia is an ocular defect (rather than an abnormality of cerebral function, which is probably the problem in most children with dyslexia), once the defect has been rectified there should be no further problems in learning to read.

VISUAL PROCESSING
Deficits at a cortical level may result in disorders of visual or auditory processing (Gordon and Ward 1995). Using magnetoencephalography Salmelin et al. (1996) studied adults with dyslexia and control subjects during passive viewing of single words. A difference was found in the left inferior temporo-occipital cortex, no doubt linked to histological abnormalities in the left planum temporale. Whereas the controls showed a sharp activation in this area about 180 ms after word presentation, the adults with a history of developmental dyslexia had no or late activation in this area. Such an impairment, in the perception of words as specific units, would interfere with language processing. Difficulties can also occur with respect to efference, as in articulatory–motor problems (Heilman et al. 1996).

The left hemisphere is specialized for temporal processing and the right is devoted to static spatial analysis, which may be why the left is favoured for linguistic analysis and the right for perception, including the visual functions under discussion (Stein 1994). As already mentioned, it must always be remembered that if there have been difficulties in language development these will very likely be followed by problems in learning to read (Poeppel and Rowley 1996).

Defects in the visual pathways, particularly at a subcortical level, lead to difficulties in learning to read. There may be an association between dyslexia and abnormalities in the magnocellular pathways of both the visual and auditory systems. The magnocellular visual pathways arise from large retinal ganglion cells, and rapidly convey black-and-white information, particularly about the timing of events, to the visual cortex via the dorsal lateral geniculate nucleus, particularly the timing of visual events. The parvocellular system starts from smaller retinal cells and more slowly transmits colour and accurate fine-detailed, point-to-point spatial information to the cortex, also via the geniculate nucleus (Guyton 1991).

Eden et al. (1996) found a deficit in the magnocellular system of adults with dyslexia, resulting in impaired detection of visual motion. Their subjects also had phonological problems and abnormalities in processing visual movement; so that in these subjects visual and auditory disorders coexisted. Frith and Frith (1996) think that the visual defects do not directly cause the reading difficulties, but that the most interesting possibility is that both types of disorder could be related to a cognitive deficit in timing affecting all modalities – for example in the auditory field a failure to discriminate between different phonemes. Be that as it may, the deficit in the magnocellular system identified by Eden et al. (1996) could be used as a biological marker for dyslexia.

Children with dyslexia perform badly in tasks requiring fast sequential processing (Eden et al. 1995). Cornelissen et al. (1995) found that children with dyslexia were less sensitive to motion than other children. This insensitivity could be due to abnormalities in the magnocellular input pathways or, just as easily, to cortical dysfunction. The link with reading could be a 'shift effect', in which the detection of a foveal target can be reduced by movement in the periphery, and an abnormal interaction between foveal and peripheral vision affects reading, especially the detection of letters. This may result in a timing disorder that prevents the rapid, smooth integration of detailed visual information needed for efficient reading. This hypothesis has not yet been proved. Also, the response to visual evoked potentials in the magnocellular pathways has been found to be slowed in children with reading disability, who did not, however, have a general slowing of the visual response (Lehmkuhle et al. 1993).

The two pathways, magnocellular and parvocellular, are most clearly distinguished in the lateral geniculate nucleus, and functional MRI has shown anomalies in the magnocellular visual system of children with dyslexia (Eden et al. 1996). In addition, disorders of the magnocellular layers in this nucleus can be seen post mortem (Livingstone et al. 1991). This may explain why individuals with dyslexia have been found to have lowered sensitivity to flicker and motion. Anatomical abnormalities in the nucleus of the medial geniculate body of individuals with developmental dyslexia were confirmed by Galaburda et al. (1994). Post mortem examination of five subjects and of seven control children with no difficulties in reading showed that in the former the nucleus on the left was smaller than that on the right. Also there were more small neurons and fewer large ones, which could account for a phonological defect. It may be that the observed defects were secondary to cortical abnormalities resulting in changes in cortical targets for axons arising in the medial geniculate nucleus during development.

These findings may also correlate with the finding that the left Wernicke's area, or planum temporale, is larger than that on the right in normal children but not in children with dyslexia. This asymmetry has been confirmed by positron emission tomography (Rumsey et al. 1992) and by MRI studies (Filipek 1995, Peterson 1995). There is suggestive evidence that normally the left planum receives more magnocellular input than the right; but when this input is reduced the planum will obviously be smaller on the left side. Other research has failed to confirm a defect in fast processing of the magnocellular versus the parvocellular system (Victor et al. 1993, Nass 1994), although there could be technical reasons for this.

Another anatomical finding that may well be relevant is the size of the corpus callosum. The genu may be smaller in individuals with dyslexia (Hynd et al. 1995), suggesting a defect in interhemispheric transmission and in the development of connections. However, disconnection of one cerebral hemisphere from the other does not necessarily lead to significant cerebral dysfunction (Jinkins 1991).

Polikoff et al. (1995) found by experiment that lesions in the right posterior parietal lobe leading to poor oculomotor control and visual neglect of the left side of space are not a significant cause of dyslexia, as some have suggested. Finally, even an unrecognized refractive error can cause problems in the processing of visual information. Children with dyslexia who cannot analyse a word linguistically have to try and remember the shape of the word as a pictogram.

AUDITORY INPUT

If reading difficulties most often arise from a basic disorder of language development, information received through the auditory channel is obviously important. Faulty language development may stem from even such a simple disorder as serous otitis media. Eaton and Nowell (1983) compared 55 children who attended schools for learning-disabled children with a cohort of 59 children from a normal school. All were from comparable backgrounds and aged between 7 and 11 years. Findings on impedance bridge testing were abnormal in 14 of the children with reading problems and in only 4 of the control children without reading problems, suggesting a correlation between middle ear problems and dyslexia.

AUDITORY PROCESSING

There are many causes of impaired hearing, involving pathways up to and including auditory processing at a cortical level, and all of them can affect the development of reading skills (Gordon and Ward 1995). Pure tone audiometry and auditory evoked responses may exclude deafness, but what of auditory discrimination? If this is impaired, difficulties with reading are likely. Disorders of central auditory processing certainly affect the development of spoken language – a good example is the Landau–Kleffner syndrome (Gordon 1997a) – and in turn this may impair reading ability because of incomplete verbal images in the central areas of reception and auditory skills (Welsh et al. 1983).

Reading is a learned skill: as recently as a few hundred years ago there were few people in the world who could read. The age when a child starts to read depends on many factors, including intelligence and the effectiveness of cerebral integration underlying visual and auditory memory, so that failure of these functions will inevitably delay reading ability. Lack of neurons is obviously a primary factor in limiting learning, but, as has been stated, learning must depend to a great extent on linking the various input and output channels. This linking cannot be achieved if the connections are not there. It is rightly accepted that dyslexia is basically a phonological defect (Das et al. 1995), so no wonder children who have suffered from delays of language development are at risk of having difficulties in learning to read. There is therefore a continuum of language disorders (Cowden 1996), and teachers of reading must give attention to boosting phonological skills (Hatcher et al. 1994). However, even if dysfunction of the visual system is only a contributing factor (Fletcher-Flinn et al. 1997), both visual and auditory impairments must always be considered.

Using functional MRI in 29 adults with dyslexia, compared with 32 normal readers, SE Shaywitz et al. (1998) recently found evidence of relative underactivity in the posterior regions (Wernicke's area, the angular gyrus, and the striatal cortex) and relative overactivity in the anterior region (inferior frontal region). They considered their results to be evidence that the impairment in dyslexia is phonological; but these results also point to the combined contribution of auditory and visual defects in difficulties in learning to read. If the visual or auditory system is extensively disrupted by whatever cause, particularly in the region of the association areas around the angular gyrus, there will be difficulties in, for example, converting print into sounds. The different patterns of activation in the posterior and anterior regions seemed to be due not to increased effort on the part of the subjects with dyslexia, but to a functional disruption of the system underlying phonological analysis.

Disconnection or non-connection syndromes

Evidence from cases in which brain insults result in acquired dyslexia in adults lends support to the concept of a neurological dysfunction. Studies of adults with acquired dyslexia mainly due to vascular lesions have suggested explanations for observed neurological symptoms and signs (Geschwind 1965). For example a patient could not name colours, but could match them by hue and could identify the figures in tests for colour vision. It was maintained that this was due to a loss of visual–auditory association resulting from the destruction of the cortical association area or the connections between the visual and auditory areas, as colours have no smell, taste, or feel, only a name (Geschwind and Fusillo 1966). If such disconnection syndromes occur, it can be hypothesized that the same type of phenomenon can result if such connections never form in the first place – that is, specific learning disorders can be regarded as disconnection or non-connection syndromes.

This theory is lent further weight by the recognition that there is a distinction between children who are slow to read when they start school due to a developmental lag and those who have difficulty in learning to read at an older age because of a specific learning disorder (Badian 1996); among the latter group there will be some who continue to show this disability in adult life, in spite of average or above average intelligence and good teaching (Korhonen 1995). This finding must surely be evidence in favour of a structural deficit in the brain, which may be compensated for but sometimes cannot be entirely overcome, such as a lack of connections between two parts of the brain.

Learning must involve the integration of sensory input from the ears, eyes, and other channels, as well as the influence of other factors such as the emotional content of the information, past experiences, and other qualities such as attention and concentration. If these associations are dependent on the connection of one part of the brain with another, then an absence of axons and dendrites, or of the neurons themselves, will have a profound effect. Such connections may never be formed, may be destroyed, or may not be used.

Connections may not be formed in the first instance, because of interference with the growth of the brain – for example when malnutrition occurs during the main spurt of brain growth. In human beings this occurs in the second half of pregnancy and continues during the first 2 years of life and is due mainly to the proliferation of the glial tissues of the brain and their myelination. Any interference with their development at this time is bound to have a profound effect on the formation of synaptic connections and, later, on learning. Such malnutrition before birth may well be one of the main reasons why dysmature babies are more likely to suffer from these disabilities as they grow older. The evidence (Dobbing 1970) suggests that if malnutrition does occur during the main spurt of brain growth, complete recovery may be impossible.

Neurons and association fibres linking them can well be destroyed by such agents as anoxia during pregnancy and birth, although a combination of adverse factors rather than anoxia alone seems to be of importance. This phenomenon is described by Hagberg et al. (1976) as 'fetal deprivation of supply'; and, as they suggest, this means that although postnatal preventive measures have been well developed and perinatal brain damage syndromes have decreased significantly, prenatal mechanisms, which now predominate, are still sometimes unresolved.

If connections are not used, this can have a profound effect on functional organization at a cortical level. There is evidence that if neurons do not connect with their target they will die – a case of 'use them or lose them' (Gordon 1995). This possibility is supported by animal experiments, such as occluding one eye or producing a squint that interferes with the interaction of stimuli from the two eyes (Gaze 1970). When this occurs at a critical stage of development, cells normally associated with afferent stimuli from one eye may be permanently linked to those from the other eye, even if normality is restored. Among humans the so-called amblyopic eye is a similar example. Double vision resulting from a squint in early childhood can be resolved by suppression of one of the images, as can happen to any stimulus that does not have any particular meaning or interferes with perception. If such inhibition goes on for long enough, it may become permanent (Gordon 1997b).

Recognition, assessment, and management
RECOGNITION
There are several ways in which dyslexia may be recognized. Dyslexia can be suspected relatively easily when a child fails to start reading at the expected age, but as this age varies widely there may be some delay before the teacher recognizes that there is a problem needing further assessment and intervention. Overall the class teacher is best placed to identify the child with dyslexia. Early detection can be enhanced by examination of children at school entry. Bax and Whitmore (1973, 1987) found that over half of the children with low scores on their assessment were exhibiting learning difficulties 3 or 4 years later. Parents may also become concerned if they observe that their child reads less well than peers or siblings at a similar age. The condition may also come to light when coexisting behaviour problems or other specific learning problems are identified and the child's overall performance is scrutinized more closely. The family doctor may well be the first of the medical personnel to see the child. One frequent mode of presentation is with such symptoms as headache, abdominal pain, and bed-wetting, due to the stress that can affect the child both at school and at home.

ASSESSMENT
In the assessment, management, and treatment of children with dyslexia no one person can supply all the answers; only a multidisciplinary team can hope to solve them. A neurodevelopmental and physical assessment by the school doctor or paediatrician is a valuable starting point in building up a picture of the nature and context of a child's difficulties. Medical assessment will need to be augmented by a full educational and psychological assessment.

History-taking
A comprehensive medical and social history must be taken from the parents, including details of the pregnancy and the child's birth, in view of the correlation between difficulties at these times and the later incidence of specific learning disorders (Brown 1976). Certain postnatal illnesses can be particularly significant, such as meningitis leading to deafness that may not even have been recognized, or asthma leading to a serious loss of

schooling. The outstanding example is epilepsy in childhood, which can affect development in several ways: through a cerebral lesion causing fits and learning difficulties, through the side effects of antiepileptic drugs, through associated emotional and behavioural disorders, and through the effects of the fits themselves. It should be remembered that epileptic activity, demonstrated in the electroencephalogram, can disrupt the processes of learning whether overt seizures occur or not (Gordon 1997b).

A family history of reading difficulty or other learning problems should be sought, in both first- and second-degree relatives. A developmental history may reveal delayed or disordered language, which is significantly associated with dyslexia (Snowling et al. 1994). A history of delayed motor development and clumsiness suggests a coexisting motor disorder.

Very occasionally the child, and sometimes the parents, may deny the presence of any kind of learning difficulties, especially if the child has presented with symptoms of stress such as headache, abdominal pain, or bed-wetting. This possibility points up the importance of obtaining a report of the child's progress in school or, better still, of a direct discussion with the teacher, preferably with the parents' permission.

Both the parents and the teacher may well be able to give useful information about the child's behaviour and emotional state. This information can be essential for effective management, whether the state is the cause or the result of the learning difficulties. A recent change in behaviour can be of particular significance.

Examination

The examiner should aim for a comprehensive assessment of the child, looking at neurodevelopmental status including fine and gross motor functions, speech and language ability, and reading, spelling, and writing ability, together with a physical and neurological examination and assessment of vision and hearing. Whitmore and Bax (1986) described such a comprehensive assessment of 5-year-olds which has been shown to be predictive of learning difficulties at age 10 (Bax and Whitmore 1987). In practice a child with reading difficulties may be referred for assessment at any age rather than at a standard age as in Whitmore and Bax's assessment. Therefore the battery of tests needs to be appropriate for the child's age.

Assessment of speech and language looks at three elements of communication: the semantic, the syntactic, and the transmission system. Picture naming, defining use, and the concepts of opposites and relative positions in space (on, under, beside, etc.) are all helpful in the assessment of speech and language ability. Syntax and understanding can be evaluated during informal conversation and using Renfrew Action Pictures and 'The Bus Story'. Articulation can be checked during vocabulary testing with pictures: the consonant sounds most frequently mispronounced are *l, k, r, s, sh,* and *th.*

Depending on the child's developmental age a simple reading test can be given. The tests described by Boder (1973) are convenient and simple to administer. The reading test consists of a Word Recognition Inventory presented in two ways: flash and untimed. The former determines sight vocabulary and the latter, the child's ability to analyse unfamiliar words phonetically. The child's reading level is derived from the sight-vocabulary score, and comparison of the number of correctly read words in the 'flash' and 'untimed' columns indicates whether the child is reading through whole-word and phonetic analysis or predominantly through one or the other. Boder (1973) also describes a spelling test that is complementary to the reading test.

If a slightly more formal approach is desired, it can be helpful to use tests such as the Frostig Developmental Test of Visual Perception and the Stott Test of Motor Performance, more as an extension of the neurological examination than as a strictly standardized assessment. When it comes to the more detailed analysis of the affected child's disability, special standardized scales may well be needed. The Extended Griffiths Mental Developmental Scale and the Wechsler Intelligence Scale for Children (WISC), which both have separate performance and verbal scales, are of particular value. The Reynell Developmental Language Scales (Reynell 1977) can give a more accurate measurement of to what extent linguistic comprehension and expression are involved.

Assessment of motor function may reveal clumsiness, which can coexist with dyslexia and may signal an underlying neurological impairment responsible for the condition. Traditional fine manipulation tasks that are a measure of eye–hand coordination include bridge and step construction using 1-inch shapes, fastening buttons, and tying shoelaces. Asking the child to copy a circle, a square, and a triangle allows observation of not only the ability to distinguish and reproduce shapes but also the maturity of pencil grip and hand preference, the latter providing evidence of lateralization and hemispheric dominance. An older child can be asked to write letters, for the evaluation of motor executive skill in writing.

Gross motor function can be examined by observing the child's gait and by asking the child to hop on each leg in turn and to walk heel-to-toe. It is worth stressing that one of the best predictors of language disorders is impaired motor development (Owen and McKinlay 1997).

Neurological examination needs to be detailed, because any positive findings are likely to be subtle. With impairment of fine motor function and coordination in mind, useful tests include those for motor impersistence (mouth held open wide and tongue protruded for 20 seconds), hand patting, finger–nose pointing, pronation–supination movements of the hand, and Bergès–Lézine imitation of gestures (Bergès and Lézine 1965). The latter items draw on several CNS functions including visual perception, concept of body image, muscle and joint senses, and motor organization and control. Muscle tone, muscle power, and limb reflexes should also be tested.

The head and face should be examined to detect abnormal facies or head shape and to assess the cranial nerves and identify any motor asymmetry or oromuscular dysfunction. Head circumference should be charted, together with height and weight, as flattening of the head-growth line may be the first indicator of failure of brain development.

Visual and auditory function should be examined with particular care. Examination of visual function should include checking not only for refractive errors and squint, but also for eye movements, nystagmus, and colour vision (as colour is sometimes used in teaching techniques [Gordon 1998]). Tests for hearing should include tests for pure tones and tests for auditory discrimination and comprehension, speaking to the child from a distance of 6 feet.

Throughout the examination, observation of the child's behaviour and the quality of the child's interaction with their parents and the examiner can give a valuable picture of coexisting behavioural or emotional problems. Features such as short attention span, high activity level, uncooperativeness, or lack of eye contact can point to disorders such as attention-deficit/hyperactivity disorder, behaviour problems secondary to learning difficulties, or social or emotional dysfunction. Teachers' and parents' accounts of behaviour in the classroom and at home can help to determine the context of these observations and to indicate the pervasiveness and seriousness of the problem.

MANAGEMENT

Children with dyslexia are not a homogeneous group, so some specialist approaches to remediation, such as Alpha to Omega (Hornsby and Shear 1975), may be suitable only for certain children. The planning of remedial teaching programmes is the responsibility of the psychologist and teacher, and their choice will depend on the nature of the disorder and their detailed analysis of the child's difficulties, with teaching geared to these, as in the Aston Portfolio (Aubrey et al. 1981). It would seem logical to use the least affected input channel (whether visual or auditory), as in Boder's method (1973), and Leatherbarrow (1986) discusses such an approach. For instance, with a predominantly phonic difficulty a 'look and say' approach might be best, but when there are perceptual problems a phonic approach might work. Bradley and Bryant (1985) have shown that children's experience of rhyme and alliteration before they come to school does make a difference to their ability to learn to read and write, and they can be trained in these. However, there are many possible methods (Hicks 1986).

One of the most successful methods is Reading Recovery (Hurry 1996), designed by Clay (1985). It is an intervention for children who have been in formal schooling for a year and are in the bottom 20% of their class for reading. Part of its success may be due to early intervention, which is likely to be more effective than remediation at a later stage. It is not only the amount of time given to remedial sessions that is important, but their frequency. If teaching is not given daily, the children will tend to forget what they have learned, so it is difficult to build on previous progress. The closer to one-to-one the teaching situation is, the more successful it may be, as shown recently by the results of summer schools in the UK for children with reading difficulties. However, just giving intensive help may not teach poor readers to read (Pinnell et al. 1994), and the success of this method rests on the selection of the children to be taught; the detailed assessment on the basis of which each child's programme is individually developed and subsequently monitored at regular intervals; and a carefully planned curriculum. Equally important may be how the method is taught, and teachers can require special training lasting a year; to ensure that their skills are maintained these may have to be checked from time to time.

The effectiveness of drugs, such as piracetam, in the treatment of dyslexia remains unproved (Bakker et al. 1987), but in such a complex disorder it seems unlikely that they would have more than a minimal effect. Life is not that simple.

Various aspects of management can affect the outcome for children with dyslexia, beneficially and adversely. Many children will be most effectively helped if clinics are held in the school, so that discussions can take place as soon as possible with the teacher and cooperation between all those trying to help the child can be encouraged; quite often these discussions should include the parent and the child (Gordon 1997b). Sometimes the teacher can be unaware of the problems, especially if physical or behavioural symptoms are dominant. Once the problem has been defined and remedial help has been arranged, the doctor's role may be limited, but there is still a role as a questioner. For example remedial teaching is not always successful: why not?

If the child's progress is not satisfactory, a number of questions may have to be asked about possible problems at home or at school which have not been resolved: about the child's health, vision, and hearing; about the treatment of associated difficulties, such as coordination disorders; about the effectiveness of management, especially of emotional and behavioural problems; about the attitudes of the parents to their affected children (parents can be unreasonable – for example if their efforts to help are excessive they can be counterproductive); and, no doubt, about many other matters. In view of the complexity of the problem the whole family is likely to be involved, and then referral to a psychiatrist for family therapy may be needed (Goodyer 1986).

Delinquency

Lack of self-esteem, so common among those with learning disorders, can easily lead to abnormal behaviour. For a start it can cause a child to act in an unacceptable manner in order to get attention or to gain the approval of peers (Gordon 1993). Poor self-esteem can contribute to bullying at school. In order to try to give themselves a higher status, children may dominate others who are younger and weaker than they are. No doubt this gives them a sense of power and counteracts feelings of failure.

Reading difficulties are frequently found among juvenile delinquents (Grande 1988). Brier (1988) considered three hypotheses that may help to explain why some individuals with learning difficulties develop unacceptable behaviour but the majority do not.

The 'susceptibility' hypothesis maintains that the effects of learning difficulties contribute directly to the abnormal behaviour. These effects include aggression and poor attention, concentration, judgement, and social perception. It is not unusual for a child who has repeatedly failed to give up trying, thus reinforcing the impression of low intelligence and perhaps causing the child to be labelled dull and difficult. Then the child's behaviour can deteriorate and lead to delinquency.

Brier's second hypothesis concerns school failure, which would start a sequence of events leading to delinquency. Criticism and rejection will certainly lead to a poor self-image and frustration, and maybe absenteeism from school. There is evidence that children with learning difficulties are seen by their peers and teachers as less attractive and acceptable, which can result in rejection. Frustration can also arise from a strong desire to achieve in the absence of the ability to do so. However, it must be remembered that some children seem to be prone to delinquent behaviour for no particular cause, and that school failure can result from this.

Brier's third hypothesis is that of differential treatment of affected children. It may be that children and adolescents with learning difficulties are more likely to be dealt with severely by the police and the courts, because they fail to comprehend the proceedings - (Dudley-Marling 1985).

Even if some of the early findings (Robins 1978, Zoccolillo et al. 1992) of a link between dyslexia and delinquency were due to defects of methodology (Williams and McGee 1994), there is nevertheless considerable scope for prevention if these disorders are recognized and intervention is instigated. Williams and McGee (1994) examined the possible relation between early reading attainments and antisocial behaviour at 7 and 9 years of age, and subsequent reading achievement and delinquent behaviour in adolescence. Reading difficulties as such did not seem to affect later delinquency, but antisocial behaviour, possibly related to these difficulties during early school years, was strongly predictive of delinquency at 15 years of age, especially for boys; and reading disability at 9 years of age foreshadowed conduct disorder at age 15. Accepting the complexity of these links, and how individual they can be, it would be surprising if occasionally they did not apply.

Case descriptions
- CD was referred at age 11 years with behavioural difficulties. It was thought that he would have difficulty when he moved to a larger secondary school (in the UK; for children aged 11 years and over). Therefore, at referral attentional problems were also mentioned. A family history revealed that C's 20-year-old brother had been in a special school and was reported not to be able to read. His mother stated that she had had some reading difficulties at school. On examination C was found to be left-handed but, curiously, had some coordination difficulties with the left hand, so that diadochokinetic movements were very clumsy on the left side but not on the right. A Fog test (walking on the outer sides of his feet) also revealed some abnormal posturing on the left side. On the Boder reading test he was found to have a 'mixed' dyslexia, with a reading age more than 3 years behind his chronological age. One wondered whether an MR scan might be justified to see if C had some evidence of a right-sided lesion to account for what might be described as very minimal hemiplegia. On the other hand the family history of reading difficulties seemed so strong that it seemed better to regard C as having a genetically based dyslexia. No further investigation was undertaken, and the child was provided with a specific reading programme.
- PQ presented at age 7 years with difficult behaviour in school – running around in the classroom – and an expected diagnosis of attention-deficit/hyperactivity disorder. The situation was complicated by the fact that the parents' relationship was known to be difficult and they were having psychotherapy. The child's problem was strongly suspected to be behavioural. However, there was no history of previous overactivity nor was the child overactive at home; in fact he played happily with the toys he was interested in. There was no family history of learning difficulties and there were no abnormal physical findings. PQ's educational history revealed that his behaviour had been reasonable in the first years at school, when he had learned to read quite readily, and that his difficult behaviour had developed over the preceding 6 months of the school year. His reading age proved to be above average, but it was easily demonstrated that he had great difficulty with writing. His copying skills were appropriate for his age, but he had very specific problems with spelling. After a remedial approach to his spelling problem, discussion with him, and recognition that his problems stemmed from his spelling difficulties, his school behaviour rapidly improved despite his parents' decision at that time to divorce. Strictly speaking this child did not have dyslexia but rather had the commonly associated problem of a spelling difficulty.

Conclusions
Successful remediation of dyslexia depends on accurately identifying the problem at an early stage, assessing the nature of the child's difficulties, and implementing an appropriate,

individually tailored programme. The doctor can play a fundamental role in this process and there is a strong argument for all doctors involved in the care of children to be taught more about the complex problems of specific learning disorders.

It seems that a disturbance of both auditory and visual functions can play a part to varying degrees in causing reading difficulties. Failures of intracerebral connections can explain many of the findings reported in this disability. Therefore, when it comes to helping dyslexic children overcome their disability, the possibility both of auditory and of visual disorder should be taken into account, and methods geared to individual needs.

Much research is still needed into many aspects of dyslexia, and one of the most promising, and exciting, medical contributions to solving the disorders underlying dyslexia is likely to be the unravelling of the mysteries of cerebral function with the use of such techniques as cerebral blood flow studies, magnetic resonance spectroscopy, and positron emission tomography (see above). In the final analysis success in learning to read depends on the proficiency of cerebral integration.

ACKNOWLEDGEMENTS

I am grateful to Drs J K Brown and R A Minns for the section on the normal development of reading, and to Dr M Bax for the case histories.

REFERENCES

Annett M, Eglington E, Smythe P. (1996) Types of dyslexia and the shift to dextrality. *Journal of Child Psychology and Psychiatry* **37**: 167–80.

Aubrey C, Evans J, Hicks C. (1981) *The Aston Portfolio: Learning Development Aids.* Cambridge: Wisbech.

Badian NA. (1996) Dyslexia: a validation of the concept at two age levels. *Journal of Learning Disabilities* **29**: 102–12.

Bakker DJ, van Leeuwen HMP, Spyer G. (1987) Neurophysiological aspects of dyslexia. In: Bakker D, Wilsher C, Debruyne H, Bertin N, editors. *Developmental Dyslexia and Learning Disorders: Diagnosis and Treatment.* Basel: Karger.

Bax M, Whitmore K. (1973) Neurodevelopmental screening in the school-entrant medical examination. *Lancet* **ii**: 368–70.

— — (1987) The medical examination of children on entry to school. The results and use of neurodevelopment assessment. *Developmental Medicine and Child Neurology* **29**: 40–55.

Bergès J, Lézine I. (1965) *The Imitation of Gestures.* Clinics in Developmental Medicine No. 18. London: Spastics International Medical Publications/William Heinemann Medical Books.

Boder E. (1973) Developmental dyslexia: a diagnostic approach based on three typical reading–spelling patterns. *Developmental Medicine and Child Neurology* **15**: 663–87.

Bradley L, Bryant P. (1985) *Rhyme and Reason in Reading and Spelling.* Ann Arbor [MI]: University of Michigan Press.

Brier N. (1988) The relationship between learning disability and delinquency: a review and reappraisal. *Journal of Learning Disabilities* **22**: 547–53.

Brown JK. (1976) Infants damaged during birth: perinatal asphyxia. In: Hull ID, editor. *Recent Advances in Paediatrics. Vol 5.* Edinburgh: Churchill Livingstone. p 35–56.

Bryant P, Bradley L. (1985) *Children's Reading Problems: Psychology and Education.* Oxford: Blackwell.

Cardon LR, Smith SD, Fulker DW, et al. (1994) Quantitative trait locus for reading disability on chromosome 6. *Science* **226**: 276–9.

Childs B, Finucci JM. (1983) Genetics, epidemiology, and specific reading disability. In: Rutter M, editor. *Developmental Neuropsychiatry.* Edinburgh: Churchill Livingstone. p 507–19.

Clay MM. (1985) *The Early Detection of Reading Difficulties: A Diagnostic Survey with Recovery Procedures.* 3rd ed. Auckland: Heinemann.

Cornelissen P, Richardson A, Mason A, et al. (1995) Contrast sensitivity and coherent motion detection measured at photopic luminance levels in dyslexics and controls. *Vision Research* **35**: 1483–94.

Cowden J. (1996) Dyslexia: a hundred years on. *British Medical Journal* **313:** 1096–7.

Critchley M. (1961) Inborn reading disorders of central origin. Doyne Memorial Lecture. *Transactions of the Ophthalmological Society* **81.**

— (1970) *The Dyslexic Child.* Springfield [IL]: Charles C Thomas.

Das JP, Mishra RK, Pool JE. (1995) An experiment on cognitive remediation of word-reading difficulty. *Journal of Learning Disabilities* **28:** 66–79.

Dobbing J. (1970) Undernutrition and the developing brain. In: Hendrick WA, editor. *Developmental Neurobiology.* Springfield [IL]: Charles C Thomas.

Dudley-Marling C. (1985) The pragmatic skills of learning disabled children: a review. *Journal of Learning Disabilities* **18:** 193–9.

Eaton DM, Nowell H. (1983) Reading disability and defects of the middle ear. *Archives of Disease in Childhood* **58:** 1010–2.

Eden GF, Stein JF, Wood HM, Wood FB. (1995) Temporal and spatial processing in reading disabled and normal children. *Cortex* **31:** 451–68.

— VanMeter JW, Rumsey JM, et al. (1996) Abnormal processing of visual motion in dyslexia revealed by functional brain imaging. *Nature* **382:** 66–9.

Filipek PA. (1995) Neurobiologic correlates of developmental dyslexia: how do dyslexics' brains differ from those of normal readers. *Journal of Child Neurology* **10:** 862–9.

Fletcher-Flinn C, Elmes H, Strugnell D. (1997) Visual-perceptual and phonological factors in the acquisition of literacy among children with congenital developmental coordination disorder. *Developmental Medicine and Child Neurology* **39:** 158–66.

Flowers DL. (1993) Brain basis for dyslexia: a summary of work in progress. *Journal of Learning Disabilities* **26:** 575–82.

Fowler MS, Mason AJS, Richardson A, Stein JF. (1991) Yellow spectacles to improve vision in children with binocular amblyopia. *Lancet* **338:** 1109–10.

Frith C, Frith U. (1996) A biological marker for dyslexia. *Nature* **382:** 19–20.

Galaburda AM, Sherman GF, Rosen GD, et al. (1985) Developmental dyslexia: four consecutive patients with cortical anomalies. *Annals of Neurology* **18:** 222–33.

— Menard MT, Rosen GD. (1994) Evidence for aberrant auditory anatomy in developmental dyslexia. *Proceedings of the National Academy of Sciences of the USA* **91:** 8010–3.

Gaze RN. (1970) *The Formation of Nerve Connections: A Consideration of Neural Specificity, Modulation and Comparable Phenomena.* London: Academic Press.

Geschwind N. (1965) Disconnection syndromes in animals and man. *Brain* **88:** 237–94, 585–652.

— Fusillo M. (1966) Color-naming defects in association with alexia. *Archives of Neurology* **15:** 137–46.

— Behan P. (1982) Left-handedness: association with immune disease, migraine, and developmental learning disorder. *Proceedings of the National Academy of Sciences of the USA* **79:** 5097–5100.

Goodyer IM. (1986) Family therapy and the handicapped child. *Developmental Medicine and Child Neurology* **28:** 247–50. (Annotation).

Gordon N. (1986) Left handedness and learning. *Developmental Medicine and Child Neurology* **28:** 656–61. (Annotation).

— (1993) Learning disorders and delinquency. *Brain and Development* **15:** 169–72.

— (1995) Apoptosis (programmed cell death) and other reasons for elimination of neurons and axons. *Brain and Development* **17:** 73–7.

— (1997a) The Landau–Kleffner syndrome: increasing understanding. *Brain and Development* **19:** 311–16.

— (1997b) Specific disorders of learning: motor skills, language and behaviour. In: Brett EM, editor. *Paediatric Neurology.* 3rd ed. Edinburgh: Churchill Livingstone. p 445–76.

— (1998) Colour blindness. *Public Health* **112:** 81–4.

— Ward S. (1995) Abnormal response to sound, and central auditory processing disorder. *Developmental Medicine and Child Neurology* **37:** 645–52. Review.

Goulandris N. (1994) Word recognition in developmental dyslexia: a connectionist interpretation. *The Quarterly Journal of Experimental Psychology* **47A:** 895–916.

Grande CG. (1988) Delinquency: the learning disabled student's reaction to academic school failure? *Adolescence* **23:** 209–19.

Guyton AC. (1991) *Textbook of Medical Physiology.* Philadelphia: W B Saunders.

Hagberg G, Hagberg B, Olow I. (1976) The changing panorama of cerebral palsy. III. The importance of foetal deprivation of supply. *Acta Paediatrica Scandinavica* **65:** 403–8.

93

Hatcher PJ, Hulme C, Ellis AW. (1994) Ameliorating early reading failure by integrating the teaching of reading and phonological skills: the phonological linkage hypothesis. *Child Development* **65:** 41–57.

Heilman KM, Voeller K, Alexander AW. (1996) Developmental dyslexia: a motor-articulatory feedback hypothesis. *Annals of Neurology* **39:** 407–12.

Hermann K. (1959) *Reading Disability.* Copenhagen: Munksgaard.

Hicks C. (1986) Remediating specific reading disabilities: a review of approaches. *Journal of Research in Reading* **9:** 39–55.

Hornsby B, Shear F. (1975) *Alpha to Omega: The A to Z of Teaching Reading and Spelling.* London: Heinemann.

Hurry J. (1996) What is so special about Reading Recovery? *The Curriculum Journal* **7:** 93–108.

Hynd GW, Hall J, Novey ES, et al. (1995) Dyslexia and corpus callosum morphology. *Archives of Neurology* **52:** 32–8.

Ingram TTS. (1969) Disorders of speech in childhood. *British Journal of Hospital Medicine* **4:** 1608–25.

— (1971) Specific learning difficulties in childhood. *British Journal of Educational Psychology* **41:** Part 1.

Jariabkova K, Hugdahl K, Glos J. (1995) Immune disorders and handedness in dyslexic boys and their relatives. *Scandinavian Journal of Psychology* **36:** 355–62.

Jinkins JR. (1991) The MR equivalents of cerebral hemispheric disconnection: a telencephalic commissuropathy. *Computerized Medical Imaging and Graphics* **15:** 323–31.

Keys MP. (1993) The pediatrician's role in reading disorders. *Pediatric Clinics of North America* **40:** 869–79.

Korhonen TT. (1995) The persistence of rapid naming problems in children with reading disabilities: a nine-year follow-up. *Journal of Learning Disabilities* **28:** 232–9.

Leatherbarrow A. (1986) Remedial teaching for literacy. In: Gordon N, McKinlay I, editors. *Neurologically Handicapped Children: Treatment and Management.* Oxford: Blackwell Scientific Publications.

Lehmkuhle S, Garzia RP, Turner L, Hash T. (1993) A defective visual pathway in children with reading disability. *New England Journal of Medicine* **328:** 989–96.

Livingstone MS, Rosen DG, Drislane FW, Galaburda AM. (1991) Physiological and anatomical evidence for a magnocellular defect in developmental dyslexia. *Proceedings of the National Academy of Sciences of the USA* **88:** 7943–7.

Luria AR. (1973) *The Working Brain.* Harmondsworth [UK]: Penguin Books.

Mason AW. (1967) Specific (developmental) dyslexia. *Developmental Medicine and Child Neurology* **9:** 183–90.

McManus IC, Shergill S, Bryden MP. (1993) Annett's theory that individuals heterozygous for the right shift gene are intellectually advantaged: theoretical and empirical problems. *British Journal of Psychology* **84:** 517–37.

Metzger R, Werner D. (1984) Use of visual training for reading disabilities: a review. *Pediatrics* **73:** 824–9.

Nass R. (1994) Advances in learning disabilities. *Current Opinion in Neurology* **7:** 179–86.

Nicolson RI. (1996) Developmental dyslexia: past, present and future. *Dyslexia* **2:** 190–207.

Njiokiktjien C, de Sonneville L, Vaal J. (1994) Callosal size in children with learning disabilities. *Behavioural Brain Research* **64:** 213–8.

Olsen R, Wise B, Conners F, et al. (1989) Specific deficits in component reading and language skills: genetic and environmental influences. *Journal of Learning Disabilities* **22:** 339–48.

Owen SE, McKinlay IA. (1997) Motor difficulties in children with developmental disorders of speech and language. *Child: Care, Health and Development* **23:** 315–25.

Pavlidis GT. (1979). How can dyslexia be objectively diagnosed? *Reading* **13:** 3–13.

Peterson BS. (1995) Neuroimaging in child and adolescent neuropsychiatric disorders. *Journal of the American Academy of Child and Adolescent Psychiatry* **34:** 1560–76.

Pinnell GS, Lyons CA, DeFord DE, et al. (1994) Comparing instructional models for the literacy education of high-risk first graders. *Reading Research Quarterly* **20:** 9–39.

Poeppel D, Rowley HA. (1996) Magnetic source imaging and the neural basis of dyslexia. *Annals of Neurology* **40:** 137–8.

Polikoff BR, Evans BJW, Legg CR. (1995) Is there a visual deficit in dyslexia resulting from a lesion of the right posterior parietal lobe? *Ophthalmic and Physiological Optics* **15:** 513–7.

Rae C, Lee MA, Dixon RM, et al. (1998) Metabolic abnormalities in developmental dyslexia detected by ^{1}H magnetic resonance spectroscopy. *Lancet* **351:** 1849–52.

Reynell J. (1977) *Manual for the Reynell Developmental Language Scales.* Revised. Windsor: NFER.

Rickards AL, Kitchen WH, Doyle LW, et al. (1993) Cognition, school performance, and behaviour in very low birth weight and normal birth weight children at 8 years of age: a longitudinal study. *Developmental and Behavioural Pediatrics* **14**: 363–8.

Robins LN. (1978) Sturdy predictors of adult antisocial behaviour: replication of longitudinal studies. *Psychological Medicine* **8**: 611–22.

Rumsey JM, Andreason P, Zametkin AJ, et al. (1992) Failure to activate the left temporoparietal cortex in dyslexia. *Archives of Neurology* **49**: 527–34.

Rutter M, Yule W. (1976) The concept of specific reading retardation. *Journal of Child Psychology and Psychiatry* **16**: 181–7.

Salmelin R, Service E, Kiesila P, et al. (1996) Impaired visual word processing in dyslexia revealed with magnetoencephalography. *Annals of Neurology* **40**: 157–62.

Shapira YA, Jones MH, Sherman SP. (1980) Abnormal eye movements in hyperkinetic children with learning disability. Neuropädiatrie **II, 1**: 36-44.

Shaywitz BA, Fletcher JM, Shaywitz SE. (1995) Defining and classifying learning disabilities and attention-deficit/hyperactivity disorder. *Journal of Child Neurology* **10** Suppl. 1: 550–7.

Shaywitz SE, Escobar MD, Shaywitz BA, et al. (1992) Evidence that dyslexia may represent the lower tail of a normal distribution of reading ability. *New England Journal of Medicine* **326**: 145–50.

— Shaywitz BA, Pugh KR, et al. (1998) Functional disruption in the organization of the brain for reading in dyslexia. *Proceedings of the National Academy of Sciences of the USA* **95**: 2636–41.

Slaghuis WL, Lovegrove WJ, Davidson JA. (1993) Visual and language processing deficits are concurrent in dyslexia. *Cortex* **29**: 601–15.

Slobin DI. (1971) *Psycholinguistics.* Glenview [IL]: Scott Foresman and Co.

Snowling M, Hulme C, Goulandris N. (1994) Word recognition in developmental dyslexia: a connectionist interpretation. *The Quarterly Journal of Experimental Psychology* **47A**: 895–916.

Stanovich KE. (1994) Annotation: does dyslexia exist? *Journal of Child Psychology and Psychiatry* **35**: 579–95.

Stein JF. (1994) Developmental dyslexia, neural timing and hemispheric lateralisation. *International Journal of Psychophysiology* **18**: 241–9.

Stein J, Fowler S. (1982) Diagnosis of 'dyslexia' by means of a new indicator of eye dominance. *British Journal of Ophthalmology* **66**: 332–6.

Stein J, Fowler S. (1985) Effects of monocular occlusion on visuo-motor perception and reading in dyslexic children. *Lancet* **ii**: 69–73.

Tonnessen E, Lokken A, Hoien T, Lundberg I. (1993) Dyslexia, left-handedness, and immune disorders. *Archives of Neurology* **50**: 411–6.

Victor JD, Conte MM, Burton L, Nass RD. (1993) Visual evoked potentials in dyslexics and normals: failure to find a difference in transient or steady-state responses. *Visual Neuroscience* **10**: 939–46.

Welsh LW, Welsh JJ, Healy MP. (1983) Effects of sound deprivation on central hearing. *Laryngoscope* **93**: 1569–75.

Whitmore K, Bax M. (1986) The School Entry Medical Examination. *Archives of Disease in Childhood* **61**: 807–17.

Williams S, McGee R. (1994) Reading attainment and juvenile delinquency. *Journal of Child Psychology and Psychiatry* **35**: 441–59.

Wolff PH, Melngailis I. (1994) Family patterns of developmental dyslexia: clinical findings. *American Journal of Medical Genetics* **54**: 122–31.

Yule W, Rutter M. (1976) Epidemiology and social implications of specific reading retardation. In: Knight RM, Baker DJ, editors. *The Neuropsychiatry of Learning Disorders.* London: University Park Press.

Zoccolillo M, Pickles A, Quinton D, Rutter M. (1992) The outcome of childhood conduct disorder: implications for defining adult personality disorder and conduct disorder. *Psychological Medicine* **22**: 971–86.

4
DYSGRAPHIA AND DYSCALCULIA

Anne O'Hare

DYSGRAPHIA

Competence at writing – using a tool to record and transmit linguistic information – is one of the most important educational skills a child can acquire. To become competent at writing, children have to learn the forms and functions of letters and how to make the complex movements required to produce them. These movements are among the most sophisticated skills of the human hand, and the more knowledge and practice children have in writing, the better consolidated are the necessary motor patterns (Martlew 1992). Once the movements have been mastered and can be performed without conscious effort, children can go on to enhance their written language through the cognitive processes of composing (Berninger and Rutberg 1992). To understand the difficulties some children have in learning to write it is necessary to know how the skill is normally acquired.

The normal development of writing
Young children entering school show no strong relation between pencil grip and their knowledge of letters, although both are relevant to the acquisition of writing. Berninger and Rutberg (1992) proposed three stages in the normal acquisition of writing. The first stage is that of 'orthographic coding – fine motor function and orthographic motor integration'. Those authors found a correlation between the complex fine motor movement of successive finger/thumb appositions and handwriting fluency. They suggested that the task of handwriting is one of planning and programming fine motor movements, and not just executing them. There is a far stronger relation between motor coordination problems and the academic skills of writing and mathematics than there is in reading (Maeland and Sovik 1993).

Normal children develop the mature grasp required for optimum use of a writing tool between the ages of 4 and 6 years. The resultant grip, whereby the thumb, index finger, and middle finger come to function together as a tripod in order to make small, highly coordinated movements, has been termed the 'dynamic tripod grip' (Rosenbloom and Horton 1971). In their study of normal children those authors found that the definitive establishment of hand dominance for the use of a pencil proceeded in parallel with establishment of the dynamic tripod grip, and that no child without this established dominance had a mature finger posture. Children who have a tripod grip early in school have a slight advantage in handwriting accuracy and children can be amenable to changing grip at this stage, which may be beneficial. In addition to the normal changes seen in the developing distal motor function, changes are seen in shoulder movements, so that the shoulder joint

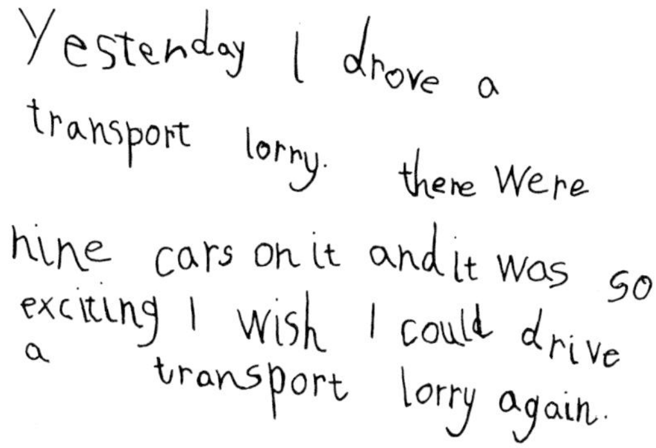

Yesterday I drove a transport lorry. there were nine cars on it and it was so exciting I wish I could drive a transport lorry again.

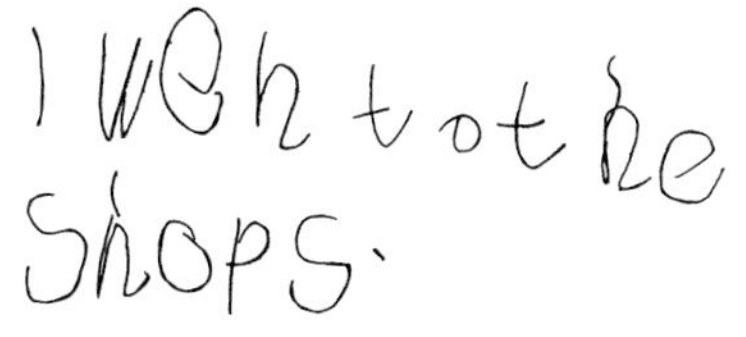

I WQh t ot he Shops.

Fig. 4.1. 'Good' *(left)* and 'poor' *(above)* handwriting in 6-year-olds.

moves upwards and outwards with maturity during writing. Neuromuscular disorders can seriously impede the normal development of the grip on the writing tool. Rosenbloom and Horton (1971), however, cautioned against overzealousness in stabilizing shoulder girdle movements in children with neuromuscular disorders, as they may be displaying a normal but delayed pattern of development of the dynamic tripod grip.

Writing movements gradually become more coordinated and the child gradually writes faster; the rate of increase is greatest between 7 and 9 years of age, after which it tapers off until about age 14 years (Ziviani and Elkins 1984). Girls maintain an advantage over boys in writing speed, even in secondary school, with the gap closing only towards the end (Dutton 1992). Speed and legibility are positively correlated ($R=0.41$) (Ziviani and Elkins 1984). There is a wide range of legibility and accuracy of letter formation in normal children (Figs 4.1 and 4.2). Letter size, position, and definition all improve during early schooling (Martlew 1992).

The second stage of writing proposed by Berninger and Rutberg (1992) is that of increasing verbal memory and increasing ability to generate and spell words, sentences, and text-level structures. When children first begin to spell, they use a predominantly phonological strategy in which they attempt to transcribe what they hear. With time and increasing exposure to printed text through reading, they increasingly incorporate visual memories for letter strings into their spelling strategies (Cornelisson et al. 1994). Oddly spelled words may be recalled almost as logotypes, and spelling is enhanced by an increasing grasp of rules such as '*i* before *e* except after *c*'. A knowledge of word structure is required so that children can increasingly apply the correct rules of spelling to their writing.

Once these stages of writing acquisition are in place, the third stage involves children's increasing cognitive skills in planning, revising, and composing in their written text. These processes continue to evolve throughout secondary school and can be measured using criteria such as mean sentence length (Dutton 1992).

Definition and incidence of dysgraphia
According to DSM-IV (American Psychiatric Association 1994) the diagnostic criteria for a disability of written expression in a child are a discrepancy between writing skills and

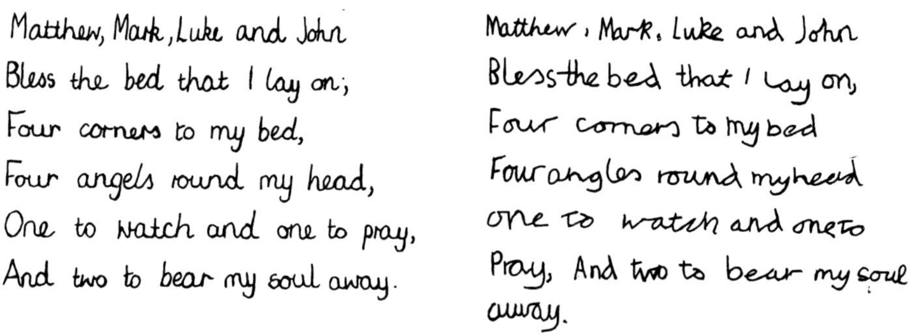

Fig. 4.2. 'Good' *(left)* and 'poor' *(right)* handwriting in 11-year-olds.

the child's age, either on functional analysis or on a standardized test, and significant interference by the writing impairment with aspects of daily living that require expressive writing skills.

Objective assessment of spelling competence in writing is straightforward. Increasingly there is also information on normal writing speeds and legibility (Ziviani and Elkins 1984, Dutton 1992, Martlew 1992). Gubbay and De Klerk (1995) surveyed normal school children to establish the neurological characteristics of handwriting impairments in those with the poorest handwriting skills. Those authors defined the children in the lowest 10% as having handwriting impairment. However, the prevalence of dysgraphia in a geographical cohort, as defined both by children's objectively assessed level of handwriting skills and also by their disability due to their handwriting difficulties, is not known. Since most children with dyslexia have at least problems with spelling in primary school, even if their reading improves, and since in addition to children with dyslexia there are children with writing difficulties predominantly relating to penmanship skills, developmental dysgraphia is probably at least as common as the figures quoted for dyslexia, namely 3 to 4% of the normal childhood population (Benton 1975).

Clinical subtypes of dysgraphia
Children with dysgraphia have difficulties either with the penmanship-related aspects of writing – motor control, or execution – or with such linguistic aspects of writing as spelling and composing, or with both aspects (O'Hare and Brown 1989a). Different authors use different terms for these subtypes, but the clinical features described are similar (Table 4.1).

LANGUAGE-BASED DYSGRAPHIA, INCLUDING SPELLING DYSGRAPHIA
In a normal population of children, most children described as having poor handwriting also have other difficulties with their written language (Gubbay and De Klerk 1995), and in particular with spelling. Often these children have (or have had) reading difficulties.

Reading is predominantly a process of visual recognition, which in the initial stages is greatly assisted by the ability to discern a correspondence between phoneme and grapheme. Spelling, however, is predominantly an auditory retrieval process, and children who are

TABLE 4.1
Features of clinical subtypes of dysgraphia

Reference	Subtype		
	Language-based	*Motor–executive*	*Visual–spatial*
O'Hare and Brown 1989	Aphasia Semantic difficulties Spelling difficulties Syntactical difficulties	Incoordination Dyspraxia	Visual–spatial difficulties
Martlew 1992	Spelling difficulties	Poor motor control	
Gubbay and De Klerk 1995	Aphasia (i) Phonological (ii) Lexical (iii) Dyslexic	Motor apraxia Mechanical agraphia	Constructional apraxia
Deuel 1995	Dyslexia	Motor clumsiness	Defect in understanding space

good readers can be poor spellers. However, normal children increasingly incorporate visual memories of letter strings into their spelling strategies, so poor readers have an additional disadvantage at spelling, over and above any problems of auditory retrieval. Although penmanship may also be immature in poor spellers, it is not invariably so, and some poor spellers nevertheless write very neatly.

The difficulties these children have in the auditory retrieval processes required for spelling can be explained by temporal processing deficits and may be open to amelioration by training with acoustically modified speech (Merzenich et al. 1995, Tallal et al. 1996). Such children find it hard to repeat or spell non-words, and assessments have been developed to measure this difficulty (Gathercole 1996).

Some children with dysgraphia make spelling errors that correlate with the degree of orthographic ambiguity and word infrequency. Two such adolescents, described by Thomas-Anterion et al. (1994), could follow phoneme-to-grapheme conversion, and those authors concluded that their subjects had a selectively poor visual memory for irregular words, because of a developmental graphemic–logemic impairment. The authors suggested that their subjects could read better than they could spell because their phonological system was intact and therefore could perform the grapheme-to-phoneme conversion needed for reading, even of irregular words. Although MRI images from these two subjects were normal, the clinical presentation was similar to that of adults with acquired lexical dysgraphia due to damage to the left angular gyrus.

Above a level of 6 years 4 months on a Schonell Graded Word Spelling Test, the target words are more complex and require more than just phonetic strategies (Cornelisson et al. 1994). There is evidence that cognitive spelling mechanisms are multidimensional structures and encode separately for aspects such as letter position, letter identity, letter doubling, and consonant/vowel positions (McCloskey et al. 1994).

Thus, although good phonological awareness is crucial for reading and spelling, impairments of other processes in orthographic processing can result in the individual being able to spell phonologically appropriate words and to experience only minimal difficulty

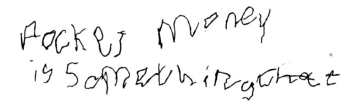

Pocket money is something that always
interest little boys, and Barney was nd
exeeption.. He thought of many ways in
which he couRd earn some pennies to spend
in the nearby toyshop. How he ldved to g
go and look at the window add see all

Fig. 4.3. Amounts of writing and typing produced in a given time by a child with incoordination dysgraphia.

in learning to read and yet to meet a barrier in the form of a spelling dysgraphia (Hanley et al. 1992).

MOTOR-EXECUTIVE DYSGRAPHIA

Children with dysgraphia who have motor-executive difficulties affecting penmanship may have either predominantly incoordination or predominantly dyspraxia. If coordination is defined as a measure of the accuracy of judging the distance, force, speed, and direction of muscle movement required to execute a planned movement and praxis is seen as the actual planning of the movement, such a distinction can be applied differentially to children with developmental or acquired dysgraphia (O'Hare and Brown 1989a). Smooth, coordinated execution of a planned movement depends not only upon the precentral motor cortex but also upon the extrapyramidal and cerebellar systems, and these two systems in turn receive extensive afferent information from the parietal, temporal, and occipital cortices (Paillard 1990).

When there are pyramidal lesions the child may be able to plan but not to execute the movements required. The degree of distal weakness correlates well with the loss of function. Movement is slower, and the loss of speed also correlates well with the loss of the skill.

Incoordination dysgraphia can follow impairment of the extrapyramidal system which regulates the natural speed of a movement and so the cadence of speech, gait, and writing. Such impairment can result in hyopkinetic dyskinesia, in which the writing is small (micrographia) and slow (bradygraphia). In hyperkinetic dyskinesia (Fig. 4.3), involuntary movements may cause sudden unexpected jerks, angulation of letters, blotching, or drawing of the pen across existing script, as in choreoathetosis. The incoordination produces

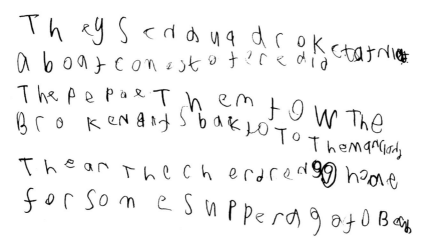

Fig. 4.4. Handwriting of a 9-year-old boy with dyspraxic dysgraphia. See case 1.

difficulties with fine motor skills besides writing. The difficulties with writing occur in copying, writing to dictation, and spontaneous composition, and many affected children have some form of cerebral palsy. Although the incoordination does affect typing speeds, a keyboard can still offer many advantages for these children (see Fig. 4.3).

Praxis is essentially the cognitive aspect of motor learning and it increases in an orderly fashion as the brain develops and as environmental experience and practice allow skills to be learned. Writing is one skill that is learned in this way, as are many other fine motor skills such as cutting with scissors, using a knife and fork, or tying shoelaces. Dyspraxia relates to inability to learn a motor skill that is commensurate with the child's age. The learning of motor skills depends also upon a normal sensory system, so that cortical sensory skills such as kinaesthesia contribute to learning an engram, or motor memory, for a learned skill, although how kinaesthesia contributes and whether it can be successfully targeted in interventions is debated (Laszlo and Bairstow 1988). Children with dyspraxic dysgraphia may have an isolated difficulty or they may also have problems in learning movement in other areas. Many children with dyspraxic dysgraphia also have difficulty with spelling.

A child with dyspraxic dysgraphia can copy single letters and can write them to dictation, but when writing words will alter the position and the direction of the letters. Such alteration can be pronounced even in copying or dictation but is exacerbated in spontaneous composition. This type of dygraphia can be particularly perplexing for both child and teacher. If children can write individual letters it seems inexplicable that they cannot write those same letters consistently within words. Such children will often seek to correct their writing, as they can see their mistakes, and yet they repeat them, so that the finished result shows crossing out and looks 'messy' (Fig. 4.4).

A child with a purely dyspraxic dysgraphia can carry out motor-free visual–spatial tasks at an age-appropriate level. This phenomenon has also been described in an adult with

101

ideomotor apraxic agraphia who had normal intellectual linguistic and visuoconstructional abilities. His reading was intact and his oral spelling and assembling of block letters were flawless. He could write single letters and digits but was severely impaired in writing words and numbers. Most errors consisted of incomplete and poorly formed letters and letter substitutions, and the number of errors increased with the length of the stimulus. Copying words was as impaired as writing to dictation. The authors concluded that this man's pattern of performance was consistent with a specific impairment of the temporal buffer in which the graphic motor patterns are maintained for neuromuscular execution (Zettin et al. 1995). There have now been a number of reports of adults with dysgraphia who have impairments of particular graphemic output 'buffers', to the extent that there may be relative sparing of lower-case compared with upper-case writing (Troijano and Chiacchio 1994, Zesiger et al. 1994) or even an acquired, selective signature dysgraphia (Regueiro et al. 1992).

A child with dyspraxic dysgraphia writes inconsistently and, as with motor-executive dysgraphia, can often be greatly helped by the introduction of a keyboard to bypass the writing difficulty.

VISUAL–SPATIAL DYSGRAPHIA
Visual–spatial dysgraphia is probably the least well defined subtype of dysgraphia. When children start to write they learn their letters visually before they start to link the phoneme and grapheme and to develop the motor engram needed for writing.

In the developmental form of visual–spatial dysgraphia, the affected child has difficulties with motor-free visual–spatial tasks that give rise to constructional dyspraxia and defects in understanding space (Deuel 1995). Such children, in contrast to some children with dyspraxic dysgraphia, have difficulties with drawing as well as with writing (Fig. 4.5). When writing they leave variable margins, tend to slope lines of writing down diagonally from left to right, run lines into one another, omit letters, misjudge the end of the line (so that they run off the page in the middle of a word), and space words badly. The difficulties occur in copying (which gives the greatest difficulty), writing to dictation, and original composition.

Aetiology of dysgraphia
AETIOLOGY OF DEVELOPMENTAL DYSGRAPHIA IN CHILDREN
Developmental dysgraphia is a failure of the normal acquisition of writing skills, but little appears to be known about its aetiology.

Delayed speech development is a frequent precursor of developmental spelling dysgraphia (O'Hare and Brown 1989a). Genetic influences have been described in instances of - comorbidity of hyperactivity and spelling disability: the two conditions have a common genetic influence (Stevenson 1993). Since the cognitive phenotype of inherited forms of learning disability is highly complex (Elbert and Seale 1988), prognostication on the basis of a child's difficulties with written spelling is very difficult. Even children who can make good grapheme-to-phoneme correspondence, and thus learn to read, may reach a ceiling in their orthographic knowledge, frustrating their ability to learn spelling that does not conform to phonemic rules.

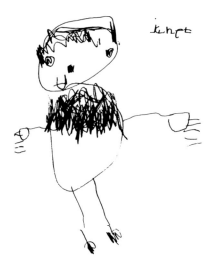

Fig. 4.5. Drawing by a 9-year-old with visual–spatial dysgraphia.

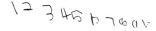

Gubbay and De Klerk (1995) proposed that their model of testing handwriting skills could be used in future studies to pinpoint the anatomical abnormality underlying the developmental dysgraphias, which to date have not been undertaken.

AETIOLOGY OF ACQUIRED DYSGRAPHIA

Whereas developmental dysgraphia is a failure of the normal acquisition of writing skills, acquired dysgraphia denotes the loss of a previously intact ability to write. Because writing competence changes during childhood, even when an acquired dysgraphia is non-progressive the writing behaviour is likely to alter over time. It is therefore difficult to assess the contribution of acquired neurological disorders to writing in young children in the early stages of learning the skill. Because there is a continuum of development between spoken language, reading, writing, and spelling, sequelae of acquired dysphasia in writing may be observed even after other features of the condition have resolved in childhood (Haecan 1976).

Acquired phonological dysgraphia is associated with anteriorly placed lesions of the supramarginal gyrus, close to the auditory cortex. Acquired lexical dysgraphia is associated with posterior parietal lesions of the angular gyrus, close to the visual cortex. Abnormalities in neurophysiological and neuroanotomical development in children with developmental dysgraphia are often inferred from clinical findings, even when MRI scans are normal (Thomas-Anterion et al. 1994).

Visual–spatial dysgraphia may also result from a range of acquired visual agnosias in children. Dejerine syndrome follows ischaemic infarction in the territory of the left posterior cerebral artery (in right-handers), with involvement of the mesial occipital and

Language   In the swim.

1.   No Mark Spits wun the most
mwdel   ✓
2,   He shavwd because hw could
slid thruww the water   eseley ᵥ
3.   The longgist is Flordir to
Qubur.   ✓
4.   .No because the children werent
a No because they werent alive in
1603 ✓

5.   No they werent held there. ✓

6.   A swimer will swim half a
length...   ✓

Fig. 4.6. Spelling errors made by a child

occipitotemporal structures, i.e. the lingual and fusiform gyrus. If the damage extends anteriorly the affected individual may experience colour agnosia or anomia for minor forms of associative visual agnosia (Bub et al. 1993). In a child the syndrome results not only in alexia but also in spelling dysgraphia, because the child is developing writing skills and cannot utilize the visual memory for orthographically irregular words (Fig. 4.6) and can develop spelling only by using letter-to-letter transformation (Table 4.2).

Bilateral temporoparietal dysfunction gives rise to impaired short-term verbal and visual memory, dysgraphia, dyscalculia, and various degrees of dysnomia and dyslexia. Neurobehavioural profiles of children with persistent hyperinsulinaemic hypoglycaemia of infancy have been consistent with the known vulnerability of these areas in the neonate to hypoglycaemia (Gross-Tsur et al. 1994).

Recognition, assessment, and management of dysgraphia

In general the professional best placed to recognize a child's specific underachievement in writing skill is the class teacher. The school should respond to concerns about underachievement in writing skill by offering additional writing instruction, and if the difficulties persist the school may look to outside agencies for a further assessment of the child. The specific learning disability of dysgraphia is increasingly recognized at this level, and cross-professional interest in the disability is fostered by organizations such as the Handwriting Interest Group, with their journal, *Handwriting Review.**

Unfortunately, however, there are some children in whom the dysgraphia is not recognized and they are referred because of secondary consequences. They may be first referred to the educational psychology service because of behavioural problems that later are seen to stem

Handwriting Review. 6 Fyfield Road, Ongar, Essex CM5 0AH, UK.

TABLE 4.2
Examples of phonetic and non-phonetic spelling errors made by children with dysgraphia

Phonetic		Non-phonetic	
Target word	*Misspelling*	*Target word*	*Misspelling*
apple	apul	apple	albl
catalogue	catalog	puppy	paap
contented	contentid	adventure	adner
packet	pacit	refreshment	rathfisth
instructed	instrukted	finger	farer
working	wurcing	plastic	patre
any	ene	bump	bute
other	uther	packet	pent
kidnapped	cidnapt	kitten	kendin
recapture	recapcher	kitten	keintt

from specific learning difficulties. Even when the poor attainments are recognized, the referring authorities may describe accompanying problems including inattention, distractibility, laziness, immaturity, or even defiance. The children themselves report 'feelings of embarrassment, humiliation, anxiety and guilt. They can feel stupid, useless, frustrated and angry. They lose confidence in themselves and often they lose their friends' (Biggar and Barr 1993). The extent to which a dysgraphic child's difficulties can be misunderstood is illustrated by the following quotation from a learning-support teacher: 'This lad made an absolute hash of this piece of work until I gave him a rocket and rubbed everything out. His second attempt is so much better. I have told him I don't think his work has to be nearly so untidy. He has just made up his mind that we will all accept any old writing from him and doesn't try any more.'

A number of findings in the paediatric history are of particular relevance to a child presenting with a dysgraphia. Information should be elicited about the child's speech and language development and reading development. There should be an enquiry to establish whether there are additional academic problems in mathematics and in fine and gross motor coordination in classroom activities such as craft and gym. A note should also be made of peer relationships and interests and of any behavioural traits suggesting a condition such as Asperger syndrome. A detailed family history is important, as is an enquiry about past medical history with particular reference to preterm birth, intrauterine growth retardation, epilepsy (particularly left temporal lobe seizures), and any insults to the central nervous system. Recurrent conductive hearing loss can make a minor contribution to a spelling difficulty, and it is also important to establish that the child's near and distance vision are normal, although this is rarely the explanation for dysgraphia.

It is helpful in formulating a response to the child's difficulties to know what the response has been from the school and whether the child has received additional writing instruction. It is also necessary to explore the child's own response to the difficulties and to the help given in school.

Examination should include an assessment of the child's writing abilities. The child should be asked to both copy and write to dictation individual letters in upper and lower case. The reading level should be established and the child should be asked to copy a piece of text at a comfortable reading level (this should be timed), to write to dictation a paragraph at a similar level, and to write a spontaneous composition. Besides speed of writing, legibility (both to the child and to the examiner) should be noted. Spelling level should be determined and a note made of errors and whether they display any phonetic pattern (see Table 4.2). Speech and language development should be investigated. Assessments such as the British Picture Vocabulary Scale (Dunn et al. 1997) and the Crichton Active Vocabulary Scale (Raven 1997) can be very helpful, as can speech and language assessment using the Griffiths Mental Development Scales (1997) and the Renfrew Action Picture Test (Renfrew 1993). Short-term auditory memory can be assessed from the Aston Index (Newton and Thomson 1997). The dysgraphia may be secondary to a speech and language disorder or to a reading difficulty, and extended assessment may be required to determine whether one of these is the underlying cause. During the assessment the child's social interaction and pragmatic use of language should be noted.

An analysis of penmanship involves an assessment of fine motor coordination, which is the accuracy of fast repetitive movements. This can be measured using tools such as Annett's pegboard (Annett 1970a,b), which will also give a measure of the discrepancy between the function of the right and left hands. Poor function of the non-dominant hand is of particular interest and may indicate that the child has transferred hand dominance from that which would have been genetically determined (Bishop 1980). A note should be made of involuntary movements: these may show up as jerks and angulations in the child's writing or as smudging of the writing produced when the hand jerks across the page. The child may grip the pen inadequately, producing shaky, tremulous writing that slopes across the page and does not conform to the lines, and micrographia or macrographia may be present. Successive finger movements should be assessed (Denckla 1973).

An assessment of the child's development of praxis should include praxis both in the task of writing and also in everyday tasks such as tying shoelaces, using a padlock, and pouring a cup of juice. Praxis refers to the ability to perform gestures and to use tools (Roy et al. 1990). Performing complex movements such as sequential tapping of the fingers in a predetermined, fixed order activates not only the ipsilateral motor cortex and supplementary motor area but also the bilateral premotor and somatosensory cortex (Yousry 1997). Imagining movement results from the utilization of stored representations of action that is subject to the same constraints as real movement. Children can mentally rehearse doing something only if they have done it before and only as they experienced it in practice (Cramond 1997). A note should be made of the type of errors that the child makes in attempting these everyday tasks. The dyspraxia may affect only writing, and letters may be drawn satisfactorily on their own but may, when put into a word sequence, be reversed either mirrorwise (static reversal) or in their position in the word (kinetic reversal). Such children may display difficulties with block design that may be reported from the psychologist's assessment or can be explored in younger children using the Griffiths Mental Development Scales (1997).

Although many children with the above-mentioned forms of dysgraphia can draw satisfactorily, some cannot, and it is important to test some perceptual–motor skills, such as block construction, and also some motor-free tasks, such as Raven's Matrices (Raven 1997), to assess visual–spatial cognitive development.

A more general test of motor impairment, such as the ABC Test of Motor Impairment (Henderson and Sugden 1992) or the Quick Neurological Screening Test (Stirling et al. 1997), may be required to assess neurodevelopmental difficulties, particularly in survivors of preterm birth who are experiencing difficulties with writing and mathematics (Jongmans 1977, Marlow et al. 1989, Hall et al. 1995).

The management of a child with dysgraphia is interdisciplinary and should address three main questions: how does one reduce the child's anxiety and frustration relating to writing, how should areas of strength be promoted to build self-esteem, and how does one remediate the dysgraphia itself? The answer to the first question may involve discontinuing writing for a time and reducing reliance on writing through scribing, audio taping, and word processing. Use of a keyboard and word processor may be particularly motivating for the child, who experiences the pleasure of a neat finished product (Davidson 1988). Enhancing self-esteem by promoting areas of strength can represent a challenge, particularly for the child with developmental incoordination disorder. Paediatric occupational therapy assessment can clarify the profile of the child's motor skills, and therapy may help the child recover confidence and improve function. The paediatric occupational therapist may also have a role in keyboard instruction and direct remediation of the dysgraphia.

The child's writing skills may improve through attention to the posture of the pencil grip, use of modified pencil grips, lined paper, right-angle boards, and the introduction of cursive writing (Tasker 1991). The management of children with a spelling dysgraphia overlaps in many respects with the management of dyslexia, as many affected children have both problems. It may be appropriate to refer such a child to a speech and language therapist with an interest in literacy, as definition of a child's difficulties in phonological awareness and auditory processing may indicate areas that the learning support teacher could usefully target in the child's educational plan.

Case descriptions – dysgraphia
CASE 1 – DYSPRAXIC DYSGRAPHIA

A 9-year-old boy was referred with a recognized writing problem because he was felt not to be applying himself satisfactorily to learning support (see the quotation from his learning-support teacher). He had no medical history or family history that might have accounted for his problems. His speech and language development before he started school had been accelerated, but he had had difficulty learning to tie his shoelaces and ride a bicycle and showed no interest in physical activities such as football. He was a very competent reader.

On assessment his IQ on the British Ability Scales (Elliot et al. 1983) was in the range 101 to 109 but his ability on the block-design test was relatively poor: at the 28th centile for power and the 34th centile for level. His figure-copying ability on the British Ability Scale was at 7.3 to 7.5 years. His oral spelling was normal. He had a fine motor dyspraxia affecting everyday skills and a fluctuant ability to write individual letters. He confused upper- and lower-case letters and could not write his name legibly. Letters were in particular vertically and horizontally reversed when written within words, and he did not leave space between words (see Fig. 4.4). He would notice that the reversed letters were wrong, but when he tried to correct them he would reverse them once again. He could not read back his own writing. At the time of the assessment he said that he was 'no good at anything'. A decision was made to discontinue handwriting entirely for 6 months and to introduce him to the use of a keyboard and word processor, which he readily learned to use. Afterwards he was given additional tuition for his handwriting, which gradually became more legible. Towards the end of his primary schooling he chose to write more than to use his keyboard. At high school (from age 12 years), however, because he still wrote only slowly and the legibility of his handwriting deteriorated markedly if he was under pressure to produce a large volume of writing, he consistently chose to use his word processor throughout his 5 years of follow-up there.

CASE 2 – VISUAL–SPATIAL DYSGRAPHIA
A 9-year old girl presented with a reluctance to write in the classroom. She had been born at 32 weeks gestation, of good birthweight and in good condition, but at age 3 days had developed an acute illness with septicaemia and had required 10 days of IPPV respiratory support. The ventricles appeared normal on ultrasound scans. On follow-up at 3 years of age she had seemed normal and was discharged. There was no significant family history of any relevant disorders.

On assessment the girl had difficulty in copying shapes and in trying to make representational drawings. Her distance acuity and near visual acuity were normal. She had learned to read without difficulty but her development in mathematics was somewhat delayed, in that she was competent at computation using single integers but in written computations in which there were digits representing 10s she would confuse the positions and columns of the numbers. She was found to be of average intelligence on the WISC–R but within this had particular difficulties with block design. She had normal fine and gross motor coordination. Her performance on the Children's Embedded Figures Test (Witkin et al. 1971) was below 2 standard deviations and that on a visual–spatial cognitive test on Raven's Matrices was below the 5th centile. Her performance on language tests was appropriate for her age. She wrote diagonally across the page, even on lined paper. She would also write off the page and onto the desk. She had difficulty in forming individual letters and showed visual confusions of letters, interchanging *o* and *a,* for example. Her spacing between words was poor, letters were omitted, and the ends of lines were misjudged. These difficulties were particularly pronounced in copying but also occurred in writing to dictation and in original composition. Her writing difficulty was alleviated to some extent by the use of a keyboard and word processor, as this assisted with some of the difficulties such as writing off the page and misjudging lines. However, her visual–spatial difficulties meant that she was quite slow to recognize and press the letter keys and so a decision was made to assist her by letting her dictate some of her work and thus benefit from her strong language skills.

DYSCALCULIA

The normal development of arithmetic

Resnick (1989) coined the phrase 'pre-verbal protoquantitative schemata' for the phenomenon whereby young preschool children, on the basis of perception, learn to appreciate the principles of something being 'more' or 'less' and those of division and merging. Verbal protoquantitative schemata are essential for comprehending what number-words denote. These schemata lay the foundation for the spatial–numerical mental imagery and the developing abilities needed for the rapid comparison and approximation of numerical quantities.

Number-words have different meanings in different contexts and children gradually acquire these different meanings and thus gradually discover their interrelations. There is approximately a 1-year lag between a child's knowledge of number-words and the appreciation that they refer to certain numerical quantities. Preverbal quantification works in parallel with, and to some extent guides, verbal and written computation. The first computational strategies are based on counting. In addition to linguistic skills, spatial skills are important for counting, as they are used to scan items already counted, as well as those to be counted later. Ultimately, spatial skills are used in the mental representation of imagined items such as fingers. Conceptual development, attention allocation, memory span, speed of processing, and computational accuracy all contribute to the development of computational strategies and to the consolidation of the long-term-memory representation of arithmetic (Lyytinen et al. 1994).

Children are considered to have considerable conceptual knowledge before they acquire automaticity in number processing and calculation processes. They implicitly know the principles of counting before they can count correctly, they judge arithmetic transformations correctly before they can resolve them, and they resolve problems of arithmetic fact by back-up strategies such as counting. Thus they have conceptual knowledge about arithmetic operations before they can retrieve arithmetic facts from memory. Similarly the process can break down differentially in adult life, with the knowledge of arithmetic facts beginning to break down while the conceptual knowledge supporting them remains intact. In one reported case an adult who had dissociative loss of arithmetic facts but who had maintained conceptual knowledge lost the ability to solve arithmetic problems but continued to be able to solve algebraic problems, as this could be done without resorting to the numerical system (Hittmair-Delazer et al. 1995). Children tend to judge algebraic expressions predominantly by referring them to the numerical system and inserting numbers into the algebraic equation and thus calculating the result.

There is a wide range of development of arithmetical skills, particularly for computation, in normal children (O'Hare et al. 1991, O'Hare and Brown 1992). By $3^1/2$ to 4 years of age children can count four bricks correctly if they are placed in a linear array, and they can count 15 by the age of 5 years. Later they learn to appreciate quantity associated with counting. The average child understands a quantity of 3 by the age of 4 years and a quantity of 4 by the age of 5 years.

One-third of 6-year-olds reverse single integers when they write them. Seven-year-olds insert extra place zeroes after three-digit numbers, whereas by the age of 8 years children can write three-digit numbers correctly. By the age of 7 years the child will have learned the operator signs. There is a wide range in calculation abilities, but in general children of 7 years or more can be regarded as displaying significant difficulty in acquiring arithmetical skills if they cannot do simple addition and subtraction without concrete materials. Similarly, children who cannot multiply single integers by age $10^{1}/_{2}$ or who cannot divide by the age of 13 are displaying significant delay.

Definition and incidence of dyscalculia

The tenth revision of the *International Statistical Classification of Diseases and Related Health Problems* (ICD-10) (World Health Organization 1992) defines dyscalculia as a specific disorder of arithmetical skills. When it occurs as a developmental disorder it can be regarded as a primary cognitive disorder of childhood affecting the ability of an otherwise intelligent and healthy child to learn arithmetic (Gross-Tsur et al. 1993).

Dyscalculia may occur either as an isolated disability or, as is often the case, as part of a mixed disorder of scholastic skills. Some definitions include deficits in the area of language and motor function as well as attention-deficit disorder and reading and spelling disorder (von Aster 1994).

The prevalence of dyscalculia was found to be 6.5% (Gross-Tsur et al. 1996) in a two-stage study. In that study, a large group of children attending mainstream schools was initially screened for arithmetical achievement, and then the children in the lowest 20% were individually tested with a standard arithmetic battery. Children with an IQ of less than 80 were excluded from the figures. One-quarter of the children with dyscalculia had attention-deficit-hyperactivity-like symptoms and 17% had dyslexia (Gross-Tsur et al. 1996). Dyscalculia affects both sexes equally – in contrast to other specific learning disabilities, in which boys are over-represented – and it is more prevalent in lower socioeconomic groups.

Clinical subtypes of dyscalculia

The developmental lag in the acquisition of numerical skills can be manifested in a variety of ways: by inability to recognize number symbols, by strephosymbolia or mirror writing, by a failure to recognize the basic mathematical operations or the use of operator and separator symbols, by an inability to recall tables and to carry numbers in multiplication, or by a failure to maintain the proper order of numbers in calculation (Gordon 1992).

As various cognitive mechanisms have been proposed to explain the acquisition of arithmetical skills, McCloskey (1992) proposed a systematic assessment of cognitive mechanisms in numerical processing and supported this with evidence from acquired dyscalculia (McCloskey et al. 1991). His model distinguishes between the number-processing system, which encompasses mechanisms for comprehending and producing numbers, and the calculation system, which consists of mechanisms involved specifically in calculation. Within the subsystems for comprehending and producing numbers, a further distinction is made between components for processing Arabic numbers ('32') and verbal numbers ('thirty-two'), and these are further subdivided into lexical and syntactic processing mechanisms. The calculation system distinguishes between mechanisms for comprehending operation symbols, retrieving facts of an arithmetic table, and executing calculation procedures.

Badian (1983) proposed three types of developmental dyscalculia: developmental anarrhythmia, in which the child confounds computational procedures such as addition, subtraction, and multiplication; attentional sequential dyscalculia, in which the child experiences great difficulty in learning and recalling multiplication tables; and spatial dyscalculia, in which the child experiences difficulties in handling multicolumn arithmetic problems and place values.

Dehaene (1992) proposed a 'triple code model', in which one component is an auditory, verbal word frame, comprising skills (for example, counting and retrieval of arithmetic fact such as those in tables) founded on general language information processing. The second component is the 'visual Arabic number forms': the numerical operations within the special syntax of the Arabic notation system, which is represented visually and organized spatially. The third component is 'analogue magnitude representation', or the skills for comparing and approximating numerical quantities.

Within a group of adolescent and pre-adolescent children with dyscalculia, described by Shalev et al. (1988), memorization and retrieval of calculation facts were the most severely impaired and it was particularly the ability to calculate division that was affected. In contrast, comprehension and production of numbers in these children with developmental dyscalculia was virtually intact. The children displayed various degrees of dyslexia, dysgraphia, anomia, and graphomotor impairments, and the authors concluded that developmental dyscalculia was the most severe manifestation of a wider range of cognitive disorders in these children. The children in the study had been referred because of the selected deficit in learning arithmetic. The assessment of arithmetical skills was based on McCloskey's (1991) cognitive framework. Many of the tasks presented to the children are similar to those in psychometric assessment of arithmetical development, such as the tasks in the British Ability Scales testing basic number skills. Such tasks include matching written Arabic numbers to quantities, appreciating relative quantities, comprehending quantities, comprehending numerical values, ordering numbers serially, counting, and calculating. Arithmetical skills such as comprehension of operator signs and oral fact retrieval and number production were explored more directly. Although clearly all these skills have a bearing on the ability to undertake the written calculations in some parts of the basic number skills of the British Ability Scales, Shalev and colleagues separated out these different skills in making their assessment. Children with scores below the 5th centile on these assessments were considered to be significantly delayed in their acquisition of arithmetical skills (Shalev et al. 1993). Further studies in children with dyscalculia, using devised batteries of tests to evaluate number comprehension, number production, and calculation processing, have similarly found the most marked weakness to be in the areas of number facts and complex calculation, with relative sparing of number production and comprehension (Gross-Tsur et al. 1996).

LEFT HEMISPHERE DYSFUNCTION AND THE DEVELOPMENTAL GERSTMANN SYNDROME

Gerstmann syndrome of right/left confusion, finger agnosia, dyscalculia, and dysgraphia in association with left hemisphere lesions of the angular gyrus in adults is thought to exist in a developmental form in some children with dyscalculia. In a study of children presenting to a child psychiatry service, Von Aster (1994) described developmental Gerstmann syndrome both in children with specific arithmetical disabilities and in children with combined disorders of arithmetical skills. Shalev et al. (1995) considered that subjects who had dyscalculia in which all four elements of the developmental Gerstmann syndrome were present did not constitute a homogeneous behavioural group; such subjects were found among samples both of good and of poor readers. Shalev and colleagues used the criteria of right hemisphere dysfunction for children with dyscalculia by eliciting left-sided soft neurological signs, impaired visuospatial function, and normal language skills, accompanied by a higher Verbal than Performance IQ. Those authors inferred left hemisphere dysfunction from the criteria of right-sided body signs, higher Performance than Verbal IQ, dyslexia, and intact visuospatial function. The authors concluded that dysfunction of either hemisphere hampered the acquisition of arithmetical skills but that impairment was more profound in the children with left hemisphere dysfunction. They identified children below the 20th centile on a standard assessment of arithmetical development and divided them into poor and good readers. Dysgraphia occurred predominantly in the children who were poor readers, and both groups of children showed evidence of construction dyspraxia and had below-normal performance on tasks such as an Embedded Figures Test (Witkin et al. 1971). Both groups were also notably poor in auditory and visual discrimination and motor coordination.

DYSCALCULIA AND THE RIGHT HEMISPHERE SYNDROME
Developmental dyscalculia can occur in association with features suggesting right hemisphere dysfunction (O'Hare et al. 1991, Gross-Tsur et al. 1995). The developmental right hemisphere syndrome encompasses emotional and interpersonal difficulties, paralinguistic communication problems, impaired visual–spatial skills, and either dyscalculia or neurological signs on the left side of the body. Similar clinical findings have been described in adults (Weintraub and Mesulam 1983). Children with developmental dyscalculia and the right hemisphere syndrome may have no structural abnormality visible on brain scans either by computed tomography or magnetic resonance imaging. The children described by Gross-Tsur et al. (1995) had additional graphomotor impairments and a number of them were extremely slow in their cognitive and motor performance, though their reading development was normal. Their emotional and interpersonal difficulties were quite handicapping. They adapted badly to new situations and had difficulty in maintaining friendships. They were withdrawn and excessively shy, and avoided eye contact. Their neuropsychological profile was compatible with a dysfunction of the medial posterior areas of the right hemisphere, which are important for spatial perception and imagery. In addition some children had features of attention-deficit/hyperactivity disorder; this may arise as a secondary effect of right hemisphere dysfunction or related diencephalic and brain stem difficulties, as the non-dominant hemisphere has preferential involvement with the frontal striatal systems. In other series perceptual–motor and attention deficits have characterized children who have learning disability specifically for arithmetic (Rosenberger 1989).

Aetiology of dyscalculia

Developmental dyscalculia is commoner in children of lower socioeconomic status and is equally represented in the sexes. Through associated clinical features as previously discussed, left or right hemisphere dysfunction is invoked. However, interpretation of neuroanatomical findings in the setting of specific learning disabilities is problematic. Our understanding is likely to improve with the use of functional brain imaging. Functional magnetic resonance imaging disclosed predominantly left hemisphere activation involving the frontal and parietal regions in a 17-year-old boy with dyscalculia and dyslexia after right hemisphere injury in infancy, whereas bilateral activation of the supramarginal gyrus was demonstrated in seven of nine controls. This boy had normal visual–spatial skills and intelligence. The combination of dyscalculia and dyslexia raised the question of left parietal dysfunction as a consequence of competition between verbal and visual–spatial functions for left hemisphere representation after the damage to the right hemisphere in infancy (Levin et al. 1996).

Complications of prematurity may predispose to difficulties with number skills. Measurement of school attainment, cognitive ability, and motor functioning in survivors of very low birthweight revealed particular difficulties with number skills. Although these children's auditory verbal subskills were less than in control subjects, the greatest difference was in Visual IQ. Screening for soft neurological signs proved useful (Hall et al. 1995) for picking out children with learning difficulties at the age of 8 years who had survived very low birthweight and who were doing poorly both on teacher assessment and on the number skills of the British Ability Scales.

Dyscalculia is also more prevalent in girls with sex chromosome aneuploidies and Turner syndrome and in female carriers of fragile X syndrome (Gross-Tsur et al. 1996). Difficulties with arithmetic in girls with Turner syndrome may be due to inadequate procedural skills combined with poor fact retrieval in timed testing situations rather than to inadequate visual–spatial ability (Rouet et al. 1994).

Children with epilepsy may have great difficulty with mathematics, particularly older children and especially 12- to 18-year-olds. SPECT scanning in children with right hemisphere epileptic foci revealed associations with visual–spatial difficulties and problems with directed attention, modulated affect, paralinguistic aspects of communication, and parallel information processing (Aldenkamp et al. 1990). The earlier the age of onset of seizures and the greater total lifetime seizure frequency, the greater the underachievement in mathematics (Seidenberg et al. 1986).

Developmental dyscalculia has been described in children with a range of neurological abnormalities, including Landau–Kleffner dysphasia (Papagno and Basso 1993), Gilles de la Tourette syndrome (McGilchrist et al. 1994), familial hemiplegic migraine (Marchioni et al. 1995), and Sturge–Weber syndrome (Fritsch et al. 1986).

Recognition, assessment, and management of dyscalculia

There is such a wide range of normal development in the acquisition of arithmetical skills that children who present because they are recognized as underachieving in this area usually have quite pronounced problems. Occasionally the dyscalculia can be masked by other features such as migraine or behavioural problems. There are also certain conditions such as Asperger syndrome and Gilles de la Tourette syndrome in which the other features are clinically more dramatic and the dyscalculia will be recognized only after assessment. The breadth of assessment of arithmetical skills is to some extent dictated by the child's age, particularly with respect to a knowledge of computation, as outlined earlier in this chapter. The children should be asked to copy numbers, to write them to dictation, and to read them, in order to assess their understanding of number syntax. Their knowledge of operator signs should be tested by assessing the recognition and the production of operator signs to dictation. Their ability to count items correctly should be assessed. Certain tools such as the Basic Number Skills on the British Ability Scales can be helpful for exploring the language associated with mathematics concepts, e.g. 'greater than,' 'the smallest'. In addition there are standard assessments of computational knowledge which may be helpful for older children in particular, as they extend to concepts such as area, graphs, and fractions (France 1979).

As dyscalculia is frequently associated with other specific learning difficulties, particularly dysgraphia, the assessment outlined earlier in this chapter is relevant to the child with dyscalculia. The child should be given a careful paediatric examination, in which features of neurocutaneous stigmata and tissue asymmetry are looked for (O'Hare et al. 1991), and attention should be paid to the child's paralinguistic skills. Assessment of reading and associated neuropsychological features may be relevant. A detailed assessment of fine motor skills and visual perceptual skills is often also indicated, and referral to paediatric occupational therapy may follow if these skills are affected. Children with poor short-term auditory memory may benefit from opportunities to repeat information, such as their times tables, with additional cues such as having them set to music.

When memorizing tables proves intractably difficult, the child may benefit from having access to written tables. Children who experience difficulty in recognizing symbols can benefit from additional cues such as colour-coding of operator signs, and this approach can also be used for coding columns in tens and units to assist children with visual–perceptual difficulties. Some children may have to carry out computations using a calculator.

The paediatric occupational therapist may again prove to be a useful link with the class teacher in instances where the child has problems of perceptual–motor and fine motor coordination. Such problems can affect how well children can use concrete materials to develop mathematical concepts. Unfortunately some children have intractable dyscalculia, the effect of which needs to be addressed across the curriculum.

Case descriptions – dyscalculia
CASE 3 – DYSCALCULIA ASSOCIATED WITH RIGHT TEMPORAL LOBE EPILEPSY AND WEAKNESS IN SPATIAL REASONING
A 9-year old boy presented with underachievement in mathematics which had been recognized since he was in early primary school. Assessment by an educational psychologist established that he had an average IQ but a significant discrepancy between Verbal and Visual IQ on the British Ability Scales (101 and 89, respectively). This indicated a weakness in spatial reasoning. On a basic number test he also had difficulty in coping with the hundreds, tens, and units columns when undertaking computations.

The boy later had a brief, nocturnal generalized convulsion. Two months after that during a brief daytime event he experienced a sensation of detachment from the real world and was observed to slowly move his head from side to side; there were no postictal phenomena. Physical examination revealed a mild dysprosodia and reduced affect but no other abnormal findings. The EEG was normal. The boy's progress at school continued to give rise to concern. He was experiencing interpersonal difficulties and was being rejected by his peers. Progress in mathematics appeared to have ceased and he was experiencing episodes at school during which he would become separated from the rest of the class and would later appear in the wrong location with no recollection of how he had got there. No further medical consultation was sought at this time and the periods of confusion at school and disorientation were only recognized in retrospect. However, a year later he had one of these episodes at home and during the night he wandered into the wrong bedroom. Subsequent EEG revealed a right temporal lobe epileptic focus. A month later he had a cluster of three brief partial complex seizures and was started on carbamazepine.

A year later, at a new school to which his parents had decided to move him, it was noted at a multidisciplinary meeting that he had had no seizures for a year. However, his teachers observed that he had difficulties in relating to his peers and that he was unusually weak at very basic arithmetic operations. The weakness persisted despite learning support. His teacher commented that he appeared to be more skilled in mathematics further forward in the curriculum, where he could use his good language skills, than he was in some quite basic computations.

Assessment of this boy revealed persisting deficits in spatial reasoning on the British Ability Scales. His short-term auditory memory, production and comprehension of numbers, and comprehension and accuracy of reading were all normal. On a profile of mathematical skills (France 1979) there were very wide discrepancies between his computational skills. His scores were between the 16th and 25th centiles for subtraction, division, and multiplication but at the 2nd centile for addition. He confused the hundreds, tens, and units columns as already described. In the section on measurement and money, he had difficulty in telling the time from a clock face.

Learning support was continued in the classroom in an effort to consolidate his basic computational skills and to determine bypass strategies where the difficulties proved intractable and were interfering with success in mathematics further along in the curriculum.

CASE 4 – DYSCALCULIA AND GILLES DE LA TOURETTE SYNDROME
A 9-year old boy presented with learning difficulties in mathematics and with unusual behaviour. In his number work he was competent only when working with numbers of 10 or less. His educational attainments in reading and spelling were within the normal range. On assessment by an educational psychologist he showed a wide scatter of scores on the British Ability Scales. His scores for nonverbal reasoning on matrices and for visual–spatial ability were very low – at the 8th and 3rd centiles, respectively – whereas his speed of information processing, recall of digits, and recognition of similarities were above average. His behaviour in the classroom was disruptive: he would make sudden noises, often like a car or an aeroplane, and these appeared involuntary. He also sometimes flapped his arms and hands. Although at first this unusual behaviour was thought to be a sign of his difficulty

in coping in the classroom, paediatric referral and and occupational therapy referral were arranged. These confirmed that he had fine and gross motor difficulties with coordination and praxis. He had a preschool history of paroxysmal episodes of simulating engine and drum noises and had recently developed coprolalia. He also had a 5-year history of intermittent tics of the legs and arms, sparing the face. His father had a history of difficulty with mathematics and was also described as 'fidgety', but he was not available for examination. The boy's motor tics and vocalizations were controlled with haloperidol, and an opportunity later arose in the classroom, during a discussion about asthma, for the other children to appreciate that this child took medication to control his movements and vocalizations. When they understood that these aspects of his behaviour had not been under his control they became a great deal more tolerant and this helped the child make some friends among his peers. He continued to have severe difficulties with mathematics and could still work only with numbers 10 or less by the end of primary school (about 12 years of age). Appropriate strategies were therefore put in place at his high school for the areas of the curriculum where this limitation would hinder his progress.

REFERENCES

Aldenkamp AP, Alpherts WCJ, Dekker MJA, Overwerg, J. (1990) Neuropsychological aspects of learning disabilities in epilepsy. *Epilepsia* **31:** 9–20.

American Psychiatric Association. (1994) *Diagnostic and Statistical Manual of Mental Disorders.* 4th ed (DSM-IV). Washington, DC: American Psychiatric Association.

Annett M. (1970a) A classification of hand preference by association analysis. *British Journal of Psychology* **61:** 303–21.

— (1970b) The growth of manual preference and speed. *British Journal of Psychology* **61:** 545–58.

Badian NA. (1983) Developmental dyscalculia. In: Mykelbost HR, editor. *Progress in Learning Disabilities.* New York: Grune and Stratton.

Benton AL. (1975) Developmental dyslexia: neurological aspects. In: Freedlander WJ, editor. *Advances in Neurology.* New York: Raven Press.

Berninger VW, Rutberg J. (1992) Relationship of finger function to beginning writing: application to diagnosis of writing disabilities. *Developmental Medicine and Child Neurology* **34:** 198–215.

Biggar S, Barr J. (1993) The emotional world of specific learning difficulties. In: Reid G, editor. *Specific Learning Difficulties: Perspectives on Practice.* Edinburgh: Moray House Publications. p 394–407.

Bishop DVM. (1980) Handedness, clumsiness and cognitive ability. *Development Medicine and Child Neurology* **22:** 569–79.

Bub DN, Arguin M, Lecours AR. (1993) Jules Dejerine and his interpretation of pure alexia. *Brain and Language* **45:** 531–59.

Cornelisson P, Bradley L, Fowler S, Stein J. (1994) What children see affects how they spell. *Developmental Medicine and Child Neurology* **36:** 716–26.

Cramond DJ. (1997) Motor imagery: never in your wildest dreams. *Research News: Neuroscience* **20:** 54–7.

Davidson PM. (1988) Word processing in children with specific learning difficulties. *Support for Learning* **3:** 210–4.

Dehaene S. (1992) Varieties of numerical abilities. *Cognition* **44:** 1–42.

Denckla MB. (1973) Development of speed in repetitive and successive finger-movements in normal children. *Developmental Medicine and Child Neurology* **15:** 635–45.

Deuel RK. (1995) Developmental dysgraphia and motor skills disorders. *Journal of Child Neurology* **10:** S6–S8.

Dunn L, Whetton C, Burley J. (1997) *British Picture Vocabulary Scale.* 2nd ed. Windsor: NFER Nelson.

Dutton KP. (1992) Writing under examination conditions – establishing a baseline. *Handwriting Review* 80–101.

Elbert JC, Seale TW. (1988) Complexity of the cognitive phenotype of an inherited form of learning disability. *Developmental Medicine and Child Neurology* **30:** 181–9.

Elliot CD, Murray DJ, Pearson LS. (1983) *British Ability Scales (Revised).* Windsor: NFER-Nelson.

France N. (1979) *Profile of Mathematical Skills.* Windsor: NFER Nelson.

Fritsch G, Sacher M, Nissen T. (1986) Clinical aspects and course of Sturge–Weber syndrome in childhood. *Monatsschrift Kinderheilkund* **134:** 242–5.

Gathercole S. (1996) *Non Word Repetition Test.* Windsor: NFER Nelson.

Gordon N. (1992) Children with developmental dyscalculia [annotation]. *Developmental Medicine and Child Neurology* **34:** 459–63.

Griffiths Mental Development Scales. (1997) High Wycombe, Bucks. [UK]: The Test Agency Ltd.

Gross-Tsur V, Manor O, Shalev RS. (1993) Developmental dyscalculia gender and the brain. *Archives of Disease in Childhood* **68:** 510–2.

— Shalev RS, Wertmanelad R, et al. (1994) Neurobehavioural profile of children with persistent hyperinsulinaemic hypoglycaemia of infancy. *Developmental Neuropsychology* **10:** 153–63.

— — Manor O, Amir N. (1995) Developmental right hemisphere syndrome: clinical spectrum of the non-verbal learning disability. *Journal of Learning Disabilities* **28:** 80–6.

— Manor O, Shalev RS. (1996) Developmental dyscalculia: prevalence and demographic features. *Developmental Medicine and Child Neurology* **38:** 25–33.

Gubbay SS, De Klerk NH. (1995) A study and review of developmental dysgraphia in relation to acquired dysgraphia. *Brain and Development* **17 (1):** 1–8.

Haecan H. (1976) Acquired aphasia in children and the ontogenesis of hemispheric functional specialisation. *Brain and Language* **3:** 114–34.

Hall A, McLeod A, Counsell C, et al. (1995) School attainment, cognitive ability and motor function in a total Scottish very-low-birthweight population at 8 years: a controlled study. *Developmental Medicine and Child Neurology* **37:** 1037–50.

Hanley JR, Hastie K, Kay J. (1992) Developmental surface dyslexia and dysgraphia: an orthographic processing impairment. *Quarterly Journal of Experimental Psychology* **44:** 285–319.

Henderson SE, Sugden DA. (1992) *ABC – Movement Assessment Battery for Children.* London: Psychological Corporation.

Hittmair-Delazer M, Semenza C, Denes G. (1995) Concepts and facts in calculation. *Brain* **117:** 715–28.

Jongmans M, Mercuri E, de Vries L, Dubowitz L, Henderson SE. (1997) Minor neurological signs and perceptual-motor difficulties in prematurely born children. *Archives of Disease in Childhood* **76:** F9–14.

Laszlo JI, Bairstow PJ. (1988) Kinaesthetic sensitivity of normal and clumsy children: a reply to Lord and Hulme [letter]. *Developmental Medicine and Child Neurology* **30:** 686–8.

Levin HS, Scheller J, Rickard T, et al. (1996) Dyscalculia and dyslexia after right hemisphere injury in infancy. *Archives of Neurology* **53:** 88–96.

Lyytinen H, Ahonen T, Rasanen P. (1994) Dyslexia and dyscalculia in children – risks, early precursors, bottle necks and cognitive mechanisms. *Acta Paedopsychiatrica* **56:** 179–92.

Maeland AF, Sovik N. (1993) Children with motor co-ordination problems and learning disabilities in reading, spelling, writing and arithmetic. *European Journal of Special Needs Education* **8:** 81–97.

Marchioni E, Galimderti CA, Soragna D, et al. (1995) Familial hemiplegic migraine versus migraine with prolonged aura: an uncertain diagnosis in a family report. *Neurology* **45:** 33–7.

Marlow N, Roberts BL, Cook RWI. (1989) Motor skills in extremely low birthweight children at the age of 6 years. *Archives of Disease in Childhood* **64:** 839–47.

Martlew M. (1992) Pen grips: their relationship to letter/word formation and literacy knowledge in children starting school. *Journal of Human Movement Studies* **24:** 165–85.

McCloskey M. (1992) Cognitive mechanisms in numerical processing: evidence from acquired dyscalculia. *Cognition* **44:** 107–57.

— Aliminosa D, Macaruso P. (1991) Theory based assessment of acquired dyscalculia. *Brain and Cognition* **17:** 285–308. (Review).

— Badecker W, Goodmanschulman RA, Aliminosa D. (1994) The structure of graphemic representations in spelling – evidence from a case of acquired dysgraphia. *Cognitive Neuropsychology* **11:** 341–92.

McGilchrist I, Wolkind S, Lischman A. (1994) Dyschronia in a patient with Tourette syndrome presenting as maternal neglect. *British Journal of Psychiatry* **164:** 261–3.

Merzenich MM, Jenkins WM, Johnston P, et al. (1995) Temporal processing deficits of language learning impaired children ameliorated by training. *Science* **271:** 77–81.

Newton M, Thomson M. (1997) *Aston Index LDA.*

O'Hare AE, Brown JK. (1989a) Childhood dysgraphia part 1: an illustrated clinical classification. *Child: Care, Health and Development* **15:** 79–104.

— —. (1989b) Childhood dysgraphia part 2 - a study of hand function. *Child: Care, Health and Development* **15:** 151–66.

— (1992) Learning disorders. Section of chapter 14, Disorders of the central nervous system. In: Campbell AGM, McIntosh N, editors. *Forfar and Arneil's Textbook of Paediatrics.* Edinburgh: Churchill Livingstone. p 847–54.

— — Aitken K. (1991) Dyscalculia in children [annotation]. *Developmental Medicine and Child Neurology* **33:** 356–61.

Paillard J. (1990) Basic neurophysiological structures of eye/hand co-ordination. In Bard C, Fleury M, Hay L, editors. *Development of Eye/Hand Co-ordination.* Charleston: University of South Carolina Press. p 26–74.

Papagno C, Basso A. (1993) Impairment of written language and mathematical skills in a case of Landau–Kleffner syndrome. *Aphasiology* **7:** 451–61.

Raven J. (1997) *Crichton Active Vocabulary Scale and Raven's Progressive Matrices.* Windsor: NFER Nelson.

Regueiro AM, Segurado OG, Mata P, Regueiro JR. (1992) Acquired selective signature dysgraphia. *Annals of Neurology* **31:** 115.

Renfrew CE. (1993) *Renfrew Action Picture Test.* Oxford: CE Renfrew Language Test Publisher. [2A North Place, Old Headington, Oxford OX3 9HX.]

Resnick LB. (1989) Developing mathematical knowledge. *American Psychology* **44:** 162–9.

Rosenberger PB. (1989) Perceptual motor and attentional correlates of developmental dyscalculia. *Annals of Neurology* **26:** 216–20.

Rosenbloom L, Horton ME. (1971) The maturation of fine prehension in young children. *Developmental Medicine and Child Neurology* **13:** 3–8.

Rouet J, Szekely C, Hockenberry MN. (1994) Specific arithmetic calculation deficits in children with Turner syndrome. *Journal of Clinical and Experimental Neuropsychology* **16:** 820–39.

Roy EA, Elliot D, Dewey D, Square-Storer P. (1990) Impairments to praxis and sequencing in adult and developmental disorders. In: Bard C, Fleury M, Hay L, editors. *Development of Eye/Hand Co-ordination.* Charleston: University of South Carolina Press. p 358–84.

Seidenberg M, Beck N, Geisser M, et al. (1986) Academic achievement of children with epilepsy. *Epilepsia* **27:** 753–9.

Shalev RS, Weirtman R, Amir N. (1988) Developmental dyscalculia. *Cortex* **24:** 555–61.

— Manor O, Amir N, Gross-Tsur V. (1993) The acquisition of arithmetic in normal children: assessment by a cognitive model of dyscalculia. *Developmental Medicine and Child Neurology* **35:** 593–601.

— — — Wertmanelad R, Gross-Tsur V. (1995) Developmental dyscalculia and brain laterality. *Cortex* **31:** 357–65.

Stevenson J, Pennington BF, Gilger JW, et al. (1993) Hyperactivity and spelling disability: testing for shared genetic aetiology. *Journal of Clinical Psychology and Psychiatry* **34:** 1137–52.

Stirling HM, Muttey M, Spalding NV. (1997) *Quick Neurological Screening Test.* Novato [CA]: Academic Therapy Publications.

Tallal P, Miller SL, Bedi G, et al. (1996) Language comprehension in language learning impaired children improved with acoustically modified speech. *Science* **271:** 81–4.

Tasker DM. (1991) Lined paper: a personal view. *Handwriting Review* 65–8.

Thomas-Anterion C, Laurent B, Le Henaff H, et al. (1994) Spelling impairments: neuropsychological study in 2 adolescents with developmental dysgraphia. *Revue Neurologique* **150:** 827–34.

Troijano L, Chiacchio L. (1994) Pure dysgraphia with relative sparing of lower case writing. *Cortex* **30:** 499–501.

Von Aster M. (1994) Developmental dyscalculia in children: review of the literature and clinical validation [review]. *Acta Paedopsychiatrica* **56:** 169–78.

Weintraub S, Mesulam MM. (1983) Developmental learning disabilities of the right hemisphere. *Archives of Neurology* **40:** 464–8.

Witkin HA, Oltman PK, Raskin E, Karp SA. (1971) *Children's Embedded Figures Test.* Palo Alto [CA]: Consulting Psychologists Press Inc.

World Health Organization. (1992) *International Statistical Classification of Diseases and Related Health Problems. Tenth Revision.* Geneva: World Health Organization.

Zesiger P, Pegna A, Rilliet B. (1994) Unilateral dysgraphia of the dominant hand in a left-hander: a disruption of graphic motor pattern selection. *Cortex* **30:** 673–83.

Zettin M, Cubelli R, Perino C, Rago R. (1995) Impairment of letter formation: the case of idiomotor apraxic agraphia. *Aphasiology* **9:** 283–94.

Ziviani J, Elkins J. (1984) An evaluation of handwriting performance. *Educational Review* **36:** 249–61.

5
DEVELOPMENTAL COORDINATION DISORDER (DCD): ALIAS THE CLUMSY CHILD SYNDROME

H J Polatajko

A significant proportion of school-aged children, about 6% according to international estimates (American Psychiatric Association 1994), have developmental coordination disorder (DCD), alias clumsy child syndrome. To put it simply, the clumsy child has difficulty with movement. However, as the term *clumsy* implies, the difficulties experienced in movement are different in kind from those experienced by individuals with paraplegia, cerebral palsy, or muscular dystrophy. The movement characteristics of children with a developmental coordination disorder (DCD) distinguish such children both from individuals with very severe motor impairments, such as those mentioned above, and from individuals with normal motor movements. What distinguishes children with DCD from the former group is a matter of severity. What distinguishes them from individuals with normal motor movements is more difficult to identify: as implied by the inclusion of DCD in this book on learning disorders, the distinguishing feature may well be a *motor learning disorder*.

In this chapter I describe the distinguishing features of DCD, with particular emphasis on clinical aspects. Its place among the specific learning disorders is discussed and it is disassociated from other sources of movement differences. The best available literature describing children with developmental coordination disorder is then summarized.[1] Finally, three cases illustrate the condition. But first, a commentary on name and definition.

Name of the disorder
As has been frequently noted (Henderson 1986, Smyth 1992, Cratty 1994, Bax 1995, Missiuna and Polatajko 1995) the terms used to identify the type of movement difficulties here referred to as 'developmental coordination disorder' are as varied as the children affected and the professions concerned with understanding and assisting them. Table 5.1 lists names often used, with the authors most associated with them. As is clear from the table, there is a myriad of names, and none has enjoyed broad acceptance. They represent

---

[1]The information for this chapter was drawn from as broad a literature base as feasible. To deal with the issues of naming in the field, information was included from publications using any of the terms commonly used to describe these children or the condition (see Table 5.1), with one stipulation: a work was considered, regardless of the term used, if sufficient information was provided about the children being described to allow the presumption that they would meet the diagnostic criteria for DCD set out in DSM-IV (American Psychiatric Association 1994).

TABLE 5.1.
Terms often used to denote developmental coordination disorder or children who have it

Term	Reference
Apraxia / Agnosia / Apraxic ataxia	Orton (1937))
	Walton et al. (1962)
	Gubbay (1975)
Clumsy child / Clumsy child syndrome / Clumsiness	Orton (1937)
	Walton et al. (1962)
	Dare and Gordon (1970)
	Gubbay (1975)
	Keogh et al. (1979)
	Gordon and McKinlay (1980)
	Henderson and Hall (1982)
	Henderson (1987)
	Hulme and Lord (1986)
	Cratty (1994)
DAMP[a]	Gillberg and Gillberg (1989)
Developmental dyspraxia / Apraxia	Gubbay (1975)
	CNSTF[b] (1981)
	Denckla (1984)
	Ayres (1985)
	Cermak (1985)
	Dewey (1995)
Developmental output failure	Levine et al. (1981)
Developmental coordination disorder	American Psychiatric Association (1987, 1994)
	Henderson et al. (1992)
	Hoare (1994)
	Mon-Williams and Wann (1994)
	Missiuna (1994)
	Rösblad and von Hofsten (1994)
	Polatajko et al. (1995b)
	Willoughby and Polatajko (1995)
Motor delay	Henderson (1986)
Motor coordination problems/difficulties	Cratty (1986)
	Roussounis et al. (1987)
Motor learning difficulties	McKinlay (1987)
Movement difficulties	Bouffard et al. (1996)
Perceptual motor dysfunction /deficits	Gordon and McKinlay (1980)
	Laszlo and Bairstow (1989)
	Clark et al. (1991)
Physically awkward child	Wall et al. (1990)
Sensory integrative dysfunction	Ayres (1972)
Visuo-motor disabilities	Dare and Gordon (1970)

[a]Deficits in attention, motor control, and perception.

[b]Child Neurology Society Task Force on Nosology of Disorders of Higher Cerebral Function in Children (David et al. 1981, cited in Denckla 1984).

neither mutually exclusive categories nor the same category. Indeed, as noted by Missiuna and Polatajko (1995), even a particular name is not consistently associated with a particular set of difficulties, other than clumsiness.

In 1994 an International Consensus Meeting on Children and Clumsiness was held to discuss, as an issue of primary importance, the name to be used to identify this heterogeneous group of children (Polatajko and Fox 1995, Polatajko et al. 1995a). The assembled experts represented leaders in the field from Australia, Canada, England, Israel, the Netherlands, Scotland, Sweden, and the United States of America and included educators, kinesiologists, occupational therapists, parents, physical therapists (or 'physiotherapists'), and psychologists. Together they considered carefully the issue of naming. While they acknowledged that the term *clumsy* both was descriptive of the condition and enjoyed wide usage outside North America, they noted that it is pejorative and therefore decided that it should no longer be used. Rather, the meeting adopted the term *developmental coordination disorder* (DCD), which was introduced by the American Psychiatric Association in the revised third edition of the *Diagnostic and Statistical Manual of Mental Disorders* (DSM-III-R) (1987) (category 315.40, Motor skills disorder: Developmental coordination disorder) and appeared again in the fourth edition, DSM-IV (American Psychiatric Association 1994) (category Motor skill disorder, 315.40, Developmental coordination disorder). Those attending the meeting agreed that this term, either in full or in its abbreviated form, would be used to facilitate communication within the field, and that is the term I use in this chapter.

Definition of DCD
Many definitions have been proposed for the disorder. However, as with the name, no consensus has emerged. The experts at the 1994 International Consensus Meeting, while generally agreeing with the descriptive definition provided in DSM-IV (American Psychiatric Association 1994), felt that it needed elaboration (Polatajko and Fox 1995). However, I would argue that the DSM-IV definition is adequate as a working definition: it both captures the characteristics of these children as generally reported in the literature and is enjoying increasing use in the research literature. Therefore I use the DSM-IV definition here.

Developmental coordination disorder is one of the motor skills disorders described in DSM-IV (American Psychiatric Association 1994). Its essential feature is *a marked impairment in the development of motor coordination* that *significantly interferes with academic achievement or activities of daily living* and that is not due to a general medical condition. The diagnostic criteria for DCD outlined in DSM-IV (p 54–55) are as follows:
A. Performance in daily activities that require motor coordination is substantially below that expected given the person's chronological age and measured intelligence. This may be manifested by marked delays in achieving motor milestones (e.g., walking, crawling, sitting), dropping things, 'clumsiness,' poor performance in sports, or poor handwriting.
B. The disturbance in criterion A significantly interferes with academic achievement or activities of daily living.
C. The disturbance is not due to a general medical condition (e.g., cerebral palsy, hemiplegia, or muscular dystrophy) and does not meet criteria for a Pervasive Developmental Disorder.

D. If Mental Retardation is present, the motor difficulties are in excess of those usually associated with it.

The clinical nature of DCD

ASSOCIATIONS: THE PLACE OF DCD AMONG THE SPECIFIC LEARNING DISORDERS

At the International Consensus Meeting on Children and Clumsiness in 1994, Kalverboer (1995) noted that the era of minimal brain dysfunction (MBD), which ended in the 1960s, was followed by an era of what he called 'derivatives' of that disorder. These are conditions that have emerged from the broad grouping of MBD as distinct disorders – the specific learning disorders. DCD, alias clumsiness, was identified by Kalverboer as one of two important derivatives, the other being attention-deficit/hyperactivity disorder. A third and possibly the most important derivative, if not iteration, of MBD is learning disability (LD) (Smith 1983, Silver 1992). DCD has been and continues to be associated with both derivatives.

The term *minimal brain dysfunction* (MBD) (to look back to that era for a moment) was coined by Clements to describe the disorder in a heterogeneous group of children who were experiencing learning problems that were not easily explained (Kavale et al. 1987, Sugden and Keogh 1990, Silver 1992, Cratty 1994). These children were considered to have motor incoordination, perceptual dysfunction, and hyperactivity associated with the learning problems (Kavale et al. 1987, Cratty 1994) and these symptoms were considered to indicate some form of minimal brain dysfunction. In 1962 Kirk (quoted in Silver 1992) proposed the term *learning disabilities* (LD)[2] to replace *minimal brain dysfunction*. This was done in part to reflect a change in thinking concerning the aetiology of the condition (Smith 1983). The older term, however, continued to be used to describe children with motor incoordination, perceptual dysfunction, and hyperactivity (Kavale et al. 1987, Silver 1992).

Soon after the term *LD* was adopted, hyperactivity was identified as a distinct disorder. Initially called 'hyperkinetic reaction of childhood', this condition has since 1987 been known as 'attention-deficit/hyperactivy disorder' (ADHD; see Silver 1992 for a discussion). The essential feature of ADHD is a persistent (lasting at least 6 months) pattern of inattention and/or hyperactivity–impulsivity that is maladaptive and inconsistent with the child's developmental level (American Psychiatric Association 1994). Some children with ADHD, but not all, have learning disabilities. Conversely, not all children with LD have an attention deficit. Similarly, a significant number of children with ADHD have perceptual–motor problems and incoordination. In some instances these problems are a direct consequence of the attention deficit; in others they are evidence of the presence of a movement disorder (American Psychiatric Association 1994).

The term *LD* continued to be used for some time to describe children with learning problems who had motor incoordination and perceptual–motor problems, and many believed that remediation of these problems would alleviate the learning disability (see Lazarus

[2]Whereas the term *learning disorder* is generally assigned to a very broad spectrum of disorders in children who experience a varity of learning problems in a variety of domains, the term *learning disability* (LD) is typically reserved to describe the problems of children who, despite good potential, experience significant difficulties in acquiring and using listening, speaking, reading, writing, reasoning, or mathematical skills (Hammill et al. 1981, cited in Kavale et al. 1987).

1990 or Cratty 1994 for a discussion). After considerable research, however, it was concluded that this was not the case and that exploring the perceptual and motor function of children with learning disabilities was a fruitless line of enquiry (see Kavale et al. 1987 for a review). Thus in 1986 the Board of Trustees of the Council for Learning Disabilities issued a position statement declaring a moratorium on the assessment and treatment of perceptual–motor problems in children with learning disabilities.

With the disassociation of perceptual and motor problems from learning disabilities, LD came to be seen almost exclusively an educational problem. The essential feature of LD now is a significant discrepancy between academic achievement and potential, and the major focus is now on the academic performance of affected children (Kavale et al. 1987). Only in the context of a search for LD subtypes is the presence of perceptual or motor problems being noted at all nowadays. While it is recognized that there are children with LD who have perceptual and motor problems, there are many others who have no such problems. Conversely, there are many children who do not have LD but who do have perceptual–motor and coordination problems and these are the children who are now considered to have DCD.

While the major interest in the period since MBD has been in children with LD and ADHD, interest in other forms of learning disorders is also growing. In particular there is a growing interest in children who, like children with LD, seem to have difficulty in a particular area of development and skill acquisition in the absence of the understood causes for such difficulties, namely children who are experiencing motor learning disorders – children with DCD (Hulme and Lord 1986).

Obviously LD, ADHD, and DCD, with their common roots in MBD, often share co-morbidity. The level of overlap, while not well documented, is clearly greater than would be expected by chance alone. The estimates of overlap vary greatly. For example Kaplan et al. (1995) reported that as many as 30% of children with LD also have ADHD, 30 to 40% of children with ADHD also have LD, and a full 50% of children with either LD or ADHD also have DCD. Sugden and Wann (1987) found 29 to 33% of children with LD to have coordination difficulties, and Silver (1992) reported that approximately 20% of children with LD also have ADHD. A large metaanalysis of 1077 studies indicated that 70% of children with LD had perceptual–motor problems, and almost 75% had attention deficits (Kavale and Nye 1985–1986). Thus the comorbidity of LD, ADHD, and DCD is quite significant. Yet each is a distinct condition: for each condition there are children who have that condition but not the others. Figure 5.1 represents the comorbidity of these primary derivatives of MBD.

DISASSOCIATIONS

When children experience clumsiness or incoordination severe enough to cause concern to their parents or teachers, a professional consultation is usually sought. This can result in one of three responses. If the family physician considers the symptoms sufficiently severe, the possible presence of some medical condition is investigated. Otherwise the clumsiness is considered to be nothing more than normal variance or a maturational delay. In either case, the clumsiness is considered benign (Henderson 1994) and no further action is thought

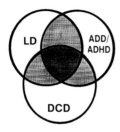

Fig. 5.1. Comorbidity of the three primary derivatives of miminal brain dysfunction.

ADD, attention-deficit disorder; ADHD, attention-deficit/hyperactivity disorder; DCD, developmental coordination disorder; LD, learning disability.

to be warranted. DCD is a condition in its own right. If children who have DCD are to receive the proper attention, it must be distinguished from other medical conditions and from normal variance or maturational delay.

Distinction of DCD from other medical conditions
Awkwardness, clumsiness, or poor coordination can be indicative of DCD. These signs can also be indicative of a neurological, intellectual, or sensory impairment (Hall 1988, Cratty 1994, Fox 1995). While the descriptors are the same, the conditions are quite different and warrant very different actions (Gordon and McKinlay 1980, American Psychiatric Association 1994, Cratty 1994). A child presenting with such signs therefore needs to be examined carefully by a developmental paediatrician to distinguish between DCD and such possible disorders as acquired brain injury, the ataxias, brain tumours, cerebral palsy, mental retardation, metabolic disorders, muscular dystrophies, myopathies, polyneuropathies, seizure disorders, Tourette syndrome, and vestibular disease (Cratty 1994, Fox 1995).

While children with DCD experience great difficulties, they do not show any of the so-called 'hard' neurological signs (that is, clear-cut evidence of neuropathology) diagnostic of a neurological condition, they are of normal intelligence, and they do not have any diagnosable sensory deficits (Hulme and Lord 1986). Indeed it was the lack of findings on neurological examination that first brought these children to attention. As Walton and colleagues (1962) commented in their paper describing 'five clumsy children': 'We thought this boy's disability appeared to be due to a congenital apraxia, but there was no clinical or other evidence of a cerebral lesion to account for it. This disorder of movement had been sufficient to cause a severe clumsiness of all voluntary activity and had led to a provisional diagnosis of mental backwardness in a child of above average intelligence' (p 604).

Children with DCD can, however, have so-called 'soft' neurological signs. Such signs are thought to be subtle evidence of otherwise undetectable abnormality (Cratty 1994). Included under the designation 'soft signs' are such features as abnormal movements, abnormal reflexes, awkwardness, associated movements, delayed motor milestones, poor coordination, and general clumsiness (Sugden and Keogh 1990, Cratty 1994). However, one or more of these soft signs are so frequently seen in children without notable problems that their significance must be interpreted with great caution (Hall 1988, Sugden and Keogh 1990, Cratty 1994).

TABLE 5.2
The three schools of thought about developmental coordination disorder, and their imperatives

School of thought	Imperative
1 Normal variance	Accept the child's limitations
2 Maturational delay	Wait – the child will outgrow it
3 Disorder	Take action, get treatment

Distinction of DCD from normal variance and maturational delay

Normal variance and maturational delay are the proposed explanations of two of the three schools of thought that have dominated the field of DCD (Table 5.2). These two explanations, unfortunately, have prevailed in the attitudes of many professionals called upon to deal with children who experience clumsiness and incoordination. DMB Hall's (1988) words in an editorial in the *British Medical Journal* reflect both of these schools of thought: 'Perhaps the notion of the clumsy child syndrome simply reflects the tendency of doctors to equate the unusual with the pathological. A more satisfactory explanation for clumsiness is biological variation. The usual distribution curve for ability predicts clumsy children as well as ultimate athletes...' (p 375). 'Motor difficulties seem to resolve in the teen years...' (p 375).

Those who hold that clumsiness and incoordination in children represent normal variation suggest that 'We do our patients no service by treating clumsiness as if it were a disease. With only rare exceptions clumsiness is a talent deficit...' (Hall 1988, p 376). I would argue that the potential exists to do great harm to children with motor difficulties if these are considered normal variation, because to consider them normal is to suggest that the children can never acquire normal, age-appropriate skills. There is ample evidence to the contrary. Orton (1937), one of the earliest authors to describe this condition, noted that with sufficient application and practice these children could master almost any skill.

Other evidence disassociating DCD from normal variation comes from the proponents of the maturational delay hypothesis. If 'clumsiness is a problem of delayed maturation and recovery is usually spontaneous' (Anonymous 1962, p 1665), then clearly it is not normal variation. The existence of the spontaneous recovery data cited by the proponents of the delay hypothesis speaks against the possibility that the signs associated with DCD simply represent normal variance in motor performance. When Hall (1988) notes that 'Motor difficulties seem to resolve in the teen years' (p 375), he is speaking against his own hypothesis of normal variance – he is implicitly invoking the maturational delay argument. These two interpretations are clearly mutually exclusive: a normal variance does not 'resolve' itself.

The contention that DCD is essentially a form of maturational delay is based on a number of observations in the literature that children with DCD generally outgrow their problems, with only the most severely affected having persistent problems (McKinlay 1987, Cantell et al. 1994). However, recent data from a number of longitudinal studies (e.g. Gillberg and Gillberg 1989, Losse et al. 1991, Cantell et al. 1994) would suggest that this is not the case: DCD does not necessarily resolve itself but, rather, has important long-term sequelae persisting into adulthood.

As Henderson (1994) has pointed out, and the International Consensus Meeting concluded (Polatajko et al. 1995a), DCD is a disorder in its own right, the condition is not benign, and children who have it require attention – that is, the experts at the meeting endorsed the third school of thought (see Table 5.2) : DCD is distinct from normal variance, maturational delay, and other medical conditions. When a child is seen for motor difficulties, DCD must be disassociated from all three of these explanations, since each demands a different response. So that the concerns of the children and their families can be alleviated and the children can receive the proper treatment, it is imperative that the condition be diagnosed correctly.

CHILDREN WITH DCD

Our understanding of children with DCD comes from two types of publications: descriptive studies and experimental studies. Descriptive studies provide an understanding of the characteristics of children with DCD. Experimental studies provide some insights into the nature of the children's motor problems. The general description of the characteristics of the children presented below is drawn both from clinical case descriptions and from group descriptions. The case descriptions found in the literature are invariably of children who were referred for assessment. The group studies found in the literature generally report on the results of standardized assessments on groups of children who either had been referred (i.e. children whose motor performance had brought them to the attention of a professional) or had been identified through some screening process or process of selection by a teacher (i.e. children whose motor performance had not caused sufficient concern to warrant their seeking professional attention). Each type of description obviously provides a somewhat different perspective and each has its inherent advantages and disadvantages. Together they provide converging validity for the general description of the characteristics of children with DCD that emerges from the literature (Hulme and Lord 1986).

Finally, drawing on the available, albeit limited, experimental literature, the nature of the movement problems is summarized.

Characteristics of the children

Perhaps the first thing that ought to be recognized about DCD, alias clumsiness, is that it is heterogeneous, as Hulme and Lord (1986) noted. Indeed work is going on to identify any subtypes of DCD (Hoare 1994). A second point to be made, which follows directly from the first, is that there is no typical clumsy child (Gordon and McKinlay 1980). Individual children with DCD vary greatly, depending on such variables as the source of the disorder, its severity, the particular areas of motor performance affected, and environmental influences. The general description that follows should be read in this light.

While each child with DCD has a set of unique characteristics, from the earliest reports common themes have emerged. Starting with the writings of Orton (1937) and Walton and colleagues (1962), most authors have described these children in much the same way (see also Dare and Gordon 1970, Gubbay 1978, Gordon and McKinlay 1980, Henderson and Hall 1982, Stephenson et al. 1990). The children generally present in clinic with awkward, clumsy movements and poor coordination, and often with complaints of falling, tripping, or bumping into things. They often have a history of delayed acquisition of motor milestones and are reported to require much more effort and take much longer than their non-clumsy peers to learn age-appropriate motor tasks. Their motor problems can affect gross motor skills, fine motor skills, or both, and any related functional skills, such as catching, throwing, batting, jumping, buttoning, tying shoelaces, writing, drawing, handling objects. Many of these children also have organizational difficulties affecting not only motor performance but also other areas of function.

Children with DCD generally cope by avoiding, when they can, those tasks that are difficult. Thus, they are often quite sedentary and may seem withdrawn. When problematic situations cannot be avoided, the children begin to experience difficulty. This often occurs first in the school years, when expectations are such that it becomes difficult to avoid situations. Problems can occur in any area of daily occupations where the task demands motor skills. In school these children may as a group have lowered academic achievement, with any or all areas of learning affected – reading, spelling, arithmetic, writing (see Smyth 1992 for a review). (However, it must be remembered that not all children with DCD have such academic problems. Indeed they may have none.) At home, dressing, feeding, and simple use of tools may be a problem (Orton 1937, Walton et al. 1962). At play, the children may be sedentary and solitary and are likely to be unpopular, having difficulty keeping up with their peers in toy use, puzzles, games, and sports (Dare and Gordon 1970). However, it is important to remember that these children demonstrate great discrepancies in motor capacities and not all skills will be problematic (Hulme and Lord 1986). A child with DCD is likely to be excellent at one motor task but poor at another.

Children with DCD are likely to have significant associated secondary emotional or behavioural problems (Hulme and Lord 1986, Kalverboer et al. 1990, Smyth 1992). The children often have low self-esteem related to their motor problems (Willoughby and Polatajko 1995) and may feel incompetent, inadequate, depressed, frustrated, or anxious. They may be withdrawn, isolated, or submissive and are often unpopular and marginal in their peer groups. They are often teased, and they often get attention by acting out or 'acting the clown'. People tend to have an unsympathetic attitude towards them because their disorder is not immediately obvious (see Smyth 1992 for a review).

DCD is generally considered a problem of school-age children, since it is early in the school years that the problem is typically identified. (In fact the problem exists much earlier and could in principle be diagnosed in the preschool years.) Furthermore it has long been considered that the problems resolve with age. In some children DCD improves spontaneously with age (Knuckey and Gubbay 1983, Roussounis et al. 1987), but for the most part studies have shown that even when it does the affected children tend always to lag behind their peers (Knuckey and Gubbay 1983, Roussounis et al. 1987). More importantly, recent longitudinal studies have shown that in many instances the repercussions are lifelong, and that not only do the motor problems persist but also other aspects of development are affected (Losse et al. 1991, Cantell et al. 1994). Longitudinal studies provide evidence that in comparison with control subjects some adolescents with DCD have lower academic achievement, fewer sparetime activities, a poorer opinion of their scholastic and athletic competence, and lower aspirations (Cantell et al. 1994). Knuckey and Gubbay (1983) found that as young adults these individuals have lower academic achievement and jobs requiring less manual skill.

Nature of the movement problems

Researchers documenting the motor performance of children with DCD have tended to use one of two basic approaches, one looking at general performance and the other at the underlying processes.

Those approaching the subject by looking at general performance have tended to describe the performance of groups of children with DCD, relative to that of normal children, on a variety of motor tasks (see Dare and Gordon 1970, Gubbay 1975, Henderson and Hall 1982, Wall 1982, Johnston et al. 1987, Wilson et al. 1995). This approach has had some prominence in the literature. Thus it is now well established that children with DCD have difficulty performing 'culturally-normative motor skills with acceptable proficiency' (Wall 1982, p 254).

Researchers using the process approach examine the *motor processes* that underlie motor performance, i.e. the *sensory, central,* and *output* processes. Using carefully constructed experiments they have begun to examine one or other of the processes underlying the motor performance of children with DCD. Unfortunately there is as yet a paucity of such research.

Most of the work on motor processes has been in the area of sensory processes. A number of researchers have investigated specific sensory systems involved in movement, arguing that the motor coordination problems of these children are due to sensory problems (see Willoughby and Polatajko 1995 for a review). Three sensory systems have been explored, both individually and in combination, i.e. cross-modally (Table 5.3). The results thus far remain inconclusive (see Willoughby and Polatajko 1995 for a discussion), although the visual and kinaesthetic systems seem promising areas of study (Hulme and Lord 1986, van der Meulen et al. 1991, Rösblad and von Hofsten 1992) while the integrative system does not (Hulme et al. 1982, Hulme and Lord 1986, van der Meulen et al. 1991). It may well be, in keeping with the heterogeneity of this syndrome, that different systems are implicated in different children.

Work in the area of the central processes is only just appearing in the literature. A few studies have investigated some discrete areas. For example, van Dellen and Geuze (1988) provided some evidence of a central processing deficiency. They found a deficiency in the cognitive decision process of motor response selection and demonstrated that this deficiency contributed to the slowness observed in children with DCD. Unfortunately there are as yet too few studies investigating central processes to form the basis for any summary. Similarly the output processes are poorly understood. While it is clear that the motor output of children with DCD is marked by movements that are less accurate, less precise, and less consistent than those of their peers (Wall 1982, Marchiori et al. 1987, Henderson et al. 1992, Missiuna 1994), the mechanisms underlying the observed awkwardness, clumsiness, and incoordination (Marchiori et al. 1987, van Dellen and Geuze 1988, Henderson et al. 1992, Missiuna 1994) remain unknown.

TABLE 5. 3
Areas of sensory processing investigated in children with
developmental coordination disorder

Area investigated	Major authors
Sensory integration	Ayres (1972)
Visual–kinaesthetic integration	Hulme et al. (1982)
	Hoare and Larkin (1991)
Kinaesthetic perception	Laszlo and Bairstow (1983, 1985, 1989)
	Smyth and Glencross (1986)
	Hoare and Larkin (1991)
	Rösblad and von Hofsten (1992, 1994)
	Piek and Coleman-Carman (1995)
	Smyth (1996)
Vestibular function	Ayres (1972)
	Horak et al. (1988)
Vision / Visual perception	Hulme et al. (1982)
	O'Briene et al. (1988)
	Murray et al. (1990)
	van der Meulen et al. (1991)
	Rösblad and von Hofsten (1992)
	Dwyer and McKenzie (1994)
	Mon-Williams and Wann (1994)

Summary

Many school-aged children around the world have a developmental coordination disorder. These children experience a chronic impairment in their motor function that causes them difficulty in learning motor-based skills and prevents them from performing culturally normative, day-to-day motor tasks as proficiently as their peers. Frequently children with DCD experience secondary emotional and behavioural problems that are a direct result of their motor ineptness. While some children with DCD outgrow their disabilities, many do not. Many experience serious lifelong sequelae that bring them into contact with health and social services. For the sake of the children, their families, and society at large, it is imperative that this disorder be identified and that services be provided to mitigate the devastating impact of DCD.

Case descriptions[3]

JOHN

John is an 8-year-old boy of normal intelligence who has a learning disability and developmental coordination disorder. He has received speech therapy since the age of 3 years.

John lives at home with his three younger sisters and his parents. His mother reports that the pregnancy and delivery were both difficult. Both parents report that John was slow to reach normal developmental milestones and that he still appears awkward and clumsy

---

[3]Contributed by A Mandich, Research Clinician, DCD Research Group, School of Occupational Therapy, The University of Western Ontario, London, Ontario. The names used for the children are fictitious.

129

when performing many tasks. He is awkward with cutlery, has difficulty turning doorknobs, bumps into things constantly, and frequently knocks over his milk at the table.

At school John excels in reading but has difficulty in writing, displaying poor pencil grasp, poor letter formation, and difficulty in orienting letters to the baseline. He avoids most gross motor activities including gym class and playground activities. The teacher has said that John is reluctant to try new activities, especially if they require motor skill. Examination shows that he cannot hop on one foot, or skip, and that he has low muscle tone and difficulty with body stabilization and overflow movements.

SUSAN

Susan is an 8-year-old-girl of normal intelligence who is extremely clumsy. She lives at home with her parents and one older brother. Her mother reports that the pregnancy and delivery were normal but that Susan's early milestones were slightly delayed. Her mother describes her as having been an irritable young child who had difficulty settling. Susan has been receiving speech therapy because of articulation problems since she was 4 years old.

Both parents now describe Susan as a 'bull in a china shop'. She falls down, bumps into things, and has difficulty in judging body position. She trips when climbing the stairs and generally has difficulty in organizing herself. Buttoning shirts, tying shoes, and doing up zippers are all very difficult for her. Mealtimes also present a challenge. When eating soup she cannot seem to keep the liquid on the spoon, and finishing a meal seems to take a long time. At school Susan has significant difficulty with fine and gross motor skills and therefore has great difficulty in keeping up with the written work. Handwriting is a particular problem: she presses extremely hard on her pencil and works very slowly. Susan does enjoy some activities, including reading, computers, ballet, and music.

STEVEN

Steven is an 11-year-old boy and is in the programme for gifted children at his school. He has been identified as having attention-deficit disorder and developmental coordination disorder. He lives at home with his parents and a younger sister. He enjoys volleyball, basketball, skiing, and karate. His parents report that he is proficient at these activities and describe him as athletic. At school Steven is described as a motivated, energetic boy who seems to associate with younger children. He excels at reading and language and finds math his most challenging subject.

Steven's early development was unremarkable, and he achieved normal developmental milestones. While his parents reported that he had experienced some difficulty in learning to do things such as tie his shoes and button his shirts, his problems were really first identified by his kindergarten teacher, who noted that he had difficulty with activities such as cutting and printing.

Both at home and at school Steven continues to experience difficulty with fine motor skills, such tasks as writing, cutting meat, and coordinating the use of knife and fork. Although he regularly attends therapy sessions for his motor difficulties, he is reluctant to admit his difficulties.

REFERENCES

American Psychiatric Association. (1987) *Diagnostic and Statistical Manual of Mental Disorders.* 3rd ed, revised (DSM-III-R). Washington, DC: American Psychiatric Association.

American Psychiatric Association. (1994) *Diagnostic and Statistical Manual of Mental Disorders (DSM-IV).* Washington, DC: American Psychiatric Association.

[Anonymous]. (1962) Clumsy children. *British Medical Journal* , Dec 22, 1665–6.

Ayres AJ. (1972) *Sensory Integration and Learning Disorders.* Los Angeles: Western Psychological Services.

Ayres AJ. (1985) *Developmental Dyspraxia and Adult-Onset Dyspraxia.* Torrance [CA, USA]: Sensory Integration International.

Bax M. (1995) Keynote address. In: Polatajko H, Fox AM. *Final Report on the Conference Children andd Clumsiness: A Disability in Search of Definition. International Consensus Meeting.* London, Ontario. Not numbered.

Board of Trustees of the Council for Learning Disabilities. (1986) Measurement and training of perceptual and perceptual–motor functions: a position statement by the Board of Trustees of the Council for Learning Disabilities. *Journal of Learning Disabilities* 9: 247.

Bouffard M, Watkinson EJ, Thompson LP, et al. (1996) A test of the activity deficit hypothesis with children with movement difficulties. *Adapted Physical Activity Quarterly* 13: 61–73.

Cantell MH, Smith MM, Ahonen TP. (1994) Clumsiness in adolescence: educational, motor, and social outcomes of motor delay detected at 5 years. *Adapted Physical Activity Quarterly* 11: 115–29.

Cermak S. (1985) Developmental dyspraxia. In: Roy EA, editor. *Neuropsychological Studies of Apraxia and Related Disorders.* Amsterdam: Elsevier. p 225–48.

Clark F, Mailloux Z, Parham LD, Primeau LA. (1991) Statement: occupational therapy provision for children with learning disabilities and/or mild to moderate perceptual and motor deficits. *American Journal of Occupational Therapy* 45: 1069–74.

Cratty BJ. (1986) *Perceptual and Motor Development in Infants and Children.* Englewood Cliffs [NJ]: Prentice-Hall.

— (1994) *Clumsy Child Syndromes: Descriptions, Evaluation and Remediation.* Chur, Switzerland: Harwood Academic Publishers.

Dare MT, Gordon N. (1970) Clumsy children: a disorder of perception and motor organisation. *Developmental Medicine and Child Neurology* 12: 178–85.

Denckla MB. (1984) Developmental dyspraxia: the clumsy child. In: Levine MD, Satz P, editors. *Middle Childhood: Development and Dysfunction.* Baltimore: University Park Press. p 251–60.

Dewey D. (1995) What is developmental dyspraxia? *Brain and Cognition* 29: 254–74.

Dwyer C, McKenzie BE. (1994) Impairment of visual memory in children who are clumsy. *Adapted Physical Activity Quarterly* 11: 179–89.

Fox M. (1995) Management issues. In: Polatajko HP, Fox AM. *Final Report on the Conference Children and Clumsiness: A Disability in Search of Definition. International Consensus Meeting.* London, Ontario. Not numbered.

Gillberg IC, Gillberg C. (1989) Children with preschool minor neurodevelopmental disorders. IV: Behaviour and school achievement at age 13. *Developmental Medicine and Child Neurology* 31: 3–13.

Gordon N, McKinlay I. (1980) *Helping Clumsy Children.* New York: Churchill Livingstone.

Gubbay SS. (1975) *The Clumsy Child. A Study of Developmental Apraxia and Agnosic Ataxia.* London: Saunders.

— (1978) The management of developmental apraxia. *Developmental Medicine and Child Neurology* 20: 643–6.

Hall DMB. (1988) Clumsy children. *British Medical Journal* 296: 375–6. (Editorial).

Henderson SE. (1986) Problems of motor development: some practical issues. In: Keogh BK, editor. *Advances in Special Education, Volume 5.* Greenwich, CT [USA]: JAI Press. p 187–218.

— (1987) The assessment of 'clumsy children': old and new approaches. *Journal of Child Psychology and Psychiatry* 28: 511–27.

—. (1994) Editorial. *Adapted Physical Activity Quarterly* 11: 111–4.

— Hall D. (1982) Concomitants of clumsiness in young schoolchildren. *Developmental Medicine and Child Neurology* 24: 448–60.

—, Rose P, Henderson S. (1992) Reaction time and movement time in children with developmental coordination disorder. *Journal of Child Psychology and Psychiatry* **33:** 895–905.

Hoare D. (1994) Subtypes of developmental coordination disorder. *Adapted Physical Activity Quarterly* **11:** 158–69.

— Larkin D. (1991) Kinaesthetic abilities of clumsy children. *Developmental Medicine and Child Neurology* **33:** 671–8.

Horak FB, Shumway-Cook A, Crowe TK, Black FO. (1988) Vestibular function and motor proficiency of children with impaired hearing, or with learning disability and motor impairments. *Developmental Medicine and Child Neurology* **30:** 64–79.

Hulme C, Lord R. (1986) Clumsy children – a review of recent research. *Child: Care, Health and Development* **12:** 257–69.

— Biggerstaff A, Moran G, McKinlay I. (1982) Visual, kinaesthetic and cross-modal judgements of length by normal and clumsy children. *Developmental Medicine and Child Neurology* **24:** 461–71.

Johnston O, Short H, Crawford J. (1987) Poorly coordinated children: A survey of 95 cases. *Child: Care, Health and Development* **13:** 361–76.

Kalverboer AF. (1995) Clumsiness, a condition emerging from having been neglected: circumspection of the concept. In: Polatajko HP, Fox AM. *Final Report on the Conference Children and Clumsiness: Disability in Search of Definition. International Consensus Meeting.* London, Ontario. Not numbered.

— de Vries H, van Dellen T. (1990) Social behavior in clumsy children as rated by parents and teachers. In: Kalverboer AF editor. *Developmental Biopsychology: Experimental and Observational Studies in Children at Risk.* Ann Arbor: University of Michigan Press. p 257–69.

Kaplan BJ, Wilson BN, Dewey D, Crawford SG. (1995) The genetic basis of clumsiness, and its overlap with other disorders. In: Polatajko HP, Fox AM. *Final Report on the Conference Children and Clumsiness: A Disability in Search of Definition. International Consensus Meeting.* London, Ontario. Not numbered.

Kavale KA, Nye C. (1985–1986) Parameters of learning disabilities in achievement, linguistic, neuropsychological, and social/behavioral domains. *Journal of Special Education* **19:** 443–58.

— Forness SR, Bender M. (1987) *Handbook of Learning Disabilities. Volume 1, Dimensions and Diagnosis.* Boston: College Hill Press.

Keogh JF, Sugden DA, Reynard CL, Calkins JA. (1979) Identification of clumsy children: comparisons and comments. *Journal of Human Movement Studies* **5:** 32–41.

Knuckey NW, Gubbay SS. (1983) Clumsy children: a prognostic study. *Australian Paediatric Journal* **19:** 9–13.

Laszlo JI, Bairstow PJ. (1983) Kinaesthesis: its measurement, training and relationship with motor control. *Quarterly Journal of Experimental Psychology, Section A, Human Experimental Psychology* **35a:** 411–21.

— — (1985) *Perceptual Motor Behaviour: Developmental Assessment and Therapy.* New York: Praeger.

— — (1989) Process-oriented assessment and treatment of children with perceptuo-motor dysfunction. In: Loviband P, Wilson P, editors. *Clinical and Abnormal Psychology.* Amsterdam: Elsevier Science Publishers. p 311.

Lazarus JAC. (1990) Factors underlying inefficient movement in learning disabled children. In: Reid G, editor. *Problems in Movement Control.* Amsterdam: Elsevier Science Publishers. p 241.

Levine MD, Oberklaid F, Meltzer L. (1981) Developmental output failure: study of low productivity in school-aged children. *Pediatrics* **67:** 18–25.

Losse A, Henderson SE, Elliman D, et al. (1991) Clumsiness in children – do they grow out of it? A 10-year follow-up study. *Developmental Medicine and Child Neurology* **33:** 55–68.

Marchiori GE, Wall AE, Bedingfield EW. (1987) Kinematic analysis of skill acquisition in physically awkward boys. *Adapted Physical Activity Quarterly* **4:** 305–15.

McKinlay I. (1987) Children with motor learning difficulties: not so much a syndrome – more a way of life. *Physiotherapy* **73:** 635–38.

Missiuna C. (1994) Motor skill acquisition in children with developmental coordination disorder. *Adapted Physical Activity Quarterly* **11:** 214–35.

— Polatajko HJ. (1995 Developmental dyspraxia by any other name. *American Journal of Occupational Therapy* **49:** 619–28.

Mon-Williams MA, Wann JP. (1994) Ophthalmic factors in developmental coordination disorder. *Adapted Physical Activity Quarterly* **11:** 170–8.

Murray EA, Cermak SA, OBriene V. (1990) The relationship between form and space perception constructional abilities, and clumsiness in children. *American Journal of Occupational Therapy* **44:** 623–8.

O'Briene V, Cermak SA, Murray E. (1988) The relationship between visual–perceptual motor abilities and clumsiness in children with and without learning disabilities. *American Journal of Occupational Therapy* **42:** 359–63.

Orton ST. (1937) *Reading, Writing, and Speech Problems in Children.* New York: Norton.

Piek JP, Coleman-Carman R. (1995) Kinaesthetic sensitivity and motor performance of children with developmental co-ordination disorder. *Developmental Medicine and Child Neurology* **37**: 976–84.

Polatajko H, Fox AM. (1995) *Final Report on the Conference: Children and Clumsiness: A Disability in Search of Definition. International Consensus Meeting.* London, Ontario. Not numbered.

— — Missiuna C. (1995a) An international consensus on children with developmental coordination disorder. *Canadian Journal of Occupational Therapy* **62**: 3–6.

— Macnab JJ, Anstett B, et al. (1995b) A clinical trial of the process-oriented treatment approach for children with developmental co-ordination disorder. *Developmental Medicine and Child Neurology* **37**: 310-19.

Rösblad B, von Hofsten C. (1992) Perceptual control of manual positioning in children with motor impairments. *Physiotherapy Theory and Practice* **8**: 223–33.

— — (1994) Repetitive goal-directed arm movements in children with developmental coordination disorders: role of visual information. *Adapted Physical Activity Quarterly* **11**: 190–202.

Roussounis SH, Gaussen TH, Stratton P. (1987) A 2-year follow-up study of children with motor coordination problems identified at school entry age. *Child: Care, Health and Development* **13**: 371–91.

Silver LB. (1992) *The Misunderstood Child.* Blue Ridge Summit [PA]: Tab Books.

Smith CR. (1983) *Learning Disabilities.* Toronto: Little, Brown and Co.

Smyth TR. (1992) Impaired motor skill (clumsiness) in otherwise normal children: a review. *Child: Care, Health and Development* **18**: 283–300.

— (1996) Clumsiness: kinaesthetic perception and translation. *Child: Care, Health and Development* **22**: 1–9.

— Glencross DJ. (1986) Information processing deficits in clumsy children. *Australian Journal of Psychology* **38**: 13–22.

Stephenson E, McKay C, Chesson R. (1990) An investigative study of early developmental factors in children with motor/learning difficulties. *British Journal of Occupational Therapy* **53**: 4–6.

Sugden D, Keogh J. (1990) *Problems in Movement Skill Development.* Columbia, SC: University of South Carolina Press.

— Wann C. (1987) The assessment of motor impairment in children with moderate learning difficulties. *British Journal of Educational Psychology* **57**: 225–36.

van Dellen T, Geuze RH. (1988) Motor response processing in clumsy children. *Journal of Child Psychology and Psychiatry* **29**: 489–500.

van der Meulen JHP, van der Gon JJD, Gielen CCAM, et al. (1991) Visuomotor performance of normal and clumsy children. I: Fast goal-directed arm-movements with and without visual feedback. *Developmental Medicine and Child Neurology* **33**: 40–54.

Wall AE. (1982) Physically awkward children: a motor development perspective. In: Das JP, Mulcahy RF, Wall AE, editors. *Theory and Research in Learning Disabilities.* New York: Plenum Press. p 253–68.

— Reid G, Paton J. (1990) The syndrome of physical awkwardness. In: Reid G, editor. *Problems in Movement Control.* Amsterdam: Elsevier Science Publishers. p 283–315.

Walton JN, Ellis E, Court DM. (1962) Clumsy children: developmental apraxia and agnosia. *Brain* **85**: 603–12.

Willoughby C, Polatajko HJ. (1995) Motor problems in children with developmental coordination disorder: review of the literature. *American Journal of Occupational Therapy* **49**: 787–9f

Wilson BN, Polatajko HJ, Kaplan BJ, Faris P. (1995) Use of the Bruininks–Oseretsky Test of Motor Proficiency in occupational therapy. *American Journal of Occupational Therapy* **49**: 8–18.

133

6
AD(H)D, HYPERKINETIC DISORDERS, DAMP, AND RELATED BEHAVIOUR DISORDERS

Peder Rasmussen and Christopher Gillberg

In the past a number of behavioural and learning disorders have been grouped together under the uninformative label of 'minimal brain dysfunction' (MBD). *MBD* was used as a blanket term to cover the abnormality of children with overactivity and learning problems who, it was often taken for granted, had 'minimal brain damage'. Subsequent empirical study has shown that (a) overactivity is usually not a sign of brain damage and (b) brain damage does not usually lead to overactivity (Rutter 1982).

Synonyms

A comprehensive survey of all the synonyms and overlapping terms used in this field is beyond the scope of this chapter. However, a list of some of the most common diagnostic labels (Table 6.1) is useful as an introduction to a description of the patterns of signs encountered in children who were, often inappropriately, diagnosed as having minimal brain dysfunction.

The array of labels listed in the table testifies to the confusion in the field. Unfortunately no consensus has yet been reached. In North America inflectional versions of the 'attention-deficit disorder – attention-deficit/hyperactivity disorder' (ADD–ADHD) spectrum are most common. In the British Isles the concepts of 'hyperkinesis' and 'clumsy child' are more popular. In Scandinavia and Central Europe yet other concepts are emerging.

The term *attention deficit disorder* (ADD) (American Psychiatric Association 1980) became obsolete almost before it was introduced, partly because of its inherent tautology: the condition must be either attention deficit *or* attention disorder, not both. One good thing about the diagnostic category ADD was that it allowed of the presence of normoactivity and hypoactivity in children with severe problems of inattention. No study has yet shown that attention deficit is invariably associated with hyperactivity. In fact most children diagnosed as hyperactive are probably not abnormally hyperactive and do not show excessive motor activity in comparison with other children of the same age and sex. However, they are perceived as showing levels of attention and of activity that are inappropriate in a particular setting, in which attending to a task may be required.

Attention-deficit/hyperactivity disorder (ADHD) was the term used in DSM-III-R (American Psychiatric Association 1987). This term is also included in DSM-IV (American Psychiatric Association 1994), here subdivided into cases with predominant hyperactivity/impulsivity, cases with predominant attention deficit, and cases with a

TABLE 6.1
**AD(H)D, hyperkinetic disorders, DAMP, and related disorders:
synonyms and partly overlapping diagnostic labels**

Diagnostic label	Comments
MBD (minimal brain dysfunction)	Once referred to minimal brain *damage* (before about 1960), now to minimal brain *dysfunction*. Almost universally used until about 1980. Still in *clinical* use in many countries. Usually refers to various combinations of attention and motor/learning problems. Inappropriate in that it implies brain dysfunction on phenotypic grounds and in its use of the word 'minimal'.
ADD (attention deficit disorder)	DSM-III label (American Psychiatric Assocation 1980). Widely used in USA. Semantically confusing (should be 'deficit' *or* 'disorder'). Diagnostic criteria very loose and subjective. Pervasiveness not required. With or without motor/learning problems.
ADHD (attention-deficit/hyperactivity disorder)	DSM-III-R label (American Psychiatric Association 1987). Does not account for cases without clear hyperactivity. If categorized as 'severe', then pervasiveness required. With or without motor/learning problems.
ADHD (attention-deficit/hyperactivity disorder, predominantly inattentive type or predominantly hyperactive–impulsive type, or combined type)	DSM-IV label (American Psychiatric Association, 1994). Accounts for cases without clear hyperactivity but does not make it clear how the two types are interrelated (if at all).
DAMP (deficits in attention, motor control, and perception	Accepted term in Nordic countries. Umbrella term covering various combinations of motor control and perceptual problems in conjunction with attentional problems encountered in children who do not show mental retardation or cerebral palsy.
Hyperkinetic disorders	Mostly used in the UK. Usually refers to a syndrome of pervasive hyperactivity. In the past this diagnosis was often made only if there were no major associated conduct problems. The syndrome was then regarded as exceedingly rare. As used in the late 1980s it has become obvious that it is not quite so rare, that conduct disorders often coincide, and that motor/speech/learning problems are the rule.
MND (minor neurological dysfunction)	Sometimes used to describe summary score for minimal motor/neurological problems or 'soft neurological signs'.
Clumsy child syndrome	UK concept. Highlights only one aspect of what is usually a multifaceted syndrome.
Motor–perceptual handicap	Common Scandinavian concept. Attention problems are common in this group.

combination of hyperactivity/impulsivity and attention deficit (Table 6.2). *ADHD* is currently the diagnostic label most often used in the literature. However, its meaning is far from clear and there have been no in-depth population-based studies of the condition. It is generally accepted that attention-deficit syndromes are often associated with other dysfunctions, commonly including problems of motor control, perception, and learning (including memory). Unfortunately this widespread realization is rarely reflected in studies

TABLE 6.2
The DSM-IV diagnostic criteria for attention-deficit/hyperactivity disorder (ADHD)[a]

A. Either (1) or (2)

(1) six (or more) of the following symptoms of **inattention** have persisted for at least 6 months to a degree that is maladaptive and inconsistent with developmental level:

Inattention

    (a) often fails to give close attention to details or makes careless mistakes in schoolwork, work, or other activities

    (b) often has difficulty sustaining attention in tasks or play activities

    (c) often does not seem to listen when spoken to directly

    (d) often does not follow through on instructions and fails to finish schoolwork, chores, or duties in the workplace (not due to oppositional behaviour or failure to understand instructions)

    (e) often has difficulty organizing tasks and activities

    (f) often avoids, dislikes, or is reluctant to engage in tasks that require sustained mental effort (such as schoolwork or homework)

    (g) often loses things necessary for tasks or activities (e.g., toys, school assignments, pencils, books, or tools)

    (h) is often easily distracted by extraneous stimuli

    (i) is often forgetful in daily activities

(2) six (or more) of the following symptoms of **hyperactivity-impulsivity** have persisted for at least 6 months to a degree that is maladaptive and inconsistent with development level:

Hyperactivity

    (a) often fidgets with hands or feet or squirms in seat

    (b) often leaves seat in classroom or in other situations in which remaining seated is expected

    (c) often runs about or climbs excessively in situations in which it is inappropriate (in adolescents or adults, may be limited to subjective feelings of restlessness)

    (d) often has difficulty playing or engaging in leisure activities quietly

    (e) is often "on the go" or often acts as if "driven by a motor"

    (f) often talks excessively

Impulsivity

    (g) often blurts out answers before questions have been completed

    (h) often has difficulty awaiting turn

    (i) often interrupts or intrudes on others (e.g., butts into conversations or games)

B. Some hyperactive-impulsive or inattentive symptoms that caused impairment were present before age 7 years.

C. Some impairment from the symptoms is present in two or more settings (e.g., at school [or work] and at home).

D. There must be clear evidence of clinically significant impairment in social, academic, or occupational functioning.

E. The symptoms do not occur exclusively during the course of a Pervasive Developmental Disorder, Schizophrenia, or other Psychotic Disorder and are not better accounted for by another mental disorder (e.g., Mood Disorder, Anxiety Disorder, Dissociative Disorder, or a Personality Disorder).

Code based on type:

314.01 Attention-Deficit/Hyperactivity Disorder, Combined Type: if both Criteria A1 and A2 are met for the past 6 months

314.00 Attention-Deficit/Hyperactivity Disorder, Predominantly Inattentive Type: if Criterion A1 is met but Criterion A2 is not met for the past 6 months

314.01 Attention-Deficit/Hyperactivity Disorder, Predominantly Hyperactive-Impulsive Type: if Criterion A2 is met but Criterion A1 is not met for the past 6 months

Coding note: For individuals (especially adolescents and adults) who currently have symptoms that no longer meet full criteria, "In Partial Remission" should be specified.

[a]American Psychiatric Association (1994).

of ADHD, and concomitant neuropsychological and motor coordination problems are often overlooked or not reported at all.

Further complication stems from the fact that many other neuropsychiatric syndromes (autism, many of the mental retardation syndromes, and Tourette syndrome, to mention a few) often include elements of the 'MBD synonym group'. At present the most common practice seems to be to diagnose only one syndrome. For instance if a 10-year-old boy has a combination of multiple motor and vocal tics, pervasive attention-deficit problems, and dyslexia, it is quite common to diagnose only Tourette syndrome, even though a case could be made for diagnosing ADHD and dyslexia also. This failure of diagnosis should become less of a problem once there is a general clinical acceptance that comorbidity is common (possibly the rule) in child neuropsychiatry, just as in child neurology.

Attention deficits
ATTENTION-DEFICIT/HYPERACTIVITY DISORDER

Impulsive, distractible, and (sometimes) hyperactive children with normal (or slightly subnormal) intelligence have long been a burdensome problem to themselves, parents, and teachers. More recently school health officers, child psychiatrists, pediatricians, and psychologists have taken an interest in this group. Even so, there is still no consensus as to what should be regarded as the boundaries, much less the aetiology, of syndromes associated with impulsivity and distractibility. At present the label most widely used for syndromes in this field is 'ADHD', the diagnostic criteria of which are shown in Table 6.2. Note that (a) it is not clear that 'attention deficits' (whatever problems this term implies) constitute the basis of the syndrome and (b) hyperactivity is not a salient feature of the behavioural cluster usually associated with so-called attention deficits. In a recent Swedish study ADHD was subdivided into 'clinical' and 'subclinical' variants (Kadesjö and Gillberg 1998), the clinical variant, in individuals meeting the full DSM-IV criteria for ADHD, and the subclinical variant being diagnosed in individuals meeting most but not all of those criteria. Clinical and subclinical ADHD were found in, respectively, 3.7% and 10.3% of 7-year-olds, regardless of any comorbidities.

Disturbances of attention are implied in the syndrome of ADHD. Most of the brain is involved in subserving attentional functions (Colby 1991). Dysfunction of frontal control (Chelune et al. 1986), of the locus coeruleus (Mefford and Potter 1989), and of the striatal (Lou et al. 1990b) and cortico-striato-nigro-thalamo-cortical loop (Voeller 1991) have all been proposed to account for the behavioural and functional problems of affected individuals. An imbalance between dopamine and noradrenaline (norepinephrine) (see e.g. Voeller 1991) and generalized resistance to thyroid hormone (Ciaranello 1993) have also been suggested to be at the neurochemical root of at least some cases of ADHD. So far there is limited evidence for any one of these models.

There is neuropsychological evidence that impulsivity in cognitive functioning may be a salient feature of so-called ADHD. In several experiments Trommer et al. (1991) examined the hypothesis that performance on the go/no-go test is abnormal in ADHD. This test requires the subject to make a simple motor response to one cue (the 'go' stimulus) while inhibiting this response in the presence of another cue (the 'no-go' stimulus). When there are frontal tumours or other frontal brain lesions, results on this test are poor, the most common error being one of commission, resulting from failure to inhibit the response to the 'no-go' stimulus. Omission errors (failure to respond to the 'go' stimulus) suggest inattention. The rate of commission errors may be particularly high in the attention-deficient group without hyperactivity, but it appears to be high in the ADHD group also. The central stimulant methylphenidate in moderate doses (0.15 to 0.30mg/kg) appears to improve performance on the go/no-go test (Trommer et al. 1991).

HYPERKINETIC SYNDROME

In the UK, *hyperkinetic syndrome* or, more recently, *hyperkinetic disorder* (ICD-10 [World Health Organization 1993) has been the preferred term and object of study in the field of disorders associated with motor overactivity, inattentiveness, and impulsivity (Table 6.3). Motor overactivity, as the term *hyperkinetic disorder* suggests, is conceptualized as the most salient feature of this disorder.

In a study by Taylor et al. (1991) a high score on Conners' Classroom Rating Scale (Conners 1969) together with a high score on the Parental Account of Children's Symptoms (PACS) interview (Taylor et al. 1986) provided the basis for a diagnosis of hyperkinetic disorder. In a two-stage epidemiological study of all (*N*=2462) 6- to 7-year-old boys without learning disability in one school district in the UK, using the Rutter teacher and parent scales (Rutter and Graham 1966; Rutter 1967) scales for initial screening, they found a point prevalence for hyperkinetic disorder (roughly equivalent to the ICD-10 diagnosis) of 1.7%. Similarly, Gillberg C et al. (1983) found persistent pervasive hyperkinesis in 1.3% of all 7-year-old boys (*N*=1750) in Göteborg, Sweden. More than 40% of the UK group of children met criteria for conduct disorder whereas fewer than 20% of the boys in the Swedish group met such criteria; the difference might well be accounted for by the stricter criteria for diagnosing conduct disorder in the Swedish study. The findings are also similar to those of another Swedish group studying a population cohort of small-town 6- to 7-year-olds and finding a prevalence of 2.4% with ADHD (Landgren et al. 1996).

DISTINGUISHING ATTENTION DEFICITS WITH OR WITHOUT HYPERACTIVITY FROM CONDUCT DISORDER

In most studies so far ADHD/hyperkinetic disorder/hyperkinetic syndrome and conduct disorder have not been separated well enough to make a decision regarding the extent of overlap of the two 'syndromes' or the nature of any link between them.

Reviewers of research on attention deficits and hyperactivity often conclude that there may not be enough validation of ADHD (or similar constructs) as a separate syndrome, and that attention deficit may better be thought of as a dimensional problem cutting across a number of other syndromes (e.g. autism, anxiety disorders) that may or may not in themselves have considerably better validation (Thorley 1984, Gillberg C and Hellgren 1996).

In many studies symptoms of 'conduct disorder' (verbal and non-verbal aggressiveness, destructiveness, and problems interacting with peers) are not clearly separated from those of 'attention deficits'. Even in DSM-IV some of the symptoms included in the diagnostic set for ADHD are suggestive of problems of conduct rather than of inattention/hyperactivity. It seems clear that much of the literature on ADHD and conduct disorder is confounded by this failure to distinguish the two and to provide accounts of the extent of possible overlap.

TABLE 6.3
The ICD-10 diagnostic criteria for F90 hyperkinetic disorders[a]

Note: The research diagnosis of hyperkinetic disorder requires the definite presence of abnormal levels of inattention, hyperactivity, and restlessness that are pervasive across situations and persistent over time and that are not caused by other disorders such as autism or affective disorders.

G1. *Inattention.* At least six of the following symptoms of inattention have persisted for at least 6 months, to a degree that is maladaptive and inconsistent with the developmental level of the child:
  (1) often fails to give close attention to details, or makes careless errors in schoolwork, work, or other activities;
  (2) often fails to sustain attention in tasks or play activities;
  (3) often appears not to listen to what is being said to him or her;
  (4) often fails to follow through on instructions or to finish schoolwork, chores, or duties in the workplace (not because of oppositional behaviour or failure to understand instructions);
  (5) is often impaired in organizing tasks and activities;
  (6) often avoids or strongly dislikes tasks, such as homework, that require sustained mental effort;
  (7) often loses things necessary for certain tasks or activities, such as school assignments, pencils, books, toys, or tools;
  (8) is often easily distracted by external stimuli;
  (9) is often forgetful in the course of daily activities.

G2. *Hyperactivity.* At least three of the following symptoms of hyperactivity have persisted for at least 6 months, to a degree that is maladaptive and inconsistent with the developmental level of the child:
  (1) often fidgets with hands or feet or squirms on seat;
  (2) leaves seat in classroom or in other situations in which remaining seated is expected;
  (3) often runs about or climbs excessively in situations in which it is inappropriate (in adolescents or adults, only feelings of restlessness may be present);
  (4) is often unduly noisy in playing or has difficulty in engaging quietly in leisure activities;
  (5) exhibits a persistent pattern of excessive motor activity that is not substantially modified by social context or demands.

G3. *Impulsivity.* At least one of the following symptoms of impulsivity has persisted for at least 6 months, to a degree that is maladaptive and inconsistent with the developmental level of the child:
  (1) often blurts out answers before questions have been completed;
  (2) often fails to wait in lines or await turns in games or group situations;
  (3) often interrupts or intrudes on others (e.g. butts into others' conversations or games);
  (4) often talks excessively without appropriate response to social constraints.

G4. Onset of the disorder is no later than the age of 7 years.

G5. *Pervasiveness.* The criteria should be met for more than a single situation, e.g. the combination of inattention and hyperactivity should be present both at home and at school, or at both school and another setting where children are observed, such as a clinic. (Evidence for cross-situationality will ordinarily require information from more than one source; parental reports about classroom behaviour, for instance, are unlikely to be sufficient.)

G6. The symptoms in G1–G3 cause clinically significant distress or impairment in social, academic, or occupational functioning.

G7. The disorder does not meet the criteria for pervasive developmental disorders (F84.–), manic episode (F30.–), depressive episode (F32.–), or anxiety disorders (F41.–).

[a]World Health Organization (1993).

For instance, many of the follow-up studies in the USA of children with ADHD who have been treated with stimulants may have included disproportionate numbers of individuals with a proclivity for criminal activity (Gittelman et al. 1985, Mannuzza et al. 1989), making it difficult to tease out the extent to which treatment has affected the attentional dysfunction

TABLE 6.4
The DSM-IV diagnostic criteria for 315.4 developmental coordination disorder[a]

A. Performance in daily activities that require motor coordination is substantially below that expected given the person's chronological age and measured intelligence. This may be manifested by marked delays in achieving motor milestones (e.g., walking, crawling, sitting), dropping things, "clumsiness", poor performance in sports, or poor handwriting.

B. The disturbance in Criterion A significantly interferes with academic achievement or activities of daily living.

C. The disturbance is not due to a general medical condition (e.g., cerebral palsy, hemiplegia, or muscular dystrophy) and does not meet criteria for a Pervasive Developmental Disorder.

D. If Mental Retardation is present, the motor difficulties are in excess of those usually associated with it.

Coding note: If a general medical (e.g., neurological) condition or sensory deficit is present, code the condition on Axis III.

[a]American Psychiatric Association (1994).

or the conduct problems or both. Similar lines of reasoning may well account for some of the discrepant findings in the follow-up literature, in which children from New York who have 'ADHD' seem to have a greater risk of criminal behaviour than children in Canada who have 'ADHD' (Klein and Mannuzza 1991, Weiss 1991).

Deficits in attention, motor control, and perception (DAMP)
DEFINITION OF DAMP

In a survey of the literature on so-called MBD (Gillberg C and Rasmussen 1982) it became apparent that the problems included were mostly various combinations of perceptual, motor, and attention deficits in children without mental retardation or cerebral palsy. The concept of DAMP (deficits in attention, motor control, and perception) was therefore introduced in the mid-1980s to cover most of the syndromes previously referred to as MBD but without implying any aetiology (Gillberg IC 1987). DAMP has now been accepted as an umbrella label in the Nordic countries (Airaksinen et al. 1990).

DAMP is the combination of pervasive attention deficit (ADD, or attention-deficit disorder) – roughly equivalent to 'clinical' or 'subclinical' ADHD – and motor-coordination/perception dysfunction (MPD, motor–perception dysfunction) – equivalent to developmental coordination disorder (DCD) (Table 6.4) – in any child of normal or low-normal intelligence who does not meet the criteria for cerebral palsy. This syndrome is referred to as ADDMPD in Table 6.5. There are also children with ADD only and MPD only. Such children, who do not have DAMP, may present diagnostic problems (Fig. 6.1).

To be classified as an attention deficit, a problem has to be present in several observational settings, such as home, school, and peer group. Reliable and valid rating scales are available. The most widely used is that of Conners (1969). The minimum requirement for diagnosing attention deficit is that the child is rated as abnormal on a scale of this kind by at least two independent observers (e.g. parent and teacher) and that the developmental history and clinical examination yield findings consistent with the diagnosis. Not all children with attention deficit are hyperactive. Some are rather hypoactive and many fluctuate between

TABLE 6.5
Diagnosis of DAMP and its components

DAMP

MPDADD   A. ADD as manifested by
                (a) severe problems in at least one or moderate problems in at least two of the following areas: attention span, activity level, vigilance, and ability to sit still, and
                (b) cross-situational problems in the areas mentioned under (a), documented at two or more of the following: psychiatric, neurological, or psychological evaluation, and maternal report.
        B. MPD as manifested by marked
                (a) gross motor dysfunction according to detailed neurological examination (see Rasmussen et al. 1983), or
                (b) fine motor dysfunction according to detailed neurological examination (see Rasmussen et al. 1983) or
                (c) perceptual dysfunction according to testing with SCSIT (Ayres 1974, and defined in Gillberg C and Rasmussen 1982).
        C. Problems not accounted for or associated with MR or CP.
        All of A–C have to be met.
        Severity is rated as follows: severe MPDADD (s-MPDADD) is diagnosed in a child who meets all of the criteria A–C and in addition meets all of the subcriteria (a)–(c) under B, and in addition shows specific language disorder; mild to moderate MPDADD (m-MPDADD) is diagnosed in all other cases meeting criteria for MPDADD.

ADD   A. ADD as for MPDADD
      B. Problems not accounted for or associated with MPD, MR, or CP.
      Both A and B have to be met.

MPD   A. MPD as for MPDADD
      B. Problems not accounted for or associated with ADD, MR, or CP.
      Both A and B have to be met.

ADD, attention-deficit disorder; CP, cerebral palsy; DAMP, deficits in attention, motor control, and perception; MPD, motor–perception dysfunction; MR, mental retardation; SCSIT, Southern California Sensory Integration Test.

hyper- and hypoactivity. Many are best described as disorganized in their activity. This is one of the many reasons why the label *hyperactivity* as a blanket term is inadequate.

The problems of motor coordination are usually best described as immature performance on a number of different neurological/neuromotor tests such as diadochokinesia, finger tapping, alternating movements, standing and skipping on one leg, walking on the sides of the feet, and various tests of fine motor performance such as tracing in a maze, cutting out paper, etc. These problems show up in everyday settings and are evident as overall clumsiness, poor table manners, difficulties dressing and tying shoe-laces, and difficulties learning to draw, write, ride a bicycle, swim, ski, and skate. Many children with such motor-coordination problems are poor at games, particularly ball games and especially if the balls used are small. The Touwen manual for examination of the child with minor neurological dysfunction (Touwen 1979) is helpful to the clinician wanting to acquire the skills necessary to perform an age-adequate neuromotor evaluation in this field. However, exact age norms are not available in this manual. There are a number of different other guides available (Denckla 1985, Whitmore and Bax 1986, Gillberg IC 1987, Michelsson and Ylinen 1987), all of which have some validity.

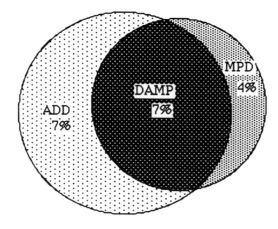

Fig. 6.1. Relation between ADD (attention-deficit disorder) and MPD (motor–perception dysfunction [roughly equivalent to DCD; see Table 6.4]). Percentages refer to approximate prevalences in the total population (Gillberg C 1983). (After Gillberg C 1997, by permission.)

Diagnosing ADD/ADHD and MPD presents some problems. One of the most important is the difficulty of mapping the behavioural descriptions onto relevant neurological substrates and behaviours. Thus, for example, a neurological model would discriminate locomotor hyperactivity, akathisia, and stereotypy, all of which could 'result' in behavioural hyperactivity. Akathisia is characterized by restless, fidgety, overactive movements and is accompanied by an inner restlessness. Exploratory locomotor hyperactivity, on the other hand, is characterized by a high level of walking about (perhaps even running), particularly in a new environment. Stereotypy involves high-frequency repetitive movements. This is just one of many possible examples of the ways in which attention-deficit/hyperactivity signs and syndromes may elude objective definition and remain in the realm of subjectively defined clinical syndromes, in spite of ever more specific requirements for diagnosis in the diagnostic manuals.

The perceptual problems appear on formal tests (such as the performance part of the WISC [Wechsler 1967] [block design, picture completion, and object assembly are often problematic], the SCSIT [Southern California Sensory Integration Test] [Ayres 1974], and specific tests of perception that may vary from country to country). There are often perceptual problems in several domains (visual, auditory, tactile, etc.), but most tests focus on visual-perceptual tasks and it is sometimes difficult to determine whether one is dealing with a pure visual-perceptual problem, a fine motor problem, a dysfunction of eye–hand coordination, or some combination of these. Clinically the perceptual problems often show up in impaired perception of form, space, and shape; in immaturity in drawing and writing; and in severe problems acquiring automatic reading skills. Disturbance of body image (with difficulty judging the location of the body and its parts in space, possibly contributing to problems such as difficulty judging the appropriate distance from other people during social interactions) is also a common consequence of various perceptual deficits.

Children with DAMP often also show various types of speech and language problems, some of which can be regarded as motor problems (some articulation problems, hypotonia of the mouth, and certain kinds of stuttering), others of which can be regarded as minor auditory perceptual problems (some articulation problems, failure to adjust volume and pitch

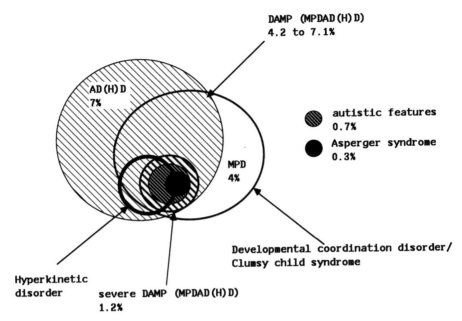

DAMP (MPDAD(H)D)
4.2 to 7.1%

AD(H)D
7%

MPD
4%

● autistic features
0.7%

● Asperger syndrome
0.3%

Developmental coordination disorder/
Clumsy child syndrome

Hyperkinetic
disorder   severe DAMP (MPDAD(H)D)
1.2%

Fig. 6.2. Overlap of (mild to moderate, and severe) DAMP (AD[H]D + MPD), autistic features, and Asperger syndrome (data from Gillberg C 1983 and Gillberg IC and Gillberg C 1989) and possible overlap with hyperkinetic syndrome and clumsy child syndrome.
(From *Clinical Child Neuropsychiatry,* Gillberg C, 1995, Cambridge: Cambridge University Press, by permission.)

of voice to auditory feedback demands), and still others of which must be seen as being related to some more basic and specific language deficit (overall delay in language development, semantic–pragmatic disorder).

DAMP (ADDMPD) can be subdivided into *severe cases* – namely those in which there are dysfunctions in all five of the following areas: (1) attention, (2) gross motor, (3) fine motor, (4) perceptual, and (5) speech/language – and *mild cases* – namely those in which only some of these dysfunctions are present.

It is quite common for children with severe DAMP to show comorbid features of autism and even the full-blown clinical picture of Asperger syndrome. The interrelations between (mild and severe) DAMP, AD(H)D, MPD, and autistic features (including Asperger syndrome) are shown in Figure 6.2.

An adequate working diagnosis in severe cases (i.e. a formulation in diagnostic terms that can serve as a basis for intervention suggestions) requires the collaboration of the paediatrician (or a child psychiatrist) with a clinical neuropsychologist and, optimally, a speech therapist, all of whom should make independent evaluations and then combine their data to reach a consensus. In mild to moderate cases, the paediatrician (or school doctor) will have to do most of the diagnostic work themselves, considering the high prevalence of the disorder and the relative lack of diagnostic resources.

EPIDEMIOLOGY

Various Swedish studies (Gillberg C et al. 1983; Landgren et al. 1996; Kadesjö and Gillberg 1998) have shown that DAMP (ADDMPD) in a severe form is present in about 1.2% of all 7-year old children, and milder variants are present in another 3 to 6%. Though children with DAMP are generally of slightly lower social class and IQ than in the general population, they can come from any social class and some have very high IQs.

SEX RATIO

Many more boys than girls have DAMP. According to the longitudinal Swedish study, the overall male:female ratio is about 2:1 to 3:1, cohorts of severe cases showing an even stronger skewing (Gillberg C et al. 1983). However, boys' brains and girls' brains develop in accordance with different schemata. Thus in children not yet of school age, boys do better than girls on some skills requiring good visuomotor performance, whereas in all other respects (except sheer physical strength) girls tend to develop faster than boys. Therefore considering boys and girls as one group will inevitably lead to boys' outnumbering girls in any epidemiological study defining DAMP on the basis of a single cut-off age. If boys were compared with boys of the same age, and girls were compared with girls of the same age, the ratio of boys with the disorder to girls with the disorder might be found to be less high than is generally thought.

BACKGROUND FACTORS

According to Swedish studies, among all cases of DAMP the condition is 'idiopathic' in about a tenth, is mainly hereditary in about a third, is mainly associated with pre-, peri-, or postnatal brain damage in another third, and is due to some combination of hereditary and potentially brain damaging factors in a fifth (Gillberg C and Rasmussen 1982). A recent study of hyperactivity in twins is compatible with a model for the development of DAMP in which hereditary factors are of predominant importance (Goodman and Stevenson 1989a,b). Also, twin studies of dyslexia (Stevenson and Graham 1993) suggest high genetic loading for reading and spelling problems – and a strong link between dyslexia and hyperactivity (Stevenson 1991) – suggesting that the whole of the clinical DAMP complex might have even stronger genetic contributions than previously appreciated.

Whatever the basic cause, there is considerable direct and indirect evidence that DAMP (and some of the ADHD or hyperkinetic syndromes) is associated with a lack of or deficiency in automatization skills, both in attentional and motor domains (Lou et al. 1984, 1989, 1990a,b; Gillberg C 1992). It is not that motor functions in themselves are qualitatively abnormal (as is the case, for instance, in cerebral palsy) in most cases. The child can perform the particular motor action required (e.g. hopping on one leg), but only if conscious cognitive control is exercised (e.g. counting out loud 'one', 'two', 'three', 'four' etc. in order not to stop the repeated action of hopping up and down). Thus, it would be inappropriate to be speaking of abnormal motor function, but quite appropriate to infer abnormal *control* of motor function.

CLINICAL COURSE AND OUTCOME

According to one major Swedish study (Gillberg IC 1987 and Hellgren et al. 1993), there are about as many children with attention problems alone as there are children with DAMP, and there are only about half as many children with motor–perception dysfunction alone as in either of the other two categories. Follow-up studies suggest that it is the children with a combination of problems who require treatment and interventions of various kinds, and that broadly speaking the outcome for the other two groups is much better. Also, the identification of 'pervasively hyperkinetic' children (Sandberg et al. 1978), as opposed to 'situationally hyperkinetic' children, has revealed that motor–perceptual and speech–language problems are almost universal in the former group, a finding that argues for the clinical separation of a diagnostic category including the combination of attention and motor–perceptual dysfunction from a distinct category or categories including only one of the two types of dysfunction.

Situational attention deficit or hyperactivity can be a sign of psychological problems specific to a particular situation. Follow-up of children with situational as distinct from pervasive hyperkinesis (Gillberg IC and Gillberg C 1988) has shown that the outcome over 6 years is much better and not too dissimilar to that of children without attention deficits of any kind.

Isolated motor–perceptual difficulties sometimes cause considerable academic problems, particularly during the early school years. Nevertheless, limited systematic follow-up and clinical experience suggest that the outcome for this group, also, is usually considerably better than for children with the combination of attention problems and motor–perceptual difficulties.

In what follows we refer often to the longitudinal study of more than 100 children with DAMP (and comparison children without DAMP) followed from early childhood to age 20 years in Göteborg, Sweden (e.g. Gillberg IC 1987). However, the account also takes into consideration the considerable data bank that exists in related fields (e.g. Taylor 1986).

Infancy
Retrospective analysis of case histories of children diagnosed as having DAMP (or ADHD) at age 4 to 6 years provides important clues to the clinical picture of DAMP in infancy.

As regards infant development, there may be at least two clinically distinct subgroups of children with DAMP: (1) the hyperactive group and (2) the hypo- or normoactive group. Infants in the hyperactive group usually have sleep problems, feeding difficulties, 'colicky' stomach pains, and a generally high level of motor activity even from the first months of life. They often start walking before 10 months of age. From then on (and sometimes even before), parents often have to change their domestic habits dramatically: anything movable has to be removed not only from the level of the child's reach, but from the child's view.

Hypoactive or normoactive infants with DAMP are regarded by parents as 'good', sometimes even 'exceptionally good'. Some of them show repetitive behaviours from a very early age (head rolling, even head banging, and repetitive sounds).

Some studies have tried to relate early visual recognition memory to later cognitive functioning (Bornstein and Sigman 1986). Convincing evidence is now accumulating that visual recognition memory may indeed be a potent predictor of later cognitive and academic success (Benasich and Bejar 1992). In addition, poor auditory temporal processing (i.e. poor performance on tests designed to monitor the ability to rapidly process changing non-verbal auditory stimuli) at about 6 months of age may be related to later problems of the DAMP/dyslexia type (Benasich and Tallal 1993). These experimental findings may well be closely linked to the inability or decreased ability to attend to relevant auditory stimuli (and sometimes visual stimuli) that is very often reported by parents of young children who later develop the full-blown clinical picture of DAMP, attention disorders without motor clumsiness, or learning disorders, including so-called dyslexia.

The preschool years

From about the age when the children start to walk, the two subgroups often appear to be indistinguishable for a number of years. Children in both groups now appear hyperactive, or at least inattentive. Parents may worry because their children just do not seem to listen, and they have noticed that shouting may be the only way of attracting the children's attention. Motor-coordination problems may surface as early as age 2 to 4 years, but are often obscured by the high activity level and lack of appropriate fear, which is also very common. Speech and language are delayed in about two-thirds of affected children, but only in about half of these is the delay severe enough to warrant consultation. Towards the end of the preschool years the child's unwillingness to draw and paint and the constant clashes in games with age-peers usually become a major source of concern, and also of increasing scolding.

The early school years

Many children with DAMP manage fairly well through infancy and the preschool years, but their behavioural and academic performance almost invariably deteriorates during the first few years at school. They are likely to have difficulties concentrating, sitting still, listening, interacting in an age-appropriate fashion with peers, and participating in games and physical education, and difficulties, sometimes almost insurmountable, in acquiring basic automatic reading and writing skills. In the great majority of children with DAMP all of these problems peak at ages 7 to 10 years, upsetting the child, parents, and teachers. The problems are especially difficult to cope with if no one involved has been told that the child has a disabling condition and is not just going through a bad streak of naughtiness.

If a group of children with DAMP is identified at around age 6 years (as was done in the Göteborg studies), by definition all will have motor-control problems and all will have pervasive attention deficits at that age. By about age 10 years only about half the children in the group will still have motor difficulties, and the attentional problems will also have subsided considerably. Unfortunately, however, the proportion of children with psychiatric or behavioural problems will have increased to 80%, from just over 60%, and 80% of all the children will have dyslexia or dysgraphia. In a comparison group of age-peers without DAMP these rates will be very much lower.

Preadolescence and adolescence

Many preadolescent and adolescent children with DAMP experience persistent difficulties concentrating. Many are described by their teachers (and sometimes parents) as daydreaming. Dyslexia is a very common complaint. The motor clumsiness is often (though not always) less conspicuous than it used to be. In several studies Hadders-Algra and her group found

146

evidence that minor neurological dysfunction decreases with the onset of puberty in some children but tends to persist in the subgroup whose dysfunction was believed to be caused by perinatal (rather than constitutional) factors (Hadders-Algra et al. 1992, Soorani-Lunsing et al. 1993). Other follow-up studies have not provided support for this idea, but rather have suggested that minor neurological dysfunction may subside before puberty and not change much in adolescence (Hellgren et al. 1993). There is a considerable risk for various types of psychiatric problems. Furthermore if children with DAMP attend a clinic for the first time in their teens, there is a great risk that the psychiatric disorder will be seen as primary and as a new problem rather than being specifically associated with DAMP. If this happens the child's problems run the risk of not being seen in perspective, and inappropriate interventions may well be suggested.

COMORBID BEHAVIOURAL PROBLEMS IN DAMP

On the whole, three main groups of comorbid emotional or behavioural problems in DAMP can be discerned: (1) depression, (2) conduct disorders, and (3) autistic traits. Quite often there are other behaviour or psychiatric problems too, including tics, anxiety, and so-called psychosomatic symptoms (headaches, gastrointestinal symptoms, etc.), but these do not appear to be more common than in the general population of children without DAMP (Gillberg C 1983).

Depression and feelings of low self-esteem are common even during the earliest school years but appear to peak around age 10 years, when they often coincide with various kinds of conduct problems. The child with DAMP often becomes increasingly aware of their 'otherness' during the school years. Feeling that 'there is nobody who can provide help', the child often becomes depressed and may even contemplate suicide (which at this age is decidedly uncommon in groups without DAMP). In the midst of depression there is also often much anger and resentment, which may show outwardly as a clinical conduct disorder. The risk is then that the child's predicament is mistaken for antisocial problems that may lead to psychopathy. Personal interview alone with the child will soon reveal, however, that this is (usually) not a hardened criminal-to-be, but rather an immature and sad child who needs to have his basic learning problems recognized. Nevertheless there are also cases of children with DAMP and severe conduct problems for whom the outlook with respect to antisocial activities, including criminality, is very gloomy (Thorley 1984, Taylor et al. 1991, Gillberg C 1992).

The conduct problems encountered in DAMP can be of any kind: stealing, fire-setting, lying, bullying, running away from home, and drug or alcohol abuse. In the preschool years there is often considerable aggression towards other children in connection with inadvertent disruption of play and games. About 10% of all children with DAMP already show severe conduct disorders when they start school. The figure increases to about 50% at about age 10 years but seems to fall back to about 30% during the teenage years.

At least half of children with severe DAMP also have autistic traits: (a) motor stereotypies and stereotypic activities including hand-flapping, finger-flicking, finger-picking, body rocking, head-banging, repetitive and monotonous production of sounds (in an almost tic-like fashion); (b) preoccupations with certain topics, objects, or parts of objects; (c) peculiarities of language (pronoun reversal, repetitive questioning, and immaturities of grammar and poor sentence structure); (d) abnormalities in the production of speech (abnormalities of pitch and volume, odd prosody, and little speech); (e) nonverbal communication problems, with a restricted repertoire of gesticulation and mimicry; (f) occasionally the full-blown clinical picture of semantic–pragmatic disorder; and (g) problems of social interaction similar to those seen in autism, but milder. 'Naive' forms of empathy deficits are often prominent, with, for example, children asking embarassing questions of people they know in front of strangers. Children with mild DAMP usually do not exhibit major features of the autistic type. It is sometimes impossible to make a clear distinction between DAMP and Asperger syndrome (Ehlers and Gillberg 1993).

In adolescents with DAMP there is a high rate of personality disorder, including a number of such disorders invariably involving social withdrawal or negativism (paranoid, schizotypal, schizoid, avoidant, or obsessive–compulsive personality disorders) (Hellgren et al. 1994). It also appears that bipolar disorders may emerge at a rate considerably higher than in the general population.

LONG-TERM FOLLOW-UP

By late adolescence and early adult life quite a few individuals who once had DAMP appear to have overcome most of the severe problems. However, at this age at least half of all individuals with DAMP have severe persisting problems of some kind. Criminal offences seem to be common, as do major psychiatric problems requiring inpatient or outpatient psychiatric treatment. Reading and writing disabilities, quite uncommon in adults who have never had DAMP, may be present in 30 to 50% of all individuals who once had the condition. Even though the motor-control problems appear to have the best prognosis of all, a substantial minority of affected individuals (probably about 1 in 5) continue to have important problems with motor clumsiness well into adulthood.

Less is known about outcome in ADD, ADHD, and hyperkinetic disorder, partly because there have been no really long-term controlled *population* studies of these categories and also because most follow-up studies of children with such diagnoses have been of individuals who had received specific treatments, especially with central stimulants. There is some evidence (Gillberg C et al. 1997) that such treatment may improve the long-term outcome and that therefore follow-up studies of treated children may not reveal the natural history of the basic problems.

The hyperkinetic syndrome

In an Isle of Wight population study in the 1960s, the 'pure' hyperkinetic syndrome was encountered in fewer than 1 in 2000 10- to 11-year-olds without 'neuroepileptic' disorders who were attending normal schools (Rutter et al. 1970). In marked contrast 7% of all children with neuroepileptic disorders and children excluded from school because of severe mental subnormality were considered to have a hyperkinetic syndrome. The notion that hyperkinesis is extremely uncommon has lingered in Europe, in spite of the fact that in the USA several per cent of all school children have been described as hyperactive/hyperkinetic (Wender 1971). It was not until the early 1980s, when a reanalysis of the Isle of Wight material revealed that about 2% of the population showed hyperactive behaviour both at home and at school, that the notion that hyperactivity – even in its pervasive forms – is a common problem in school-age children became more accepted. Until then European children had tended to be diagnosed as hyperactive/hyperkinetic only if hyperactivity was their only (or at least main) problem. In clinical practice there is very often overlap between hyperactivity/attention problems and conduct disorders. It is now becoming more common to make dual and triple diagnoses in child psychiatry. As a consequence, rates of hyperkinetic syndromes reported from Europe and the USA are less discrepant, though there does still appear to be a difference, which is more difficult to account for.

The concept of hyperactivity has become linked with that of attention deficit. It is not yet clear that attention deficit underlies hyperactivity in the majority of cases. Attention deficits are quite often associated with normoactive behaviour, hypoactivity, or fluctuating degrees of activity. The hyperkinetic syndrome as a disorder of pervasive behavioural problems (Taylor et al. 1991) has come a long way from its anecdotal and flimsy status 20 years ago (see Table 6.3). In distinctiveness, reliability, and validity, it is not yet anywhere near the status of other child psychiatric diagnoses such as anorexia nervosa, elective mutism, school refusal, or autism. In the next 10 years pervasive hyperkinesis may emerge as a distinct clinical entity. However, it does not appear to be the umbrella term needed in the field of DAMP.

Other clinical entities with attention deficits as an important element in the differential diagnosis

In many neuropsychiatric disorders attention deficits constitute an important part of the dysfunction in everyday life. Epilepsy of various kinds often goes together with attention disorders, but the treatment is mainly directed at reducing the frequency of epileptic seizures. In other situations the attention deficit is such a dominating problem that the underlying disorder is diagnosed extremely late, or not at all – for example in certain chromosomal aberrations (XYY, XXY, and the fragile X syndrome) and neurocutaneous disorders (neurofibromatosis and tuberous sclerosis). Progressive neurological disorders can present with attention deficits. The clinician must decide in each individual case whether the developmental history or the clinical findings indicate a need for extended medical examination.

Many clinics follow a policy of choosing the most 'severe' diagnosis that is applicable in a given case. If, for example, a child fulfils criteria for autistic disorder, ADHD (or DAMP), and moderate mental retardation (a child with fragile X syndrome would be an example of this), the diagnosis 'ADHD' is often omitted. In a child with mild mental retardation in combination with ADHD (e.g. a child with fetal alcohol syndrome), the diagnosis 'mental retardation' is often regarded as the predominant one and ADHD not only may not be diagnosed but may even be overlooked. In clinical practice it is not uncommon that a diagnosis of DAMP/ADHD is made in the preschool or early school age with an indication that the child also has 'autistic traits', and that long-term follow-up shows that these autistic traits tend to dominate the clinical picture to the extent that a 'new' diagnosis of, for example, Asperger syndrome or high-functioning autism must be made. Clinicians must be aware of these shortcomings of diagnostic policies and also must be prepared to explain them to the parents (and the youngster), who otherwise are left puzzled and embarrassed.

TOURETTE SYNDROME

The case of overlapping neuropsychiatric diagnoses is clearly illustrated in many individuals with Tourette syndrome. The diagnosis of this syndrome rests solely on the presence of a combination of vocal and motor tics of a certain degree over a certain period of time, irrespective of cognitive level and the presence or absence of other neuropsychiatric symptoms. In fact about 60% of children with Tourette syndrome also fulfil criteria for ADHD, often with deficits of impulse control as a predominant feature (Comings 1990). In many, if not most, cases ADHD is present from infancy or early childood and the tics do not appear until late preschool or early school years. In such cases a diagnosis of ADHD may thus have to be 'changed' to a diagnosis of Tourette syndrome. The parents may ask themselves (or the physician) if the earlier diagnosis of ADHD was wrong.

Furthermore, there is a considerable overlap between the diagnoses of Tourette syndrome and obsessive–compulsive disorder. It is our clinical impression that not a few children with Tourette syndrome show signs of empathy deficit and that some of them in adolescence meet criteria for Asperger syndrome. However, most individuals with Tourette syndrome do not have the kind of severe and pervasive empathy deficit ecnountered in Asperger syndrome.

A proportion of children with Tourette syndrome exhibit learning disabilities of a kind similar to learning disabilities in ADHD and DAMP. According to some investigators difficulties with mathematics may be particularly common in Tourette syndrome (Comings 1990).

Case reports (all names have been changed)

ADAM, AGE 5 YEARS

Adam was referred to a child psychiatrist by a paediatrician because of problems of inattention, 'not listening', and 'destructiveness'.

He was the second child born to healthy parents. His mother had had reading problems in the first 3 years of school. She described Adam's father as having difficulties concentrating and as having had a history of mild to moderate problems of adjustment in adolescence. Both parents have been employed full-time for many years. A sister 3 years older than Adam has 'no problems' and is a 'child with straight As'. The pregnancy was uneventful until week 32, when Adam was born after heavy maternal bleeding. His birthweight was 1520g. He remained in hospital for 5 weeks, during which his mother spent almost all her time with him or close to him.

His first 6 months of life, including the neonatal period, were relatively uncomplicated. Thereafter he had severe sleep problems and feeding problems for more than a year. He started walking unsupported at 16 months. He was referred by the nurse at the well-baby clinic for auditory evaluation at 20 months, with a suspected severe hearing deficit. 'No spoken language and inattentiveness' were the reasons for referral. Mild bilateral hearing deficits and serous otitis media were diagnosed, but follow-up 2 months later revealed normal hearing and normal ear status. He said his first words another 2 months later. He had relatively good language development during his third year but tended not to listen when spoken to, being always preoccupied with some repetitive action or just running about. At 4 years of age he would not attend during routine visual examination.

In the year preceding referral his mother had become more concerned. She felt that something was wrong and that Adam's inability to concentrate and his tendency to bump into things and to cause things to break or come apart were his major problems. The day nursery, where he spent about 6 hours every weekday, had had to hire a special assistant in order to be able to keep him in the group. He had one good friend, with whom he would play for an hour or so but who had tended to tire of Adam in the past few months. The special assistant had suggested that the mother seek help at the local child psychiatric clinic. The mother felt that she was somehow to blame for all the problems.

On examination, though Adam was calm at first, seemingly intent and listening to the questions put to him by the child psychiatrist, some of his responses were just a little 'off', as though he had just been thinking about something else. He appeared to be of normal intelligence. After only about 5 minutes he started exploring the room, not really in a hyperactive way, but with the effect that 15 minutes later most of the things on the doctor's desk were on the floor, a curtain had fallen down, and Adam was lying on the floor staring up at the ceiling. He almost fell asleep but then rose and walked into the corridor where he could be heard exploring adjoining doors, bookshelves, and a nearby office. According to his mother this behaviour was typical.

On motor examination he was markedly clumsy and could not manage to hop, to stand on one leg, or to walk on his heels, but otherwise neurodevelopmental and neurological examination yielded normal results. His score on the brief Conners parent scale was 19 and on the brief Conners teacher scale 18 (range 0 to 30 on both), indicating clear deviance with regard to attention and hyperactivity. He did not score on the items of restlessness or overactivity.

His developmental quotient on the Griffiths scale (Griffiths 1970) was 94, with a relatively even level except that his result on the subtest for eye–hand coordination was at the level of a 3-year-old. He could only count to 3 and could not write his own name.

Adam met the criteria for DAMP (and, hence, also for DCD) (see Table 6.5). He also met full criteria for ADHD (predominantly inattentive type). He and his parents received information about the diagnosis and about the fact that neither of them was 'to blame' for the problems. At a separate meeting, his mother and the child psychiatrist informed his assistant and the head teacher at the day nursery of the diagnosis. Written information about DAMP was distributed. The need for a calm and well-structured environment was highlighted. Follow-up 6 months later by the child psychiatrist was agreed upon.

BILL, AGE 10 YEARS

Bill was referred to the child psychiatrist for overactive and disruptive behaviour. He attended fourth grade (that is, the normal level for his age) and his teacher had told Bill's mother that she felt something had to be done and that Bill might need psychotherapy for his 'acting out' behaviours. She said she had seen other children with this type of problem and that psychological trauma had often been at the root of it. The mother felt shocked by the teacher's suggestion, as she thought that Bill had an excellent relationship with his family. True, he was overactive, impulsive, and had difficulties keeping a friend because 'something' always happened to start fights, but she resisted the notion that her son was 'emotionally disturbed'.

151

Bill was an only child, born to healthy parents. His intrauterine and neonatal periods had been uneventful, and his birthweight was 3500g. His mother remembered that he had been very active in the womb, kicking constantly, but she had not found this alarming. Bill's father used to joke about how he himself had been considered the clown of his group of peers when he was at school, and that he had hated school because he felt that sitting still was extremely boring. The father now had his own firm and worked as a mason. Bill's mother, a qualified nurse, worked part-time in a geriatric day centre. Except for the father's history there were no indications of familial/hereditary problems that might be related to the boy's behaviour.

Bill came to the clinic with his mother, and they were first interviewed together. While seated, he 'nervously' moved his hands about, pulled at his fingers, swayed his left foot back and forth, and tapped his right one. His head often moved from side to side as though he were listening to the rhythm of some pop music (which he was not). He looked around the room in a jittery manner as though constantly distracted by something. He responded to all the questions and often interrupted before the doctor had had a chance to complete a question, and often also when not addressed. In spite of the restless motor activity he seemed to be able to concentrate reasonably on all the topics raised. His mother confirmed that he had some social problems, particularly when it came to taking the perspective of another person.

His motor performance was slightly immature, particularly with regard to fine motor skills, but the examining doctor did not consider that a diagnosis in this domain was warranted. Bill's scores on the Conners parent and teacher scales were 20 and 24, respectively. His scores on the items relating to attention and distractibility were not deviant. The mother brought a written report from the teacher in which she stated that Bill had such problems sitting still and was so impulsive that very little in the way of academic progress had been achieved in the past year.

His behaviour was very similar when he was examined by the neuropsychologist, who was alone with him in the room. Bill's IQ on the WISC–III (Wechsler 1992) was 110, with very poor scores on the digit span and digit symbol (coding) subtests. He had bursts of facial tics while being tested. Afterwards his morther confirmed that ever since the age of about 8 years he had shown such tics when under stress, or sometimes even when completely relaxed.

Bill was diagnosed as having ADHD (predominantly hyperactive/impulsive type) and chronic motor tic disorder. He did not meet criteria for DCD and, hence, not for DAMP. Bill and his mother were told of the diagnoses and their implications. Bill said that he felt the description of ADHD applied almost perfectly to himself and seemed relieved that his 'nervousness' and fidgetiness had some sort of 'explanation'. The psychiatrist, psychologist, and mother together drew up a preliminary rehabilitation plan. This would involve talking to the teacher at a special conference, hopefully providing some extra assistance in the school, and helping Bill with his homework. The possibility of medication with a stimulant was discussed, but the decision was postponed for several months so that any effects of a change in the educational setting could be evaluated.

CHARLES, AGE 13 YEARS
Charles's mother contacted the child psychiatrist because she felt her son was depressed.

Charles was the third child born to a father with diabetes mellitus type 1 and a mother who had been treated for hypertension in pregnancy with a beta-blocker. Charles had two elder brothers, both healthy in all respects, and a younger sister, 5 years of age, who had recently been evaluated because of overall slow development. She had been found to be just mildly delayed in most areas, but had not been diagnosed as having mental retardation. Charles had been born at term, weighing 2950g and 48 cm in length. All his siblings, also born at term, had weighed more than 3600g. Thus he was slightly light for date at birth.

Charles had always been something of a 'dreamer' and had been slower in language development than his brothers. He was described as 'cautious' and had not learned how to ride a bicycle until he was 8 years old, or to swim until he was almost 10. He had always found excuses for not participating in physical education in school and he would not go along on outing days, especially not in the winter. He had not spoken to his parents about the reasons for this, but his mother knew that he could not skate or ski and that he would not even let his brothers – who were good at both – try to teach him how. He did not have any friends and preferred to play with children several years his junior. In spite of some difficulties with spelling and 'mild concentration difficulties' according to the mother, he loved reading, mostly fiction, and he had even read quite a number of psychological thrillers that he had borrowed from his mother. His mother felt he was always 'somewhere else' and reported that he had to be addressed several times before he would respond. During the past year Charles's mother had noticed that he had gradually become more irritable and depressed and would often (especially during the last 4 weeks or so) cry over little things or for no apparent reason at all.

The physical and neuromotor examination revealed normal height and weight. There was no pubertal development. Charles seemed depressed but participated in the examination as best he could. There were no obvious indications of attentional problems, excessive motor activity, or impulsivity. He was clearly left-handed. He had bilateral dysdiadochokinesia. He could not manage to jump up and down 20 times on his right foot, but just managed on the left side. He managed to stand on one foot for only 5 seconds on the right side, 15 seconds on the left. The findings on the Fog test for associated movements (Fog and Fog 1963) showed clear bilateral abnormality. He had mild bilateral tremor and was very slow in his performance on pencil-and-paper tasks. Reflexes in his arms and legs were normal and there was no Babinski sign on either side. Charles's scores on the brief Conners parent and teacher scales were 15 and 6, respectively, indicating that there appeared to be some attentional problems at home but that the teacher had not noticed similar deficits in the classroom. On the Birleson depression inventory (Birleson 1981) (range 0 to 36, with a high score indicating depression) his score was 21, indicating considerable depressive symptomatology.

His IQ on the WISC–III was 102. His scores on digit symbol (coding), object assembly, and block design were very poor. Almost everything he did during testing he did slowly.

A diagnosis of dysthymic disorder (DSM-IV; American Psychiatric Association 1994) and DCD was made. Some mild to moderate symptoms of attention deficit were present, but these were not sufficient to warrant a diagnosis of DAMP (and certainly not of ADHD). Some of the problems of inattention might be associated with depression rather than with ADHD. A preliminary assumption was made that Charles had had DCD ever since early childhood and that although symptoms of this disorder were no longer causing major functional disability they had always made Charles feel awkward, clumsy, and even stupid (in spite of the fact that he had normal intelligence). The depressive symptoms had developed gradually as a consequence of Charles's growing awareness that he had a mild but, to most people around him, invisible disability. The child psychiatrist told Charles and his mother of the results and explained that the symptoms of DCD would probably lessen in time, but that some motor clumsiness was likely to persist. All three agreed to postpone a decision about psychopharmacological treatment for a few weeks. A month later Charles already felt happier and was talking to the other children in his classroom about DCD. On follow-up 2 months after that he did not feel a need for medication.

REFERENCES

Airaksinen E, Bille B, Carlström G, et al. (1990) Barn och ungdomar med DAMP/MBD [Children and adolescents with DAMP/MBD]. *Läkartidningen* **88**: 714. In Swedish.

American Psychiatric Association. (1980) *Diagnostic and Statistical Manual of Mental Disorders.* 3rd ed (DSM-III). Washington, DC: American Psychiatric Association.

— (1987) *Diagnostic and Statistical Manual of Mental Disorders.* 3rd ed, revised (DSM-III-R). Washington, DC: American Psychiatric Association.

— (1994) *Diagnostic and Statistical Manual of Mental Disorders.* 4th ed (DSM-IV). Washington, DC: American Psychiatric Association.

Ayres AJ. (1974) *Southern California Sensory Integration Test.* Los Angeles: Western Psychological Services.

Benasich AA, Bejar II. (1992) The Fagan test of infant intelligence: a critial review. *Journal of Applied Developmental Psychology* **13**: 153–71.

— Tallal P. (1993) An operant conditioning paradigm for assessing auditory temporal processing in 6- to 9- month-old infants. *Annals of the New York Academy of Sciences* **682**: 312–4.

Birleson P. (1981) The validity of depressive disorder in childhood and the development of a self-rating scale: a research report. *Journal of Child Psychology and Psychiatry* **22**: 73–88.

Bornstein MH, Sigman MD. (1986) Continuity in mental development from infancy. *Child and Development* **57**: 251–74.

Chelune GJ, Ferguson W, Koon R, Dickey TO. (1986) Frontal lobe disinhibition in attention deficit disorder. *Child Psychiatry and Human Development* **16**: 221–34.

Ciaranello R. (1993) Editorial. *New England Journal of Medicine* **328**: 1038–9.

Colby CL. (1991) The neuroanatomy and neurophysiology of attention. *Journal of Child Neurology* **6 (Suppl.):** S90–S118.

Comings D. (1990) *Tourette Syndrome.* Duarte, CA: Hope Press.

Conners CK. (1969) A teacher rating scale for use in drug studies with children. *American Journal of Psychiatry* **126**: 884–8.

Denckla MB. (1985) Neurological examination for subtle signs (PANESS). *Psychopharmacology Bulletin* **21**: 773–800.

Ehlers S, Gillberg C. (1993) The epidemiology of Asperger syndrome. A total population study. *Journal of Child Psychology and Psychiatry* **34**: 1327–50.

Fog E, Fog M. (1963) Cerebral inhibition examined by associated movements. In: Bax M and Mac Keith R, editors. *Minimal Cerebral Dysfunction.* Clinics in Developmental Medicine No. 10. London: Spastics International Medical Publications/William Heinemann Medical Books Ltd. p 52–7.

Gillberg C. (1983) Perceptual, motor and attentional deficits in Swedish primary school children. Some child psychiatric aspects. *Journal of Child Psychology and Psychiatry* **24**: 377–403.

— (1992) Autism and autistic-like conditions: subclasses among disorders of empathy. The Emanuel Miller Memorial Lecture 1991]. *Journal of Child Psychology and Psychiatry* **33**: 813–42.

— (1995) *Clinical Child Neuropsychiatry.* Cambridge: Cambridge University Press.

— (1997) *Ett Barn i Varje Klass: om DAMP/MBD och ADHD. [One Child in Every Classroom: about DAMP/MBD and ADHD].* Stockholm: Bokförlaget Cura. (In Swedish).

— Hellgren L. (1996) Outcome of attention disorders. In: Sandberg S, editor. *Hyperactivity Disorders.* Cambridge: Cambridge University Press.

— Rasmussen P. (1982) Perceptual, motor and attentional deficits in seven-year-old children: background factors. *Developmental Medicine and Child Neurology* **24:** 752–70.

— Carlström G, Rasmussen P. (1983) Hyperkinetic disorders in seven-year-old children with perceptual, motor and attentional deficits. *Journal of Child Psychology and Psychiatry* **24:** 233–46.

— Melander H, von Knorring A-L, et al. (1997) Long-term stimulant treatment of children with attention-deficit hyperactivity disorder symptoms. A randomized, double-blind, placebo-controlled trial. *Archives of General Psychiatry* **54:** 857–64.

Gillberg IC. (1987) Deficits in attention, motor control and perception: follow-up from pre-school to early teens. MD Thesis. University of Uppsala.

— Gillberg C. (1988) Generalized hyperkinesis: follow-up study from age 7 to 13 years. *Journal of the American Academy of Child and Adolescent Psychiatry* **27:** 55–9.

— — (1989) Asperger syndrome – some epidemological considerations: a research note. *Journal of Child Psychology and Psychiatry* **30:** 631–8.

Gittelman R, Mannuzza S, Shenker R, Bonagura N. (1985) Hyperactive boys almost grown up: I. Psychiatric status. *Archives of General Psychiatry* **42:** 937–47.

Goodman R, Stevenson J. (1989a) A twin study of hyperactivity – I. An examination of hyperactivity scores and categories derived from Rutter teacher and parent questionnaires. *Journal of Child Psychology and Psychiatry* **30:** 671–89.

— — (1989b) A twin study of hyperactivity – II. The aetiological role of genes, family relationships and perinatal adversity. *Journal of Child Psychology and Psychiatry* **30:** 691–709.

Griffiths R. (1970) *The Abilities of Young Children. A Study in Mental Measurement.* London: University of London Press.

Hadders-Algra M, van Eykern LA, Klip-van den Nieuwendijk AW, Prechtl HFR. (1992) Developmental course of general movements in infancy. 2: EMG correlates. *Early Human Development* **28:** 231–51.

Hellgren L, Gillberg C, Gillberg IC, Enerskog I. (1993) Children with deficits in attention, motor control and perception (DAMP) almost grown up: general health at 16 years. *Developmental Medicine and Child Neurology* **35:** 881–92.

— Gillberg IC, Bågenholm A, Gillberg C. (1994) Children with deficits in attention, motor control and perception (DAMP) almost grown up: psychiatric and personality disorders at age 16 years. *Journal of Child Psychology and Psychiatry* **35:** 1255-71.

Kadesjö B, Gillberg C. (1998) Attention deficits and clumsiness in Swedish 7-year-old children. *Developmental Medicine and Child Neurology* **40:** 796–804.

Klein RG, Mannuzza S. (1991) Long-term outcome of hyperactive children: a review. *Journal of the American Academy of Child and Adolescent Psychiatry* **30:** 383–87.

Landgren M, Petterssen R, Kjellman B, Gillberg C. (1996). ADHD, DAMP and other neurodevelopmental/psychiatric disorders in 6-year-old children: epidemiology and co-morbidity. *Developmental Medicine and Child Neurology* **38:** 891–906.

Lou HC, Henriksen L, Bruhn P. (1984) Focal cerebral hypoperfusion in children with dysphasia and/or attention deficit disorder. *Archives of Neurology* **41:** 825–9.

— — et al. (1989) Striatal dysfunction in attention deficit and hyperkinetic disorder. *Archives of Neurology* **46:** 48–52.

— — Greisen G, Schneider S. (1990a) Redistribution of cerebral activity during childhood. *Brain Development* **12:** 301–5.

— — Bruhn P. (1990b) Focal cerebral dysfunction in developmental learning disabilities. *Lancet* **335:** 8–11.

Mannuzza S, Klein RG, Konig PH, Ciampino TL. (1989) Hyperactive boys almost grown up. IV. Criminality and its relationship to psychiatric status. *Archives of General Psychiatry* **46:** 1073–9.

Mefford IN, Potter WZ. (1989) A neuroanatomical and biochemical basis for attention deficit disorder with hyperactivity in children: a defect in tonic adrenaline mediated inhibition of locus coeruleus stimulation. *Medical Hypotheses* **29:** 33–42.

Michelsson K, Ylinen A. (1987) A neurodevelopmental screening examination for five-year-old children. *Early Child Development and Care* **29:** 9–22.

Rasmussen P, Gillberg C, Waldenström E, Svenson B. (1983) Perceptual, motor and attentional deficits in seven-year-old children: neurological and neurodevelopmental aspects. *Developmental Medicine and Child Neurology* **25:** 315–33.

Rutter M. (1967) A children's behaviour questionnaire for completion by teachers: preliminary findings. *Journal of Child Psychology and Psychiatry* **8:** 1–11.

—. (1982) Syndromes attributed to minimal brain dysfunction in childhood. *American Journal of Psychiatry* **139:** 21–33.

— Graham P. (1966) Psychiatric disorder in 10- and 11-year-old children. *Proceedings of the Royal Society of Medicine* **59:** 382–7.

—— Yule W. (1970) *A Neuropsychiatric Study in Childhood.* Clinics in Developmental Medicine Nos. 35 / 36. London: Spastics International Medical Publications / William Heinemann Medical Books.

Sandberg ST, Rutter M, Taylor E. (1978) Hyperkinetic disorder in psychiatric clinic attenders. *Developmental Medicine and Child Neurology* **20:** 279–99.

Soorani-Lunsing RJ, Hadders-Algra M, Huisjes HJ, Touwen BC. (1993) Minor neurological dysfunction after the onset of puberty: association with perinatal events. *Early Human Development* **33:** 71–80.

Stevenson J. (1991) Which aspects of processing text mediate genetic effects? *Reading and Writing* **3:** 249–69.

— Graham P. (1993) Antisocial behaviour and spelling disability in a population sample of 13 year old twins. *European Child and Adolescent Psychiatry* **2:** 179–91.

Taylor E. (1986) Childhood hyperactivity. *British Journal of Psychiatry* **149:** 562–73.

— Schachar R, Thorley G, Wieselberg M. (1986) Conduct disorder and hyperactivity: I. Separation of hyperactivity and antisocial conduct in British child psychiatric patients. *British Journal of Psychiatry* **149:** 760–7.

— Sandberg S, Thorley G, Giles S. (1991) *The Epidemiology of Childhood Hyperactivity.* London: Institute of Psychiatry.

Thorley G. (1984) A pilot study to assess behavioural and cognitive effects of artificial food colours in a group of retarded children. *Developmental Medicine and Child Neurology* **26:** 56–61.

Touwen BCL. (1979) *Examination of the Child with Minor Neurological Dysfunction.* 2nd ed. Clinics in Developmental Medicine No. 71. London: Spastics International Medical Publications / William Heinemann Medical Books.

Trommer BL, Hoeppner J-AB, Zecker SG. (1991) The go–no go test in attention deficit disorder is sensitive to methylphenidate. *Journal of Child Neurology* **6 (Suppl)**: S128–S131.

Voeller KKS. (1991) Clinical management of attention deficit hyperactivity disorders. *Journal of Child Neurology* **6 (Suppl.)**: S51–S65.

Wechsler D. (1967) *Manual of the Wechsler Intelligence Scale for Children.* New York: Psychological Corporation.

— (1992) *Wechsler Intelligence Scale for Children - Third Edition UK. Manual.* Sidcup, Kent, UK: The Psychological Corporation Ltd.

Weiss G. (1991) Attention deficit hyperactivity disorder. In: Lewis M, editor. *Child and Adolescent Psychiatry. A Comprehensive Textbook.* Baltimore, Maryland: Williams and Wilkins.

Wender PH. (1971) *Minimal Brain Dysfunction in Children.* New York: Wiley.

Whitmore K, Bax M. (1986) The school entry medical examination. *Archives of Diseases in Childhood* **61:** 807–17.

World Health Organization. (1993) *The ICD-10 Classification of Mental and Behavioural Disorders: Diagnostic Criteria for Research.* Geneva: World Health Organization.

7
THE GENETICS OF SPECIFIC LEARNING DISORDERS

Jim Stevenson

The genetics of specific learning disorders has a chequered history. For some disorders (such as reading disability) there is a long history of studies documenting familial occurrence. For others (such as the clumsy child) there is no established body of genetic investigation. For still others (such as ADHD) there is a more recent but now burgeoning field of genetic studies. This chapter concentrates on reading disability and ADHD.

Some of the influences on any particular aspect of learning or educational attainment will also affect other abilities and general intelligence. In this chapter only studies designed to address the specific genetic influences on a particular ability are reviewed. It should be remembered that for any child these factors will be acting alongside those affecting more general characteristics. These more general factors will include both genetic and environmental influences that may tend to lead to slow development or poor final levels of attainment. It has been long recognized that genetic factors are a major influence on moderate to severe learning disabilities (i.e. when the IQ is below 70). These include genes of major effect (such as that contributing to phenylketonuria) as well as chromosomal anomalies (such as Down syndrome). Indeed it appears that learning (both general and specific) and behaviour are particularly susceptible to aberrant genetic influences. This realization has led to the development of the systematic study of the behavioural characteristics of children with known genetic abnormalities – the study of behavioural phenotypes (O'Brien and Yule 1995).

Identifying genetic and environmental influences

Quantitative genetic analysis is an attempt to identify the relative magnitudes of the influences of variation in genetic make-up and variation in environments experienced on a condition. The estimates based on such an analysis are limited by the population from which the samples have been obtained – that is, they are population-specific. Their generalisability is constrained by the extent to which the full range of genotypic and environmental variation has been sampled.

The extent of genetic variation is substantial, even though much of our DNA is identical to that in other humans and indeed even in other species. However, the extent to which we do vary in genetic make-up may be reflected in phenotypic variation. This genetic variability by and large acts additively, though there are non-additive genetic effects such as dominance (interactions between pairs of genes at the same position on a chromosome – all of our genes are paired) and epistasis (interactions between genes at different positions on a chromosome). Here I am concerned with additive genetic effects (A).

Environmental influences or experiences can be thought of in two broad categories. One type may act to make siblings within a family resemble one another, or (to put it another way) to make people from different families different. For example to the extent that the quality of housing affects a child's well-being, this will tend to affect children in the same family similarly. Parents' push towards educational achievement is also likely to act in this manner. This type of environmental influence is called the common, or shared, environment (C).

The second type of environmental influence is one that acts to make differences between members of the same family and is called a unique, or non-shared, environmental influence (E). Illnesses experienced by only one sibling, the quality of relationships with particular teachers, and friendship groups are all examples of influences likely to make brothers and sisters different from one another. It must be remembered that brothers and sisters also differ genetically from one another (except for the special case of monozygotic twins). Therefore differences within a family may be a product of both A and E.

The relative magnitudes of the effects of A, C, and E on a condition can be estimated by comparing the characteristics of people with known degrees of genetic relatedness who have or have not shared the environment of the same family. Twins are particularly useful for such comparisons, since the two classes of twin differ by the extent to which they have genes in common: identical, or monozygotic, twins have all their genes in common whereas fraternal, or dizygotic, twins have on average 50% of their genes in common. Adopted children can be compared with their biological brothers or sisters living in different families or they can be compared with their adoptive or biological parents. In both cases the known differences in the similarity of the genetic make-up or the extent of shared environments makes it possible to estimate A, C, and E. The values reported for A, C, and E reflect the proportion of the variance in a characteristic that is due to this influence and will therefore range between 0 (no effect) and 1.0 (all the variance attributed to that source).

The development of our understanding of the molecular basis of inheritance now means that it is possible to study the possible genetic influences on a condition much more directly than before. Genetic linkage studies trace whether a particular condition is inherited within a family or set of families alongside another characteristic of known genetic origin and with a known location in the genome. These markers, as they are called, are often just pieces of DNA whose location is known and which show variations in structure (their function is usually unknown and indeed some may have no function). If a condition appears to be inherited along with the marker, then linkage between the marker and a gene influencing the condition is established. Once a linkage has been established, there is then an often protracted search for the actual gene that is influencing the condition of interest.

Linkage studies require data from several generations of large families. More recent molecular genetic techniques adopt strategies that are both more straightforward to interpret and less restrictive in the range of data that need to be available. Association studies compare the genetic variation at a particular gene. Different forms of a gene are referred to as alleles. If individuals with a condition have a particular allelic form more often than controls (often unaffected family members), then that gene shows an association with the condition (Owen and McGuffin 1993). An account of how estimates for the size of genetic and environmental influences are obtained from the correlations and concordances for relatives of various types is given by Plomin et al. (1997); their book also provides an introduction to molecular genetics.

Reading disability
Defining reading disability and its subtypes is complex. A number of component skills are required for reading, making broad demands on processing of both visual and linguistic information. The task of defining such disability is made more difficult by the tendency to create complex categories of disability, such as dyslexia. Some of these complex definitions have been unsatisfactory, because they defined by exclusion, or because they could be applied only to children of average intelligence or higher, or because they took no account of the child's profile of relative ability or disability; and some definitions (e.g. Critchley and Critchley 1978) suffered from all of these inadequacies.

One approach to defining reading disability in terms of a discrepancy between reading ability and that expected from an individual's overall level of cognitive ability is to use a regression of reading attainment on IQ (Rutter and Yule 1975), but this approach has not facilitated the identification of types of disability (Stanovich et al. 1997). Both for children who fail to learn to read as part of a general low level of mental development and for those developing otherwise normally, deficits in phonological processing lie at the core of reading disability (Stanovich 1988, Stanovich and Siegel 1994). The severity of the phonological deficit is probably the determining factor for the type of reading disability the individual will show (Snowling and Nation 1997).

Early studies
Ever since the first studies of reading disability by neurologists, the familiality of the condition has been noted (Hinshelwood 1907). Whatever the evidence that a condition tends to occur in the same families more often than would expected by chance, it does not prove that there is a genetic influence. The condition could be transmitted across generations for environmental reasons. Such transmission might be particularly expected for a condition such as reading disability, in which the ability of parents with limited literacy to provide adequate early reading experience for their children and to value the attainment of literacy may well be compromised.

In order to disentangle genetic from environmental contributions, specific types of research design are required. As explained already, there are both quantitative and molecular approaches to the examination of genetic influences. The quantitative genetic studies of reading disability include segregation analysis, in which the patterns of occurrence across generations are tested against alternative genetic models, such as dominant or recessive transmission. There have been few adoption studies of reading disability to date. However, research on twins has provided some strong support for the significance of genetic influences on reading disability.

The early twin studies were based largely upon case reports of small sets of twin pairs, for whom concordance rates were estimated. The data from these early studies were consistent with a substantial genetic influence. In particular the nearly 100% concordance rate for monozygotic twins was indicative of an almost total genetic determination of the condition (see Stevenson et al. 1987 for a critique of these early twin studies).

QUANTITATIVE GENETIC STUDIES

There have been two main studies providing evidence for the role of genetic factors in reading disability. The first, undertaken in London, was based on a general population sample of 287 twin pairs (Stevenson et al. 1987). The initial analyses from this study suggested only a modest influence of genetic factors on reading disability (A=0.29) but a more marked influence on spelling disability (A= 0.73). The second major twin study was undertaken in Colorado by John DeFries and colleagues (1987). For this study a sample of twins with at least one member of the pair showing reading disability was identified from the Colorado school population; the estimated magnitude of genetic influences was somewhat larger (A=0.40) than that from the London study.

Because a significant proportion of the twins in the Colorado study were younger than those in the London study, Stevenson et al. (1987) suggested that there may be age-related changes whereby spelling but not reading maintains evidence of strong genetic influences as the child gets older. This 'developmental hypothesis' arose in part because reading disability can be remediated more easily than spelling difficulties. DeFries et al. (1997) tested this prediction within the Colorado sample – the only sample in a genetically informative study of reading and spelling that was large enough to permit comparison of age-related genetic effects. They found that for reading of single words (reading recognition) the estimated values of A were 0.64 and 0.47 for the younger ($\leq$11.5 years) and older ($>$11.5 years) twins, respectively. By contrast the age-related genetic effects for spelling disability were 0.52 and 0.68 for the younger and older groups, respectively. These findings suggest that the degree of genetic influence on aspects of literacy difficulties can be accurately assessed only if both age and the particular aspect of literacy are taken into consideration.

The second major conclusion from these twin studies is that the reading process needs to be broken down into subprocesses to examine genetic effects. In both the Colorado (Olson et al. 1989) and the London (Stevenson 1991) studies, phonological processing (as measured by non-word reading) was found to carry a significant genetic effect (A=0.46 and 0.74 in those two studies, respectively). Orthographic ability, as measured by reading of orthographically irregular words and by the ability to discriminate among pseudohomophones (i.e. to identify the real word embedded in a list of non-words that sound the same), had non-significant heritabilities.

MOLECULAR GENETIC STUDIES

In 1994 reading disability became one of the first cognitive disabilities shown to be linked to a specific genetic site, when the Colorado group (Cardon et al. 1994, 1995) found linkage to a specific locus on the short arm of chromosome 6 (6p21.3) for reading recognition. Subsequent analyses of data from 50 pairs of dizygotic twins from the Colorado study suggested that the gene at this site may not have the same magnitude of effect on different aspects of reading and spelling ability (Gayan et al. 1995).

One of the major problems with this kind of molecular genetic study is that the results are often difficult to replicate by other researchers – i.e. the linkages often seem to be sample-specific. However, in the case of reading disability a separate research group based at Yale were able to replicate the chromosome 6 linkage (Grigorenko et al. 1997). They found that the type of reading disability most closely linked to that chromosome was phonological processing and that a more general deficit, in reading single words, was linked to chromosome 15.

The research into the genetics of reading disability is therefore now moving into a phase where it will become crucial to identify the actual genes influencing phonological processing, how the products of these genes influence the developing brain both structurally and functionally, the cognitive processes that are dependent on these aspects of brain function, and to what extent these processes can be modified by carefully structured educational experience or possibly by pharmacological treatment. This will require the collaborative efforts of molecular geneticists, developmental biologists, brain imagers, and cognitive psychologists. At this stage only parts of this research programme are being put together, for example in the collaboration between brain imagers and cognitive neuroscientists (Paulesu et al. 1996). By contrast the situation with ADHD is that pharmacological treatments with some degree of efficacy are already known (Swanson et al. 1995). Here it is expected that the emerging understanding about the genetic influences on brain chemistry may lead to a more effective range of drug treatments to accompany psychologically based treatments.

ADHD and hyperactivity

There has been as much controversy over the definition of the phenotype related to undercontrolled disinhibited hyperactive behaviour in children as there has been over reading disability (Barkley 1997). The essential components of the syndrome of AHDH are impulsivity, overactivity, and inattention, and in the DSM-IV classification (American Psychiatric Association 1995) these symptoms must be present before the age of 7 years, must be pervasive (e.g. present at home and in school), and must result in a clinically significant disability.

QUANTITATIVE GENETIC STUDIES

Small-scale early twin studies showed an influence of genetic factors on activity level (e.g. Willerman 1973). The first study in which the effects of genetic and environmental influences on hyperactivity were examined systematically was that by Goodman and Stevenson (1989). That study suggested that the value of A for hyperactivity was between 0.30 and 0.40, that of C was between 0.0 and 0.3, and that of E was about 0.2. Stevenson (1992) undertook a more extensive analysis of this same data set and obtained a very high estimate for A of 0.81 based on a composite index of extreme hyperactivity. This estimate ranks hyperactivity and ADHD among the most heritable of children's mental disorders (LaBuda et al. 1993). Subsequent twin studies from the UK (Thapar et al. 1995), Norway (Gjone et al. 1996), the USA (Sherman et al. 1997), and Australia (Levy et al. 1997) have confirmed the substantial role played by genetic factors in ADHD symptomatology.

The studies by Gjone et al. (1996) and Levy et al. (1997) showed that ADHD can be conceptualized as being at the extreme of a dimension 'hyperactivity'. Variation of symptom severity along this dimension is as much genetically determined as is ADHD itself. This suggests that the genetic mechanisms influencing ADHD are likely to be polygenic (rooted in many separate genes), or at least to be the product of a number of genes none of which has a major effect. This formulation of ADHD as an extreme on a dimension contrasts with a categorical approach, which would be more appropriate if there were a single major gene that produces the condition. These studies of ADHD provide an example of how quantitative genetic research can help not only to refine our understanding of a genotype but also to clarify how a behavioural phenotype is measured and the nosology of a condition is developed.

MOLECULAR GENETIC STUDIES

Quantitative genetic studies have provided strong justification for the search for the genes that might contribute to ADHD and are making a substantial contribution to the aetiology of this condition. In addition ADHD is known to respond favourably to treatment with methylphenidate, a stimulant thought to be a dopamine agonist that increases synaptic dopamine by inhibiting reuptake (Patrick et al. 1987). It has been postulated that ADHD may be caused by an underactive dopamine system (Levy 1991).

With these considerations in mind, molecular geneticists investigating ADHD have been concentrating on genes contributing to the functioning of the dopamine system. It has been suggested that allelic variation in the dopamine transporter gene (*DAT1*) on chromosome 5 (5p15.3) might be associated with ADHD (Cook et al. 1995). There is also some suggestion that the dopamine D_2 receptor gene (*DRD2*) on chromosome 11 (11q22–23) might be implicated in ADHD as well as in Tourette syndrome and alcoholism (Comings et al. 1996). However, the strongest evidence to date concerns the dopamine D_4 receptor gene (*DRD4*), on chromosome 11 (11p15.5). Allelic variation (particularly the seven-repeat form) in this gene has been found to be more frequent in children with ADHD than in matched controls (LaHoste et al. 1996). Interestingly, this allelic variation in *DRD4* has been found to be associated with individual differences in novelty seeking in two general population samples (Benjamin et al. 1996, Ebstein et al. 1996). The interest in these latter findings is that they parallel the finding from the twin studies of Gjone et al. (1996) and Levy et al. (1997) that ADHD is an extreme of normal variation, of which the personality dimension 'novelty seeking' could be one component.

Practical implications

The advances in genetic studies of specific learning disabilities are likely to have a considerable impact in the long term on both the clinical and educational treatment of children who have these conditions. Some of these developments will be relatively uncontroversial and can simply be seen as an extension of current practice. For example it is likely that novel psychopharmacological agents can be produced as the underlying pathophysiology becomes better understood. The use of such new agents in ADHD will simply be an extension of existing practice. However, the possibility of increased understanding of underlying mechanisms also raises the possibility of increasing medicalization of disabilities that have traditionally been seen as educational. For example despite claims that piracetam may be effective in the treatment of dyslexia (Connors et al. 1987), reading disability has not been treated with drugs. The possibility that a pharmacological treatment could rationally be designed to compensate for biological deficiencies in children with reading disabilities opens up the possibility of a marked extension of drug treatments. A wider debate would then be needed about the extent to which such biologically based treatment of specific learning disabilities is appropriate.

Perhaps even more controversial would be the use of genetic knowledge to identify children who are at risk of developing specific learning disabilities. Already in relation to ADHD, as was shown above, the sevenfold repeat allele in *DRD4* might be a candidate for a genetic marker whose presence puts a child at increased risk for ADHD. If children were being routinely screened for such genetic variations, it would be feasible to think of both pharmacological and educational/psychological preventive interventions being applied. Any such initiative would be dogged by the problems of the multiplicity of genes involved in any one condition and the possibility that a child carrying such a genetic variant may only be at a moderately higher risk of developing the condition than the general population.

These issues about the clinical and educational implications of genetic studies are not restricted to learning disabilities. However, to many the questions of the abuse of genetic information may be very much highlighted when such information is applied to what are seen as less life-threatening or less handicapping conditions such as the specific learning disabilities. Equally it has to recognized that identifying a child as carrying a biological marker for a specific learning disability does not necessarily imply that a biologically based treatment should be used. Children who are biologically at risk can be provided with a socially based preventive measure. For example children carrying a genetic risk for reading disability might especially benefit from early intensive training in phonological awareness. A screen for such a genetic variant would allow such training to be provided at a beneficially earlier age than would be possible if the risk was identified only after the child had begun to fail at reading.

Conclusions

Genetic studies of specific learning disabilities are entering a new phase. These disabilities are produced not by the effects of single major genes but rather by the joint action of a number of genes and environmental influences. Quantitative genetic studies will continue to be needed to identify which important features of these conditions are affected by genetic factors. Increasingly these studies will be multivariate genetic investigations looking at the underlying architecture of genetic and environmental components influencing these conditions. One such study is that of Sherman et al. (1997), who have shown how the same genetic factors are implicated in both the 'overactive' and the 'impulsive–inattentive' components of ADHD. Molecular genetic studies will continue to identify the many genes that contribute to these conditions. Attention will then focus increasingly upon how these genes interact and their impact on the developing and functioning nervous system. Ultimately these investigations may lead to novel psychopharmacological treatments – for example drugs for the treatment of ADHD that act on a wider range of components of the dopamine system than methylphenidate. There may also be a new era of educational possibilities that will arise from the early identification (through detection of genetic risk) of children who are susceptible to the development of various educational disabilities, and from the development of psychopharmacological treatments that will make the child, and the developing central nervous system, more amenable to environmental and educational assistance.

REFERENCES

American Psychiatric Association. (1995) *Diagnostic and Statistical Manual of Mental Disorders. International Version.* 4th ed (DSM-IV). Washington, DC: American Psychiatric Association.

Barkley RA. (1997) Behavioral inhibition, sustained attention, and executive functions: constructing a unifying theory of ADHD. *Psychological Bulletin* **121:** 65–94.

Benjamin J, Li L, Patterson C, et al. (1996) Population and familial association between the D4 dopamine-receptor gene and measures of novelty seeking. *Nature Genetics* **12:** 81–4.

Cardon LR, Smith SD, Fulker DW, et al. (1994) Quantitative trait locus for reading disability on chromosome 6. *Science* **266:** 276–9.

— — — et al. (1995) Quantitative trait locus for reading disability: Correction. *Science* **268:** 5217.

Comings DE, Wu S, Chiu C., et al. (1996) Polygenic inheritance of Tourette syndrome, stuttering, attention deficit hyperactivity, conduct and oppositional defiant disorder. *American Journal of Medical Genetics (Neuropsychiatric Genetics)* **67:** 264–88.

Conners CK, Reade M, Wilsher C. (1987). Piracetam – effects on reading-achievement and evoked-potentials in dyslexics. *Pharmacology, Biochemistry and Behavior* **27:** 589.

Cook EH, Stein MA, Krasowski MD, et al. (1995) Association of attention-deficit disorder and dopamine transporter gene. *American Journal of Human Genetics* **56:** 993–8.

Critchley M, Critchley EA. (1978) *Dyslexia Defined.* London: William Heineman Medical Books.

DeFries JC, Fulker DW, LaBuda MC. (1987) Evidence for a genetic aetiology in reading disability of twins. *Nature* **329:** 537–9.

— Alarcon M, Olson RK. (1997) Genetic aetiologies of reading and spelling deficits: developmental differences. In: Hulme C, Snowling M, editors. *Dyslexia: Biology, Cognition and Intervention.* London: Whurr. p 20–37.

Ebstein RP, Novick O, Umansky R, et al. (1996) Dopamine D4 receptor (*D4DR*) exon III polymorphism associated with the human personality trait of novelty seeking. *Nature Genetics* **12:** 78–80.

Gayan J, Olson RK, Cardon LR, et al. (1995) Quantitative trait locus for different measures of reading-disability. *Behavior Genetics* **25:** 266. (Abstract).

Gjone H, Stevenson J, Sundet JM. (1996) Genetic influence on parent-reported attention-problems in a Norwegian general population twin sample. *Journal of the American Academy of Child and Adolescent Psychiatry* **35:** 588–8.

Goodman R, Stevenson J. (1989) A twin study of hyperactivity. 2. The etiological role of genes, family relationships and perinatal adversity. *Journal of Child Psychology and Psychiatry* **30:** 691–709.

Grigorenko EL, Wood FB, Meyer MS, et al. (1997) Susceptibility loci for distinct components of developmental dyslexia on chromosomes 6 and 15. *American Journal of Human Genetics* **60:** 27–39.

Hinshelwood J. (1907) Four cases of congenital word-blindness occurring in the same family. *British Medical Journal* **1:** 608–9.

Labuda MC, Gottesman II, Pauls DL. (1993) Usefulness of twin studies for exploring the etiology of childhood and adolescent psychiatric-disorders. *American Journal of Medical Genetics* **48:** 47–59.

LaHoste GJ, Swanson JM, Wigal SB, et al. (1996) Dopamine D4 receptor gene polymorphism is associated with attention deficit disorder. *Molecular Psychiatry* **1:** 121–4.

Levy F. (1991). The dopamine theory of attention deficit hyperactivity disorder (ADHD). *Australian and New Zealand Journal of Psychiatry* **25:** 277–83.

— Hay DA, McStephen M, et al. (1997) Attention-deficit hyperactivity disorder: a category or continuum? Genetic analysis of a large-scale twin study. *Journal of the American Academy of Child and Adolescent Psychiatry* **36:** 737–44.

O'Brien G, Yule W, editors. (1995) *Behavioural Phenotypes.* Clinics in Developmental Medicine No. 138. London: Mac Keith Press.

Olson R, Wise B, Conners F, et al. (1989) Specific deficits in component reading and language skills: genetic and environmental influences. *Journal of Learning Disabilities* **22**: 339–48.

Owen MJ, McGuffin P. (1993) Association and linkage: complementary strategies for complex disorders. *Journal of Medical Genetics* **30**: 638–9.

Patrick KS, Mueller RA, Gualtieri TC, Breese GR. (1987) Pharmacokinetics and actions of methylphenidate. In: Meltzey HY, editor. *Psychopharmacology: Third Generation of Progress.* New York: Raven Press.

Paulesu E, Frith U, Snowling M, et al. (1996) Is developmental dyslexia a disconnection syndrome – evidence from PET scanning. *Brain* **119**: 143–57.

Plomin R, DeFries JC, McClearn GE, Rutter M. (1997) *Behavioral Genetics.* New York: W H Freeman.

Rutter M, Yule W. (1975). The concept of specific reading retardation. *Journal of Child Psychology and Psychiatry* **16**: 181–97.

Sherman DK, Iacono WG, McGue MK. (1997) Attention-deficit hyperactivity disorder dimensions: a twin study of inattention and impulsivity–hyperactivity. *Journal of the American Academy of Child and Adolescent Psychiatry* **36**: 745–53.

Snowling MJ, Nation KA. (1997) Language, phonology and learning to read. In: Hulme C, Snowling M, editors. *Dyslexia: Biology, Cognition and Intervention.* London: Whurr. p 153–66.

Stanovich KE. (1988) Explaining the differences between the dyslexic and the garden-variety poor reader: the phonological-core variable-difference model. *Journal of Learning Disabilities* **21**: 590–612.

— Siegel LS. (1994) The phenotypic performance profile of reading-disabled children: a regression-based test of the phonological-core variable-difference model. *Journal of Educational Psychology* **86**: 1–30.

— — Gottardo A. (1997) Progress in the search for dyslexia sub-types. In: Hulme C, Snowling M, editors. *Dyslexia: Biology, Cognition and Intervention.* London: Whurr. p 108–30.

Stevenson J. (1991) Which aspects of processing text mediate genetic effects? *Reading and Writing* **3**: 249–69.

— (1992) Evidence for genetic etiology in hyperactivity in children. *Behavior Genetics* **22**: 337–44.

— Graham P, Fredman G, McGloughlin V. (1987) A twin study of genetic influences on reading and spelling ability and disability. *Journal of Child Psychology and Psychiatry* **28**: 229–47.

Swanson JM, McBurnett K, Christian DL, Wigal T. (1995) Stimulant medications and treatment of children with ADHD. *Advances in Clinical Child Psychology* **17**: 265–322.

Thapar A, Hervas A, McGuffin P. (1995) Childhood hyperactivity scores are highly heritable and show sibling competition effects: twin study evidence. *Behavior Genetics* **25**: 537–44.

Willerman L. (1973) Activity level and hyperactivity in twins. *Child Development* **44**: 288–93.

8
PRE- AND PERINATAL PRECURSORS OF SPECIFIC LEARNING DISORDERS

Mijna Hadders-Algra and Elina Lindahl

Children with specific learning disorders show problems with reading (dyslexia), spelling (dysgraphia), or arithmetic (dyscalculia) even when their intellectual capacity is otherwise normal. It is generally acknowledged that learning disabilities have a multifactorial aetiology, to which hereditary factors, social conditions, and the sex of the child all contribute (Frith 1984, Rourke and Strang 1984; see also Chapters 7 and 10). The role of pre- and perinatal risk factors has been a subject of discussion since Pasamanick and coworkers introduced the idea of 'the continuum of reproductive casualty' (Lilienfeld and Pasamanick 1955, Pasamanick et al. 1956, Kawi and Pasamanick 1958, Knobloch and Pasamanick 1959). According to their hypothesis, perinatal events can give rise to a continuum of cerebral damage, ranging from major forms of damage – resulting in perinatal death or serious disorder – to minor cerebral insults, which are followed by the development of learning and behavioural problems. Nowadays the consensus is that pre- and perinatal adversities indeed can contribute to the development of learning disorders, but opinions differ about the type of risk factors playing a role, the conditions under which those factors might affect the developing brain (e.g. in poor social situations only?), and the extent to which they induce learning problems.

In this chapter we review studies dealing with pre- and perinatal risk factors and specific learning disorders, paying special attention to comorbidity in the form of minor neurological dysfunction. The cases of five children (whose names have been changed) are presented to underline the notion that a learning disorder can be attributed only in part to perinatal morbidity. The presentation of the cases is followed by a general overview of the subject. Finally we present the results of two long-term projects in which mixed samples of high-risk infants were followed up for more than 8 years (the Helsinki Neonatal Risk Study and the Groningen Perinatal Project).

Cases
- Nine-year-old Sam was recently seen by the remedial-teaching team of his school because of reading and spelling problems. The major problem turned out to be Sam's slow reading speed. He does not have other cognitive or motor problems. An investigation into possible antecedents of Sam's dyslexia revealed no perinatal complications but revealed that his older brother and his father, a general practitioner, also have dyslexia of a type similar to Sam's.

- Jan, an 8-year-old boy, was recently admitted to a school for special education. He thinks school is very difficult, particularly arithmetic. While doing a simple addition, he shows that he lacks a concept of numbers – three fingers equally likely representing the numbers 3, 4, 5, or 6. His language development is at a low-average level. Jan was the first child of lower-class parents who married in their middle thirties. During pregnancy his mother had many minor complaints (nausea, anaemia, lack of energy, worries about the condition of the child). Jan was born at term with an appropriate birthweight, but he did not cry immediately. His neonatal period was complicated by feeding problems necessitating his admission to a paediatric ward for a few days. Always a quiet boy, he developed without apparent problems until he started school. A neurological assessment before Jan was admitted to the special school revealed hypotonia and mild problems in coordination and fine manipulative ability.

- Jim is an intelligent 10-year-old boy who is interested in biology and geography. Nevertheless he has trouble at school. His reading is fast and sloppy, and his spelling, a disaster. Besides this dyslexia, he has mild attention problems. None of his relatives has dyslexia. Jim's perinatal history revealed an uncomplicated pregnancy and delivery. During infancy and pre-school age he had eczema and asthmatic bronchitis, requiring treatment with bronchodilators and corticosteroids. A recent neurological assessment found mild problems of coordination and of fine manipulative abilities and mild motor asymmetry, consisting in strong right-handedness and asymmetric tendon reflexes, which were consistently more brisk on the left than on the right. It was concluded that Jim had the so-called L type of dyslexia (meaning that he uses mainly his left cerebral hemisphere for reading; Bakker 1984) due to a mild dysfunction of the right hemisphere. As the familial and perinatal history revealed no clues to the origin of Jim's dysfunctions, it could be argued that these were caused by his frequent illnesses when he was very young, and the drugs used to treat them. An alternative explanation for Jim's problems could be a hemispheric dysgenesis, which might be revealed by MRI.

- Linda is a slender 9-year-old girl who was recently diagnosed as having the so-called P type of dyslexia, which is characterized by slow reading and a prevailing sensitivity to the perceptual features of a text – to the form of the letters rather than to the meaning of the words. There is no family history of dyslexia. Linda's father, a truck driver, stays home often because of back complaints and the family income is therefore irregular. One of three sisters and two brothers, Linda was born at 42 weeks, weighing 2650 g (<10th centile). Her Apgar scores were excellent (10 at each of 1 and 3 minutes). She developed well and was seldom ill. When she began to have reading problems at age 8 years she was thoroughly evaluated, and no neurological dysfunction was found.

- Richard is an 8-year-old boy who despite having a low-average IQ has problems with reading, spelling, and arithmetic. In part the learning problems can be attributed to attention problems: attention-deficit/hyperactivity disorder (ADHD) was diagnosed when was he was 4 years old. Richard is the third child in a lower-class family. He was born at 31 weeks gestational age after an emergency caesarean section because of placental abruption. His neonatal records reported perinatal acidaemia, Apgar scores of 2 at 1 minute and 6 at 3 minutes, and many spells of apnoea and bradycardia. His development as an infant was satisfactory and he could walk a few weeks after his first birthday. During his preschool years his initial liveliness gradually changed into hyperactivity with attention problems. Richard started his school career at an ordinary school but after a year was referred to a school for special education. At that time neurological assessment revealed a minimal hypertonia on the right side of his body, choreiform movements, and mild problems of coordination and fine manipulative ability.

Prospective studies on pre- and perinatal risk factors and learning disabilities

Most perinatal follow-up studies focus on sequelae of three types of adversities: preterm birth, intrauterine growth retardation (IUGR), and perinatal asphyxia. These three conditions can be regarded as final common pathways of unfavourable obstetrical situations (Touwen and Huisjes 1984).

FOLLOW-UP OF INFANTS WITH LOW BIRTHWEIGHT (LBW)

During the 1960s and 1970s, most perinatal risk studies followed up children to toddler or preschool age. During the 1980s, however, concern was growing about the long-term outcome of the increasing number of infants surviving complicated pre-, peri-, and neonatal periods (Bax 1983, 1986; Touwen 1986; McCormick 1989; Volpe 1991; Nishida 1993). There has ensued a boom of studies following up for as long as 6 years the development of infants with LBW (usually considered to be <2500 g) or very low birthweight (VLBW; usually <1500 g) – categories that include infants born preterm or growth-retarded or both. Studies providing data about subsequent cognitive development and learning disorders in infants with various degrees of LBW are summarized in Table 8.1. At school age many but not all non-disabled LBW children were found to have lower Full Scale IQs than control infants born at term with normal birthweights. LBW more often affected Performance than Verbal IQ (Ornstein et al. 1991), and lower Performance IQs were related to the presence of minor neurological dysfunction (Largo et al. 1990). Jongmans and coworkers (1993) found that minor neurological dysfunction at 6 years of age was related to abnormalities on the neonatal ultrasound brain scan, namely periventricular densities persisting for more than 14 days (Jongmans et al. 1993). Of the children who had had (V)LBW, many had lower Full Scale IQs than children with normal weight at birth but the majority had IQs within the normal range.

Nevertheless high prevalences of school problems, such as needing special education or being in an inappropriately low grade for age, have been reported in LBW children (see Allen 1984, Ornstein et al. 1991). The rate of school failure found in VLBW populations ranged from 21 to 51% – 3 to 10 times as high as in children with normal birthweight (Calame et al. 1986, Edmonds et al. 1990, McCormick et al. 1990, Saigal et al. 1991, Brandt et al. 1992, Hille et al. 1994, Hall et al. 1995). For extremely-low-birthweight (ELBW) children (children whose weight at birth was <1000 g) the rates of school difficulties found were even higher, reaching 60 to 64% (Nickel et al. 1982, Hall et al. 1995). Specific learning disorders were also often found in LBW populations. Reading was the most frequently evaluated academic skill. Increased rates of poor reading were found in 8 of the 10 VLBW studies considered here (see Table 8.1). Spelling was only occasionally assessed. In three of the four studies providing data on both reading and spelling in LBW children and matched controls, the effect of LBW on reading was similar to that on spelling (Westwood et al. 1983, Saigal et al. 1991, O'Callaghan et al. 1996). In a fourth study, however, a negative effect of LBW on reading but not on spelling was found (Robertson et al. 1990). Arithmetic was the academic skill most strongly affected by LBW (see Table 8.1).

Perinatal and neonatal morbidity in LBW infants varies greatly. For instance, gestational age at birth can range from 24 to 37 weeks; birthweight can be appropriate for gestational age or much too low; perinatal asphyxia can be present; and the clinical picture can be dominated by pulmonary, circulatory, or gastrointestinal problems (Klaus and Fanaroff 1986). Each of these factors can affect the young, developing brain. Nevertheless very few consistent effects of specific perinatal risk factors, such as IUGR or asphyxia at birth, on cognitive development at school age have been found (Ornstein et al. 1991), although a trend of higher rates of school failure in ELBW children seems to emerge. The possibly increased morbidity among ELBW children is not attributable to higher rates of bronchopulmonary dysplasia in these infants: Vohr and colleagues (1991) found that bronchopulmonary dysplasia was associated with higher rates of neurological dysfunction at 10 to 12 years of age, but not with higher rates of cognitive failure. Maybe the possibly higher rate of cognitive problems in ELBW children than in VLBW children is related to the younger ages at which ELBW infants are born (mean gestational age at birth of ELBW infants 27 to 28 weeks, that of VLBW infants 30 to 32 weeks; see references in Table 8.1). The periventricular white matter is particularly vulnerable to hypoxic–ischaemic events before 29 weeks postmenstrual age, because of a paucity of penetrating cerebral and periventricular arteries (Paneth et al. 1994, Volpe 1995).

This brings us to the possible neuropathological correlates of learning disorders in LBW children. Although direct evidence is lacking (see also Chapter 2), autopsy studies have shown considerable heterogeneity of brain lesions in preterm infants. The most frequently affected sites in the brains of preterm infants are the periventricular and intrahemispheric white matter and the hippocampal gray matter, but lesions are also commonly found in the corpus callosum, the basal ganglia, and the cerebellum (Fuller et al. 1983; Paneth et al. 1990, 1994; Armstrong 1993). What is common to the affected sites is their involvement in complex neural processing: the white matter contains projection systems ensuring communication within and between the cerebral hemispheres; the hippocampus plays an important role in memory processes; and the basal ganglia and cerebellum play a role not only in sensorimotor aspects of motor programming, movement planning, program selection, and motor memory, but also in cognitive learning tasks (Alexander and Crutcher 1990, Ito 1990, Leiner et al. 1993). Therefore it could be surmised that the susceptibility of the preterm brain to lesions in areas involved in complex neural processing puts the preterm infant at risk for learning disorders.

LBW studies have shown that two additional factors are significant in the development of cognitive dysfunctions at school age: male sex and unfavourable social conditions (Ornstein et al. 1991). Eight of the 11 studies that provided information on the effect of the child's sex reported a disadvantage for males, and the other three did not find an effect of sex (see Table 8.1). Boys are reputed to be at higher risk for neurodevelopmental disorders

TABLE 8.1

Studies of cognitive development in infants with low birthweight, followed up for at least 6 years

Reference	Study group	Controls	Follow-up to age (y)	Severe disability excluded?[a]	Cognition[b] Full Scale IQ	Cognition[b] Effect on VIQ vs PIQ	School problems[b] General	School problems[b] Reading, spelling	School problems[b] Arithmetic	Minor neurological dysfunction[c]	Males vs females	Effect of socioeconomic status[d]
Bjerre and Hansen 1976	LBW <2500g	NBW classmates	7	No	–	–	Sp. ed. S>C	–	–	–	–	None
Forfar et al. 1994	LBW <2000g	NBW	9–10	Yes	S=C	–	–	–	–	–	–	Additional
Parkinson et al. 1981	Term, SGA (<10th centile)	Term, AGA	7	No	–	–	Difficulties S>C (IU head growth decreased)	–	–	–	M>F	–
Westwood et al. 1983	Term, SGA (< –2SD)	Term, AGA	13–19	Yes	S<C	–	–	S=C	S>C	–	–	Additional
Neligan et al. 1976	Preterm, SGA (<10th centile)	Term, AGA	7	No	S<C	–	–	S=C	–	–	M>F	Additional
Hadders-Algra et al. 1988a	Term, SGA, Preterm, AGA Preterm, SGA	Term, AGA	6	Yes	–	–	S>C	–	–	+	M>F	Additional
Largo et al. 1990	Preterm, AGA	Term, AGA	7 and 9	No	S=C	Effect on V < on P	Sp. ed. S>C	S>C	–	+ (PIQ)	M>F	–
McCormick et al. 1990	LBW 1500–2500g VLBW <1500g	NBW	4–17	Yes	–	–	Difficulties V>L>N	–	–	–	M>F	–
Lowe and Papile 1990	VLBW ≤1500g	Term classmates	5–6	Yes	S=C	–	– (PIVH grade 1–2)	S>C	–	–	–	–

Lloyd et al. 1988	VLBW <1500g	NBW classmates	5½–9	Yes	S<C	Poor performance S<C	S>C	S>>C	–	–	Additional
Ross et al. 1991	VLBW <1500g	Term	7–8	Yes	–	Poor performance S<C	S=C	S>C	–	–	Interaction
Kitchen et al. 1980	VLBW <1500g	NBW	8	No	S<C	Effect on V < on P	–	S>C	–	M=F	–
Calame et al. 1986	VLBW <1500g	Term, AGA	8	Yes	–	Increased sp. ed.	–	–	+	–	None
Robertson et al. 1990	VLBW ≤1500g Preterm, AGA Preterm, SGA	NBW classmates	8	No	S<C	–	read: S>C spell: S=C	S>C	–	M>F	Additional
Hack et al. 1991	VLBW <1500g	No	8	Yes	IQ related to head size at 8 mo of age	–	Related to head size at 8 mo	Related to head size at 8 mo	–	M=F	Additional
Hunt et al. 1988	VLBW <1500g	No	8 and 11	Yes	Effect on V = that on P	17% LD (related to P IQ)	–	–	–	M>F	Interaction
Hille et al. 1994	VLBW <1500g	No	9	No	–	19% sp. ed. 32% 1 yr behind 39% sp. asst.	–	–	–	M>F	Additional
Michelsson et al 1984	VLBW ≤1500g	NBW classmates	9	Yes	Effect on V < on P	S>C	S>C	–	+	–	–

Table continued on next page

–, No data given; AGA, appropriate for gestational age; ELBW, extremely low birthweight; IU, intrauterine; LBW, low birthweight; NBW, normal birthweight; P (IQ), Performance; PIVH, periventricular–intraventricular haemorrhage; SGA, small for gestational age; sp. asst., special assistance needed; sp. ed., special education needed; V (IQ), Verbal; VLBW, very low birthweight.

[a]Does paper provide data on effect of LBW on cognitive function and learning problems after exclusion of handicapped children?

[b]S=C, no significant difference between study and control groups; S>C, significantly more problems in study group than in control group; S<C, significantly worse score in study than in control group; E<V<N, ELBW scored significantly worse than VLBW, VLBW scored significantly worse than NBW.

[c]Presence (+) of relation between minor neurological dysfunction and learning problems.

[d]Interaction if any between socioeconomic status and (V)(E)LBW.

171

TABLE 8.1
(Continued)

Reference	Study group	Controls	Follow-up to age (y)	Severe disability excluded?[a]	Cognition[b]		School problems[b]			Minor neurological dysfunction[c]	Males vs females	Effect of socioeconomic status[d]
					Full Scale IQ	Effect on VIQ on PIQ vs	General	Reading spelling	Arithmetic			
Vohr et al 1991	VLBW ≤1500g	Term	10–12	No	S=C	–	–	S=C	S>C	–	–	–
Hall et al. 1995	ELBW <1000g VLBW 1000–1499g	NBW classmates	8	Yes	E<V<N	Effect on V < on P	E>V>N	S>C	S>>C	+	–	–
Nickel et al. 1982	ELBW ≤1000g	No	6–18	No	–	–	64% sp. ed.	–	Poor	–	–	–
Victorian group	ELBW 500–999g	No	8	No	–	–	13% in special school	Normal school: 23% delayed	–	–	–	–
Saigal et al 1991	ELBW 500–1000g	Term	8	Yes	S<C	Effect on V < on P	sp. ed. S>C	S>C	S>C	–	M=F	Additional
O'Callaghan et al. 1996	ELBW 500–999g	NBW classmates	8–17	Yes	–	–	–	S>C	S>C	–	M>F	None

–, No data given; AGA, appropriate for gestational age; ELBW, extremely low birthweight; IU, intrauterine; LBW, low birthweight; NBW, normal birthweight; P (IQ), Performance; PIVH, periventricular–intraventricular haemorrhage; SGA, small for gestational age; sp. asst., special assistance needed; sp. ed. special education needed; V (IQ), Verbal; VLBW, very low birthweight.

[a]Does paper provide data on effect of LBW on cognitive function and learning problems after exclusion of handicapped children?

[b]S=C, no significant difference between study and control groups; S>C, significantly more problems in study group than in control group; S<C, significantly worse score in study than in control group; E<V<N, ELBW scored significantly worse than VLBW, VLBW scored significantly worse than NBW.

[c]Presence (+) of relation between minor neurological dysfunction and learning problems.

[d]Interaction if any between socioeconomic status and (V)(E)LBW.

172

than girls, but no satisfactory explanation for the disadvantage has yet been found (Taylor 1981). The answer to the intriguing question of male vulnerability probably lies in the complex interplay of genetic factors and steroid hormones: the genetic factors directly affecting the function of individual neurons (Reisert and Pilgrim 1991) and the steroid hormones have widespread effects on the developing brain (McEwen 1992). Most of the studies that reported on social class demonstrated that unfavourable social conditions were injurious to cognitive development (see Table 8.1). In the majority of studies this effect was additional to others, but in two studies social class was found to interact directly with neonatal morbidity. This means that lower social class adversely affected cognitive development only in those neonates with LBW who were severely ill, and not in relatively healthy ones (Hunt et al. 1988, Ross et al. 1991). Sommerfelt and coworkers also reported an interactional effect of social class: in children whose fathers had low levels of edcation, the cognitive performance of LBW children at 5 years of age was the same as that of control children born at term, whereas in children whose fathers had a higher level of education the LBW children performed worse than the controls (Sommerfelt et al. 1995).

FOLLOW-UP OF ASPHYXIATED NEONATES
Surprisingly, the boom in long-term follow-up studies of at-risk neonates was restricted to those with low birthweights of various degrees. Very few studies evaluated the long-term effect of perinatal asphyxia. This is rather odd, as perinatal asphyxia or 'birth trauma' was long considered to be a major cause of minor brain dysfunction (Rie and Rie 1980). Available follow-up studies of asphyxiated neonates focused on neurological disability and rarely extended the follow-up beyond the age of 4 years (Niswander et al. 1975, Mulligan et al. 1980, Robertson and Finer 1985, Seidman et al. 1991, Shankaran et al. 1991). A few studies indicated that perinatal asphyxia increases the risk for neurological disorder only when the asphyxia is followed by neonatal encephalopathy (Mulligan et al. 1980; Robertson and Finer 1985, 1993; Shankaran et al. 1991). Whether the same holds true for the development of learning disorders remains to be seen.

FOLLOW-UP AFTER FETAL EXPOSURE TO TOXIC SUBSTANCES
Prenatal exposure to toxic substances can be another source of learning disorders (Swaab and Mirmiran 1984). Again, few studies followed up children for as long as 6 years. Some studies of fetal exposure to drugs did not find a teratogenic effect on behavioural or cognitive development (betamethasone, methyldopa: Cockburn et al. 1982, MacArthur et al. 1982, Schmand et al. 1990). Others produced equivocal results: intrauterine exposure to ritodrine, used to treat imminent preterm labour, might be associated with an increased prevalence of poor academic achievement (Polowczyk et al. 1984, Hadders-Algra et al. 1986b). A third group of studies did find significant adverse effects of prenatal exposure to toxic substances on cognitive performance when the child reached school age. Chen and Hsu (1994) found that the Full Scale IQs of 7- to 12-year-old children who had been exposed antenatally to high doses of polychlorinated biphenyls were 4 to 5 points lower than those of non-exposed, matched controls. Prenatal exposure to antiepileptic drugs was associated with lower IQs (phenytoin with or without carbamazepine: Gaily et al. 1988) or with small head size, poor

school achievement, and problems with arithmetic (phenobarbital: Van der Pol et al. 1991). Similar negative effects of antenatal exposure to alcohol were reported. Maternal patterns of binge drinking or regular drinking during pregnancy were related to lower IQ, school failure, poor spatial organization, and problems with arithmetic in their school-age offspring (Sampson et al. 1989, Streissguth et al. 1989).

FOLLOW-UP IN HETEROGENEOUS GROUPS OF INFANTS

All four research groups that evaluated long-term development in mixed groups of neonates reported a contribution of perinatal adversities to the development of learning difficulties. Werner and Smith, who followed up their 1955 Hawaii birth cohort to 18 years of age, reported that the development of learning disorders was related to the presence of 'perinatal stress' and low social class (Werner and Smith 1979). Nichols and Chen studied the development of learning disorders in the large 1959–1960 cohort of the US National Collaborative Perinatal Project. Multivariate analysis showed that the presence of learning disability was correlated with low social class, a low number of prenatal health-care visits, hospitalization during pregnancy, cigarette smoking, and a lengthened second stage of labour (Nichols and Chen 1981). The results of two major studies, the Helsinki Neonatal Risk Study and the Groningen Perinatal Project, are reported separately below.

Helsinki Neonatal Risk Study

The Helsinki Neonatal Risk Study is a long-term follow-up study of 386 infants born in a large maternity hospital in Helsinki in 1972–1973 (Michelsson et al. 1981, 1984; Lindahl and Michelsson 1986, 1987; Helenius 1987; Lindahl 1987; Lindahl et al. 1988a,b; Michelsson and Lindahl 1987, 1993). Infants who met predefined inclusion criteria at birth were followed up to age 9 years to find out how neonatal risk factors affected their development. The development of specific learning disorders was particularly looked for. Children were included in the study if they had one of the risk diagnoses listed in Table 8.2. Twenty-one per cent of the infants had more than one risk diagnosis. Nineteen had a birthweight of ≤1500g. Intrauterine growth retardation (birthweight <10th centile) was found in 53 children. Children who developed a major disability such as cerebral palsy or mental retardation were excluded from the 9-year follow-up. The effect of perinatal and neonatal risk factors was evaluated not only with the help of the original inclusion criteria, but also with a series of optimality variables (see Prechtl 1968, Kyllerman and Hagberg 1983). In addition to the children of the study group, a comparison group of 107 children without neonatal risk factors was seen at age 9 years.

The 9-year assessments were summarized as the outcome scores on five measures: a neurological and neurodevelopmental examination (NEURO) (Lindahl et al. 1988b), the Test of Motor Impairment (TMI) (Stott et al. 1972), seven subtests of the Illinois Test of Psycholinguistic Abilities (ITPA) (Kuusinen and Blåfield 1974), the Wechsler Intelligence Scale for Children (WISC) (WISC 1971), and standardized Finnish tests for reading and spelling (SCHOOL) (Ruoppila et al. 1968, 1969). These scores were dichotomized into normal and abnormal. It is important to realize that an abnormal SCHOOL score did not denote obvious school failure, as 91% of the study-group children attended mainstream school at

TABLE 8.2

**Helsinki Neonatal Risk Study: original risk diagnoses of
the children seen at 9 years of age (N=386)**

Risk diagnosis	Number of children
Low birthweight (LBW) (≤2000g)	91
Respiratory problems necessitating ventilatory support	31
Apgar score ≤6 at 5 min or later	77
Neurological symptoms*	45
Hyperbilirubinaemia	164
Hypoglycaemia	36
Septic infection	3
Maternal diabetes	30

*Including marked hypotonia, apathy, hyperexcitability, rigidity,
convulsions, apnoeic spells, or prolonged feeding difficulties.

an appropriate level. The effect of the (perinatal) risk factors was analysed with multivariate statistics (stepwise logistic regression analysis and stepwise multiple regression analysis; see Lindahl et al. 1988b).

In general the children in the study group were twice as likely to have problems as those in the comparison group. Figure 8.1 summarizes the abnormal scores on four of the tests, according to neonatal risk group. Two or more abnormal scores were found in 31% of the children in the study group and in 20% of those in the comparison group, and three or more abnormal scores, in 17% and 10%, respectively. Three or more abnormal scores were significantly more often found in the children with LBW or neonatal neurological symptoms ($P<0.05$). The ITPA and WISC tests did not significantly differ between the risk groups. The differences between the groups on the TMI were insignificant but had the same trend as was found for the NEURO.

The logistic regression analysis (Table 8.3) revealed that neurological dysfunction (as measured by the NEURO score) was correlated in particular with respiratory and neurological problems in the neonatal period. LBW was not correlated with neurological dysfunction, but IUGR and hypothermia, often found in LBW infants, were. On the TMI, only signs of cerebral depression, IUGR, and hypothermia were significant predictors of poor performance. Both the NEURO and the TMI are mainly measures of motor competence and coordination, and therefore it is not surprising that low scores on these tests are associated with problems often seen in LBW infants. Social class and hereditary factors did not play a role in neurological or motor problems.

In failure at language competence (as measured by the ITPA score), the most important risk factor was neurological dysfunction in the neonatal period. Other significant factors were reproductive failure, pregnancy problems potentially associated with deficient fetal nutrition, and low social class. Poor cognitive performance (as measured by the WISC score) was associated with hyperbilirubinaemia due to isoimmunization and – like the ITPA score – with factors associated with potential disturbances of fetal nutrition and social class. Poor reading and spelling (as measured by the SCHOOL score) were associated with neurological symptoms in the neonatal period and with hyperbilirubinaemia. Also maternal

TABLE 8.3
Helsinki Neonatal Risk Study: factors significantly associated with outcome at 9 years of age

Risk factor	Outcome on tests[a] at age 9 years				
	NEURO	TMI	ITPA	WISC	SCHOOL
Respiratory problems (not RDS)	6.1				
Cerebral irritation	2.9				
Cerebral depression	2.4	2.2	4.0		2.6
Hyperbilirubinaemia					
Due to isoimmunization				2.6	2.8
Of unknown aetiology	2.0				
Mother had previous abortion			2.6	2.6	
Mother smoked					6.1
Abnormal maternal urinary estriol			4.4	9.0	
Placental infarction					21.6
IUGR <10th centile	1.8	2.0	2.2	1.9	2.2
Diazepam during labour					2.5
Cord complication				3.0	
Hypothermia	1.6	2.8			
Base excess less than −10				2.4	
Hereditary factors	1.8				2.5
Male sex	1.7				
Social class[b]					
I			1.0	1.0	1.0
II			4.6	3.6	4.5
III			4.7	4.7	7.0
IV			7.0	4.9	7.1

Values are results of logistic regression analysis, i.e. odds ratios with a 95% lower confidence limit <1.0. (After Lindahl et al. 1988b, by permission.)

IUGR, intrauterine growth retardation; RDS, respiratory distress syndrome.

[a]NEURO, a neurological and neurodevelopmental examination; TMI, Test of Motor Impairment; ITPA, Illinois Test of Psycholinguistic Abilities; WISC, Wechsler Intelligence Scale for Children; SCHOOL, standardized Finnish tests for reading and spelling. For details of tests, see text.

[b]Social class: I, high; II, higher middle; III, lower middle; IV, low.

Fig. 8.1 *(Facing page)*: Helsinki Neonatal Risk Study: percentages of children in various neonatal risk groups who failed in four outcome measures at 9 years of age.

Tests: NEURO (a neurological and neurodevelopmental examination; see text), ITPA (Illinois Test of Psycholinguistic Abilities), WISC (Wechsler Intelligence Scale for Children), and SCHOOL (standardized Finnish tests for reading and spelling; see text).

Groups: Comp, comparison group; LBW, all low-birthweight infants, with or without other diagnoses; Resp, only respiratory problems necessitating ventilatory support; Apgar, only Apgar score ≤6 at 5 min or later; Neurol, only neurological symptoms; Bilir, only hyperbilirubinaemia; Hypogl, only hypoglycaemia; DM, only maternal diabetes; many dg, more than one diagnosis, but not LBW.

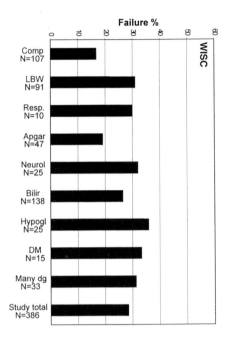

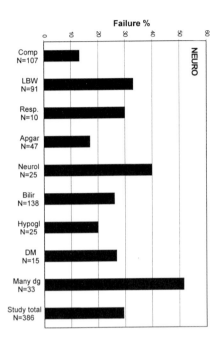

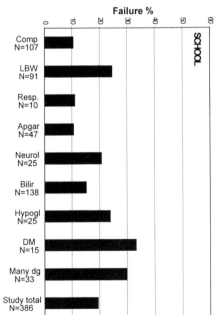

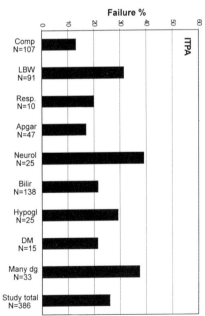

177

smoking during pregnancy, placental infarction, and IUGR played a role – all factors suggesting a disturbance of intrauterine nutrition and oxygenation. Other factors that contributed significantly to the SCHOOL score were low social class and the presence of learning disabilities in first-degree relatives. Of the children with an abnormal SCHOOL score, 67% also failed on the ITPA, 64% on the WISC, 58% on the NEURO, and 33% on the TMI.

The relative importances of the neonatal, antenatal, and biological/social factors were analysed using stepwise multiple regression (Table 8.4). The neonatal variables accounted for 1 to 7% of the variance within the five outcome scores, while combined antenatal variables accounted for 3 to 10% and social class alone accounted for 2 to 7%. Neonatal neurological abnormality was the factor most consistently associated with a poor outcome. The neurological signs were not, however, associated with low Apgar scores. The children with low Apgar scores without any other risk diagnosis were, in this study, the group with the least problems. It is hard to estimate retrospectively how many of the neurologically abnormal infants fulfilled the criteria of hypoxic–ischaemic encephalopathy – maybe most of them did. In any case the presence of neonatal neurological deviance, whether due to antenatally or to perinatally acquired pathology, appeared to be strongly associated with neurological and cognitive dysfunction.

The Helsinki study indicated that both potential hereditary and environmental factors – measured in a quite robust way – played an important role in the development of learning disabilities. This finding is in accord with the findings of others (Neligan et al. 1976, Drillien et al. 1980, Taylor et al. 1985, Naye and Peters 1987, Sameroff et al. 1987). Social class played a considerable role, even though class differences in standard of living and in the possibilities for education are considerably smaller in Finland than in many other countries.

If the data from the Helsinki Neonatal Risk Study are extrapolated to the general Finnish population – assuming that neurodevelopmental disabilities are present in about 10% of all Finnish children – the risk diagnoses of the Helsinki Study would account for one-third to one-sixth of such problems.

Groningen Perinatal Project
The Groningen Perinatal Project is a long-term follow-up of a 3-year birth cohort of 3162 infants born at the University Hospital in Groningen from 1975 to 1978. The aim of this research project is to study how pre- and perinatal events are related to neurological, cognitive, and behavioural development. To this end the pre- and perinatal condition of all infants was described extensively, not only in terms of single items, such as preterm birth or breech presentation, but also with the help of the Obstetrical Optimality Score. This score is based on 74 variables describing obstetrical conditions, ranging from the parents' socioeconomic status and matters of their health to the infant's condition immediately after birth (Touwen et al. 1980). The number of items with a value within a predefined optimal range is the infant's optimality score. All the infants in the Groningen project were examined neurologically during the neonatal period using Prechtl and Beintema's (1975) standardized technique and were classified as neurologically normal, mildly abnormal, or definitely abnormal. The classification 'definitely abnormal' signified the presence of a complete

TABLE 8.4
Helsinki Neonatal Risk Study: relative importances of neonatal, antenatal, and biological/social factors for outcome at 9 years of age

Outcome measure[a]	Background variable	r	r^2
NEURO	Social class	0.17	0.03
	Sex	0.24	0.06
	Birthweight	0.29	0.08
	Cerebral depression	0.33	0.11
	Duration of hyperbilirubinaemia	0.35	0.12
	Respiratory problems (not RDS)	0.36	0.13
TMI	Social class	0.14	0.02
	Respiratory problems (not RDS)	0.18	0.03
	Birthweight	0.22	0.05
	Cerebral depression	0.23	0.06
	Duration of hyperbilirubinaemia	0.25	0.06
ITPA	Social class	0.25	0.06
	Cerebral depression	0.30	0.09
	Urinary infection	0.33	0.11
	IUGR	0.35	0.12
	Duration of gestation	0.36	0.13
WISC	Social class	0.22	0.05
	IUGR	0.28	0.08
	Maternal parity >4	0.34	0.11
	Abnormal maternal urinary estriol	0.36	0.13
	Tachypnoea	0.38	0.14
	Blood exchange transfusion	0.39	0.15
	Placental infarction	0.40	0.16
SCHOOL	Social class	0.24	0.06
	Placental infarction	0.31	0.10
	Hereditary factors	0.36	0.13
	Abnormal maternal urinary estriol	0.38	0.15
	Cerebral depression	0.40	0.16
	IUGR	0.42	0.17
	Diazepam during labour	0.43	0.19

Values are the results of stepwise multiple regression analysis, i.e. the correlation coefficient r and the r^2, which represents the cumulative explanatory power. (After Lindahl et al. 1988b, by permission.)

IUGR, intrauterine growth retardation; RDS, respiratory distress syndrome

[a]Outcome measures: NEURO, neurological and neurodevelopmental examination; TMI, Test of Motor Impairment; ITPA, Illinois Test of Psycholinguistic Abilities; WISC, Wechsler Intelligence Scale for Children; SCHOOL, standardized Finnish tests for reading and spelling.

neonatal neurological syndrome, such as hypo- or hypertonia, or a hyperexcitability or apathy syndrome (Prechtl and Beintema 1975). 'Mildly abnormal' indicated the partial presence of such a syndrome. Definite neonatal neurological abnormality was found in 5% of the infants studied, and mild abnormality, in 23%. Neonatal deviance was related to the presence of asphyxia (indicated by the presence of acidaemia), IUGR, and preterm birth (Jurgens-van der Zee et al. 1979, Huisjes et al. 1980), especially when these events had been accompanied by a low Obstetrical Optimality Score (Touwen and Huisjes 1984).

Follow-up examinations were carried out at ages 1½, 4, 6, 9, 12, and 14 years (Bierman-Van Eendenburg et al. 1981; Touwen et al. 1982, 1988; Hadders-Algra et al. 1985, 1986a,b, 1988a,b,c; Hadders-Algra and Touwen 1990, 1992, 1998; Lunsing et al. 1991, 1992a,b; Soorani-Lunsing et al. 1993a,b, 1994), focusing on the developmental outcome of the children with neonatal neurological abnormalities. The neonatally deviant children were evaluated together with age-matched controls who had been neonatally normal or mildly abnormal. At each age Touwen's (1979) standardized, age-adequate neurological examination was carried out, with special attention to the presence of minor neurological dysfunction. Behavioural and cognitive problems were also assessed at each check-up. The cognitive evaluation consisted in the evaluation of school performance and the assessment of reading, spelling, and arithmetic at ages 9 and 12 years with short, standardized Dutch tests. At age 14 years school performance was evaluated again and a short, standardized IQ test was given. Physical health was evaluated by assessing the type and number of complications (diseases or trauma) that had occurred during the check-up interval. At ages 12 and 14 years physical signs of puberty were also appraised (Lunsing et al. 1992b).

DEVELOPMENT OF MINOR NEUROLOGICAL DYSFUNCTION (MND)

One of the major findings in the Groningen Perinatal Project was the age dependence of MND (Hadders-Algra and Touwen 1997). The low rate at preschool age (Bierman-Van Eendenburg et al. 1981, Touwen et al. 1982) increased steadily, to a peak just before the beginning of puberty (Hadders-Algra et al. 1986a, 1988b; Lunsing et al. 1992a). This age-dependent increase in MND parallels, and is presumably related to, the age-dependent increase in the complexity of brain function. The rate of MND declined dramatically at the onset of puberty. This decline may be mediated by hormonal changes (Soorani-Lunsing et al. 1993b). The age-dependent changes in MND were accompanied by changes in correlations with antecedent risk factors and by changes in concomitant cognitive problems and behavioral difficulties. In prepubertal school children the number of neurological signs turned out to be important. In 9-year-olds two types of MND were distinguished on the basis of how many clusters of neurological signs were affected – each cluster representing a subset of the neurological repertoire (Table 8.5). Children were classified as having MND-1 (dysfunction in one or two clusters) or MND-2 (dysfunction in more than two clusters) (Hadders-Algra et al. 1988b). MND-1 was not correlated with neonatal neurological condition, being found in 15% of each of the neonatally normal, mildly abnormal, and definitely abnormal groups. MND-2, however, was closely correlated with neonatal neurological condition, being present in 5, 10, and 18% of the neonatally normal, mildly abnormal, and definitely abnormal children, respectively. Multivariate analysis confirmed that the perinatal roots of MND-2, the more complex form, were considerably stronger than those of MND-1 (Table 8.6). For example, the risk of developing MND-2 was related to a lower Obstetrical Optimality Score, and this risk increased markedly when the score was decreased by more than 10 points. The relation between neonatal neurological morbidity and the eventual appearance of MND-2 was markedly affected by social class: children with neonatal abnormalities born into families of low social class were four times as likely to develop MND-2 as were children with similar neonatal neurological dysfunctions born

TABLE 8.5
Sign clusters summarizing Touwen's (1979) neurological examination

Sign cluster	Criteria for a dysfunctional cluster
1 Posture and muscle tone	Consistently present mild abnormalities in muscle tone and posture
2 Reflexes	Consistent presence of increased or decreased thresholds and/or asymmetries; presence of the Babinski sign
3 Choreiform dyskinesia	Marked presence of choreiform jerks in distal and facial muscles and/or slight or marked presence of choreiform movements of proximal body parts, eyes, and tongue
4 Coordination and balance	At least two or more tests of coordination and balance (e.g. diadochokinesis, tandem gate, standing on one leg) inappropriate for age
5 Fine manipulative ability	At least two or more tests of fine manipulation (e.g. finger opposition test, follow-a-finger test) inappropriate for age
6 Rarely occurring dysfunctions	Dysfunction of a cranial nerve (e.g. paresis of VIth or VIIth nerve) or presence of excessive amount of associated movements

(After Hadders-Algra et al. 1988b, by permission.)

TABLE 8.6
Groningen Perinatal Project: factors significantly associated with the development of minor neurological dysfunction by 9 years of age

Risk factor	MND-1	MND-2
Neonatal neurological condition according to socioeconomic status		
Low socioeconomic status		
Neurologically normal	–	1
Neurologically mildly abnormal	–	6.7
Neurologically definitely abnormal	–	16.4
Middle/high socioeconomic status		
Neurologically normal	–	1.6
Neurologically mildly abnormal	–	2.5
Neurologically definitely abnormal	–	4.1
Obstetrical Optimality Score (each point reduction)	–	1.1
Severe IUGR (birthweight percentile <2.3)	4.1	–
Male sex	1.6	2.2

Values are the results of logistic regression analysis, i.e. odds ratios with a 95% lower confidence limit >1.0. (After Hadders-Algra et al. 1988b, by permission.)
IUGR, intrauterine growth retardation; MND, minor neurological dysfunction (dysfunction in one or two [MND-1] or three or more [MND-2] clusters on Touwen's [1979] neurological examination; see text, and Table 8.5).

into families of middle or high social class. Social class, defined in this project on the basis of socioeconomic status, may reflect a complex intermingling of 'nature' and 'nurture', in which feeding practices may also play a role (Lanting et al. 1994). With respect to the development of MND-1, only severe IUGR and male sex were found to contribute significantly. Male sex was also a risk factor for the development of MND-2. In both types of MND the ratio of boys to girls was 2:1.

The alleviating effect of puberty on MND resulted in a reduction of the prevalence of MND. At age 14 years, 6% of the children who had been neurologically normal at birth had MND, in comparison with 28% of the children who had shown definite neurological abnormalities at birth. After the children reached puberty, MND-2 virtually disappeared. The majority of children with MND at this age presented with only one dysfunctional cluster, that is, they had either mild hypotonia, choreiform dyskinesia, coordination problems, or a dysfunction of fine manipulation (Soorani-Lunsing et al. 1993b). Combinations occurred, but only rarely. The qualitatively different forms of MND showed different relations with perinatal events (Table 8.7). Two types of dysfunction appeared to be clearly correlated with pre- and perinatal events: a) dysfunctions of fine manipulative ability – correlated with the neonatal neurological condition, the presence of minor physical anomalies, and low social class, and b) coordination problems – correlated with very preterm birth (<34 weeks). Choreiform dyskinesia correlated significantly with a low Apgar score, but not with acidaemia, which is a better indicator of perinatal asphyxia than is a low Apgar score. The fourth type of dysfunction, hypotonia, was not correlated with any perinatal event but instead appeared to be correlated with a family history of neurological or psychiatric disorders and with complications in the interval between ages 9 and 12 years.

In summary, in prepubertal school-age children the *quantity* of neurological signs is the most relevant neurological parameter, but after the onset of puberty the *quality* of neurological dysfunction is the most pertinent indicator of brain dysfunction. Apparently the process of puberty converts the non-specific expression of dysfunction of the prepubertal nervous system into a specific and possibly more adult-like display of dysfunction.

DEVELOPMENT OF LEARNING DISABILITY
In this chapter we focus on the development of learning disabilities by 9 years of age, that is, at prepubertal school age (Hadders-Algra et al. 1988c), and by 14 years of age, when virtually all the children examined had entered puberty (Soorani-Lunsing et al. 1994).

At 9 years of age there was a clear correlation between neonatal neurological morbidity and need for special education: 3% of the 437 children with no or mild neonatal neurological abnormalities were attending a school for special education (5% of the boys, 1.5% of the girls – a non-significant difference between the sexes), whereas of the 133 children with marked neonatal neurological dysfunction 17% needed special education (17% of both boys and girls; effect of the neonatal neurological condition: $\chi^2=26.7$, $P<0.001$). Neonatal neurological deviance was also a significant risk factor for specific learning problems, especially problems with reading and arithmetic and to a lesser extent with spelling (Fig. 8.2). The risk of spelling problems was increased only in the group of girls with definite neonatal neurological abnormalities. Many of the children with learning disabilities showed signs of MND (Hadders-Algra and Touwen 1992) (see Fig. 8.2). Twice as many boys with reading, spelling, or arithmetic problems had MND as boys whose skills at these were normal. In girls the association with MND was even stronger: the rate of MND in girls with learning difficulties was four times as high as in girls without learning difficulties. Because of the frequent comorbidity between MND and learning difficulties, we took the presence of MND into account in the multivariate analysis of risk factors in the development of learning difficulties.

TABLE 8.7
Groningen Perinatal Project: factors significantly associated with the development of minor neurological dysfunction by 14 years of age

Risk factor	Hypotonia	Choreiform dyskinesia	Coordination problems	Fine manipulative disability
Positive family history for neuropsychiatric diseases	5.8	–	–	–
Presence of minor physical anomalies	–	–	–	3.3
Very preterm birth (<34 wk)	–	–	*	–
Apgar score at 3 min <7	–	10.0	–	–
Definite neonatal neurological abnormality	–	–	–	3.5
Complications between ages 9 and 12 yr	4.1	–	–	–
Low socioeconomic status	–	–	–	5.0

Values are the results of logistic regression analysis, i.e. the odds ratios with a 95% lower confidence limit >1.0. (After Soorani-Lunsing RJ, Hadders-Algra M, Olinga AA, et al. (1993) Minor neurological dysfunction after the onset of puberty: association with perinatal events. *Early Human Development* **33:** 71–80.)
*The number of children with coordination problems was too small to perform logistic regression analysis. Univariate analysis revealed a relation between the presence of coordination problems and gestational age at birth <34 weeks (Fisher exact test, $P<0.001$).

TABLE 8.8
Groningen Perinatal Project: risk factors (including the presence of MND) significantly associated with learning disabilities

Risk factor	School failure	Poor reading[a]	Poor spelling[a]	Poor arithmetic[a]
Sex				
Male	–	–	1.6	–
Female	–	–	–	–
Preterm birth (<34 wk)	–	–	–	4.5
Definite neonatal neurological abnormality	2.0	2.0	–	–
Presence of MND				
MND-1	2.0	5.0	3.0	4.1
MND-2	6.7	6.0	6.0	10.0
Low socioeconomic status	3.0	3.3	4.5	4.5
Family adversity	–	–	1.6	–

Values are the results of logistic regression analysis, i.e. the odds ratios with a 95% lower confidence limit >1.0. (After Hadders-Algra et al. 1988c, by permission.)
MND, minor neurological dysfunction (dysfunction in one or two (MND-1] or three or more [MND-2] clusters on Touwen's [1979] neurological examination; see text, and Table 8.5).
[a]<10th centile on stardardized Dutch tests.

The risk factors that were significant in the development of learning problems at 9 years of age are presented in Table 8.8. Low socioeconomic status played an important role in all types of learning difficulties. The presence of MND was also clearly related to learning skills. MND-2, with its strong roots in the pre- and perinatal period, affected academic performance, particularly in arithmetic, more than did MND-1. Perinatal risk factors not only contributed indirectly – through MND – to the development of learning problems, but were found also to contribute directly. Neonatal neurological deviance was associated

183

POOR READING

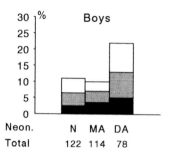

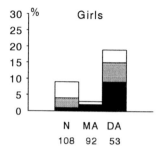

Neon.						
Total	122	114	78	108	92	53

POOR SPELLING

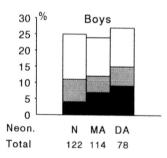

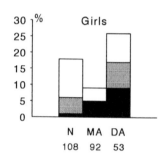

Neon.						
Total	122	114	78	108	92	53

POOR ARITHMETIC

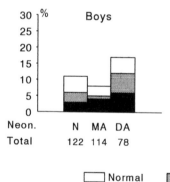

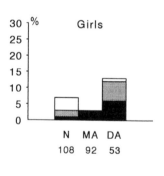

Neon.						
Total	122	114	78	108	92	53

☐ Normal　▓ MND-1　■ MND-2

Fig. 8.2: Groningen Perinatal Project: percentages of children with poor skills at 9 years of age, shown according to their neurological classification at birth.

Shading indicates the proportion of children with signs of minor neurological dysfunction (MND) at 9 years of age. Classification at birth: N, neurologically normal; MA, mildly abnormal; DA, definitely abnormal. Poor reading, spelling, arithmetic: <10th centile on standardized Dutch tests.

directly with school failure and poor reading, and likewise very preterm birth (<34 weeks) was associated with arithmetic problems. The data also indicated that the link between (neonatal) brain dysfunction and academic skills was stronger for difficulties with reading and arithmetic than for difficulties with spelling. The latter form of learning difficulty appeared to be more correlated with problems in the home environment (see Table 8.8).

The multivariate analyses of risk factors in school failure at age 14 years revealed that all risk was explained by the presence of the various forms of MND, for which the odds ratios (and 95% lower confidence limits) were as follows: fine manipulative dysfunction, 12 (4.9); coordination problems, 13 (2.3); choreiformity, 6.6 (2.1); and hypotonia, 9.5 (2.9). No significant (additional) contribution of single perinatal risk factors, social conditions, or the sex of the child was found (Soorani-Lunsing et al. 1994).

Conclusions

Perinatal risk factors do contribute to learning disorders, as is illustrated by the salient relation between neonatal neurological morbidity and learning difficulties. Specific risk factors with a distinct effect on school performance are very preterm birth (<34 weeks), severe IUGR (usually summarized as VLBW), and intrauterine exposure to alcohol. The prevalences of these risk factors are quite low. For instance, only 2 to 3% of all infants are born before 34 weeks of gestation or with severe IUGR (Verloove-Vanhorick and Verwey 1987). The effect of the low prevalence of children at high risk for learning disabilities is that such children make up only 20 to 30% of all children with learning disabilities; in other words, three-quarters of learning disabilities do not have a perinatal aetiology. Evidence is emerging that adversities occurring very early during development (prenatally) are more likely to result in a severe disorder such as cerebral palsy, whereas adversities from the last trimester of pregnancy to the age of at least 2 years are more often followed by 'minor' problems, such as MND or learning disabilities (see Nelson and Ellenberg 1986; Hadders-Algra et al. 1988a). Other explanations for the relatively low contribution of perinatal adversities to the development of learning disabilities could be our lack of knowledge about minor (genetically based?) developmental abnormalities of the brain, such as cortical heterotopias and neuronal cortical focal dysgeneses, which might be related to learning problems (Kaufmann and Galaburda 1989, Humphreys et al. 1990). This possibility begs for exploration with brain imaging techniques.

Perinatal risk factors are associated with school failure in general, but also with specific learning disorders. Arithmetic appears to be the academic skill that is most strongly correlated with perinatal adversities, as underlined by the prominent association between arithmetic failure and the presence of severe forms of MND in the children studied. Mathematical procedures may require simultaneous reasoning, that is, they require both the integrity of multiple sites in the brain and also interconnectivity of these sites, whereas verbal skills may depend more on sequential reasoning (see Roth et al. 1993).

Perinatal adversities can lead to the development of learning disorders, but it is important to realize that a single pre- or perinatal risk factor rarely results in a developmental disorder, such as learning problems. This generalization also probably holds true for perinatal asphyxia: when asphyxia occurs in isolation it probably will not induce cognitive dysfunction, but when it is accompanied by a multitude of adversities the risk of late sequelae, such as learning disorders, will increase considerably. Multifactoriality is not restricted to the pre- and perinatal period. Many factors after birth also contribute to the development of learning problems, the role of the complex variable *social class* being an example. The possibility that neonatal (neurological) morbidity and social class could interact in the development of minor brain dysfunction (such as MND or learning disorders) offers the challenging opportunity of selective intervention (see also Brooks-Gunn et al. 1994).

REFERENCES

Alexander GE, Crutcher MD. (1990) Functional architecture of basal ganglia circuits: neural substrates of parallel processing. *Trends in Neuroscience* **13:** 266–71.

Allen MC. (1984) Developmental outcome and follow-up of the small for gestational age infants. *Seminars in Perinatology* **8:** 123–56.

Armstrong DL. (1993) Preterm periventricular axonal and myelin injury. *Seminars in Perinatology* **17:** 342–50.

Bakker DJ. (1984) Hemispheric specialization and specific reading retardation. In: Rutter M, editor. *Developmental Neuropsychiatry.* Edinburgh: Churchill Livingstone. p 498–506.

Bax M. (1983) Following up the small baby [editorial]. *Developmental Medicine and Child Neurology* **25:** 415–6.

— (1986) Perinatal care – success or failure? [editorial]. *Developmental Medicine and Child Neurology* **28:** 277–8.

Bierman-Van Eendenburg MEC, Jurgens-van der Zee AD, Olinga AA, et al. (1981) Predictive value of neonatal neurological examination: a follow-up study at 18 months. *Developmental Medicine and Child Neurology* **23:** 296–305.

Bjerre I, Hansen E. (1976) Psychomotor development and school-adjustment of 7-year-old children with low birthweight. *Acta Paediatrica Scandinavica* **65:** 88–96.

Brandt P, Magyary D, Hammond M, Barnard K. (1992) Learning and behavioral–emotional problems of children born preterm at second grade. *Journal of Pediatric Psychology* **17:** 291–311.

Brooks-Gunn J, McCarton CM, Casey PH, et al. (1994) Early intervention in low-birth-weight premature infants: results through age 5 years from the Infant Health and Development Program. *Journal of the American Medical Association* **272:** 1257–62.

Calame A, Fawer CL, Claeys V, et al. (1986) Neurodevelopmental outcome and school performance of very-low-birth-weight infants at 8 years of age. *European Journal of Pediatrics* **145:** 461–6.

Chen Y-J, Hsu C-C. (1994) Effects of prenatal exposure to PCBs on the neurological function of children: a neuropsychological and neurophysiological study. *Developmental Medicine and Child Neurology* **36:** 312–20.

Cockburn J, Moar VA, Ounsted M, Redman CWG. (1982) Final report of study on hypertension during pregnancy: the effects of specific treatment on the growth and development of the children. *Lancet* **i:** 647–9.

Drillien CM, Thomson AJM, Burgoyne K. (1980) Low-birthweight children at early school-age: a longitudinal study. *Developmental Medicine and Child Neurology* **22:** 26–47.

Edmonds JE, Szymonowicz WM, Keith EP. (1990) School performance of very low birthweight (VLBW) preterm children at 8 years of age. *Infant Behavior and Development* **13:** 355. (Abstract).

Forfar JO, Hume R, McPhail FM, et al. (1994) Low birthweight: a 10-year outcome study of the continuum of reproductive casualty. *Developmental Medicine and Child Neurology* **36:** 1037–48.

Frith U. (1984) The similarities and differences between reading and spelling problems. In: Rutter, M, editor. *Developmental Neuropsychiatry.* Edinburgh, London, New York: Churchill Livingstone. p 453-72.

Fuller PW, Guthrie RD, Alvord EC Jr. (1983) A proposed neuropathological basis for learning disabilities in children born prematurely. *Developmental Medicine and Child Neurology* **25:** 214–31.

Gaily E, Kantola-Sorsa E, Granström M-L. (1988) Intelligence of children of epileptic mothers. *Pediatrics* **113:** 677–84.

Hack M, Breslau N, Weissman B, et al. (1991) Effect of low birthweight and subnormal head size on cognitive abilities at school age. *New England Journal of Medicine* **325:** 231–7.

Hadders-Algra M, Touwen BCL. (1990) Body measurements, neurological and behavioural development in six year old children born preterm and/or small-for-gestational-age. *Early Human Development* **22:** 1–13.

— — (1992) Minor neurological dysfunction is more closely related to learning difficulties than to behavioral problems. *Journal of Learning Disabilities* **25:** 649–57.

— — (1998) Perinatal events and soft neurological signs in neurobehavioral outcome studies. *Developmental Neuropsychology*. Forthcoming.

— — Olinga AA, Huisjes HJ. (1985) Minor neurological dysfunction and behavioural development: a report from the Groningen Perinatal Project. *Early Human Development* **11:** 221–9.

— — Huisjes HJ. (1986a) Neurologically deviant newborns: neurological and behavioural development at the age of six years. *Developmental Medicine and Child Neurology* **28:** 569–78.

— — —. (1986b) Long term follow-up of children prenatally exposed to ritodrine. *British Journal of Obstetrics and Gynaecology* **93:** 156-61.

— Huisjes HJ, Touwen BCL. (1988a) Preterm or small-for-gestational-age infants: neurological and behavioural development at the age of 6 years. *European Journal of Pediatrics* **147:** 460–7.

— — — (1988b) Perinatal correlates of major and minor neurological dysfunction at school age: a multivariate analysis. *Developmental Medicine and Child Neurology* **30:** 472–81.

— — — (1988c) Perinatal risk factors and minor neurological dysfunction: significance for behaviour and school achievement at nine years. *Developmental Medicine and Child Neurology* **30:** 482–91.

Hall A, McLeod A, Counsell C, et al. (1995) School attainment, cognitive ability and motor function in a total Scottish very-low-birthweight population at eight years: a controlled study. *Developmental Medicine and Child Neurology* **37:** 1037–50.

Helenius M. (1987) Writing disabilities and cognitive functions at the age of nine years in a neonatal high-risk group. *Early Child Development and Care* **29:** 69–77.

Hille ETM, Den Ouden AL, Bauer L, et al. (1994) School performance at nine years of age in very premature and very low birthweight infants: perinatal risk factors and predictors at five years of age. *Journal of Pediatrics* **125:** 426–34.

Huisjes HJ, Touwen BCL, Hoekstra J, et al. (1980) Obstetrical-neonatal neurological relationship: a replication study. *European Journal of Obstetrics, Gynaecology and Reproductive Biology* **10:** 247–56.

Humphreys P, Kaufmann WE, Galaburda AM. (1990) Developmental dyslexia in women: neuropathological findings in three patients. *Annals of Neurology* **28:** 727–38.

Hunt JV, Cooper BAB, Tooley WH. (1988) Very low birth weight infants at 8 and 11 years of age: role of neonatal illness and family status. *Pediatrics* **82:** 596–603.

Ito M. (1990) A new physiological concept on cerebellum. *Revue Neurologique* **146:** 564–9.

Jongmans M, Henderson S, De Vries L, Dubowitz L. (1993) Duration of periventricular densities in preterm infants and neurological outcome at six years of age. *Archives of Disease in Childhood* **69:** 9–13.

Jurgens-Van der Zee AD, Bierman-Van Eendenburg MEC, Fidler VJ, et al. (1979). Preterm birth, growth retardation and acidemia in relation to neurological abnormality of the newborn. *Early Human Development* **3:** 141–54.

Kaufmann WE, Galaburda AM. (1989) Cerebrocortical microdysgenesis in neurologically normal subjects: a histopathological study. *Neurology* **39:** 238–44.

Kawi AA, Pasamanick B. (1958) Association of factors of pregnancy with reading disorders in childhood. *Journal of the American Medical Association* **166:** 1420–3.

Kitchen WH, Ryan MM, Rickards A, et al. (1980) A longitudinal study of very low-birthweight infants. IV: An overview of performance at eight years of age. *Developmental Medicine and Child Neurology* **22:** 172–88.

Klaus MH, Fanaroff AA. (1986) *Care of the High-Risk Neonate.* 3rd ed. Philadelphia, London: W B Saunders.

Knobloch H, Pasamanick B. (1959) Syndrome of minimal cerebral damage in infancy. *Journal of the American Medical Association* **170:** 1384–7.

Kuusinen L, Blåfield L. (1974) *Illinois Test of Psycholinguistic Abilities, Finnish edition.* Institute of Educational Research, Report No. 234. Jyväskylä, Finland: University of Jyväskylä.

Kyllerman M, Hagberg B. (1983) Reduced optimality in pre- and perinatal conditions in a Swedish newborn population. *Neuropediatrics* **14:** 37–42.

Lanting CI, Fidler V, Huisman M, et al. (1994) Neurological differences between 9-year-old children fed breast-milk or formula-milk as babies. *Lancet* **344:** 1319–22.

Largo RH, Molinari L, Kundu S, et al. (1990) Intellectual outcome, speech, and school-performance in high risk preterm children with birthweight appropriate for gestational age. *European Journal of Pediatrics* **149:** 845–50.

187

Leiner HC, Leiner AL, Dow RS. (1993) Cognitive and language functions of the human cerebellum. *Trends in Neurosciences* **16:** 444–47.

Lilienfeld AM, Pasamanick B. (1955) The association of maternal and fetal factors with the development of cerebral palsy and epilepsy. *American Journal of Obstetrics and Gynecology* **70:** 93–101.

Lindahl E. (1987) Motor performance of neonatal risk and non-risk children at early school age. *Acta Paediatrica Scandinavica* **76:** 809–17.

— Michelsson K. (1986) Neurodevelopmental significance of minor and major congenital anomalies in neonatal high risk children. *Neuropediatrics* **17:** 86–93.

— — (1987) Prognosis of neonatal 'at risk' infants at early school age. *Early Child Development and Care* **29:** 23–41.

— — Donner M. (1988a) Prediction of early school-age problems by a preschool neurodevelopmental examination of children at risk neonatally. *Developmental Medicine and Child Neurology* **30:** 723–34.

— — Helenius M, Parre M. (1988b) Neonatal risk factors and later neurodevelopmental disturbances. *Developmental Medicine and Child Neurology* **30:** 571–89.

Lloyd BW, Wheldall K, Perks D. (1988) Controlled study of intelligence and school performance of very low-birthweight children from a defined geographical area. *Developmental Medicine and Child Neurology* **30:** 36–42.

Lowe J, Papile L-A. (1990) Neurodevelopmental performance of very-low-birth-weight infants with mild periventricular, intraventricular hemorrhage. *American Journal of Diseases of Children* 144: 1242–5.

Lunsing RJ, Hadders-Algra M, Touwen BCL, Huisjes HJ (1991) Nocturnal enuresis and minor neurological dysfunction at 12 years: a follow-up study. *Developmental Medicine and Child Neurology* **33:** 439–45.

— — Huisjes HJ, Touwen BCL. (1992a) Minor neurological dysfunction from birth to 12 years. I: Increase during late school-age. *Developmental Medicine and Child Neurology* **34:** 399–403.

— — — — (1992b). Minor neurological dysfunction from birth to 12 years. II: Puberty is related to decreased dysfunction. *Developmental Medicine and Child Neurology* **34:** 404–9.

MacArthur BA, Howie RN, Dezoete JA, Elkins J. (1982) School-progress and cognitive development of 6-year-old children whose mothers were treated antenatally with betamethasone. *Pediatrics* **70:** 99–105.

McCormick MC. (1989) Long-term follow-up of infants discharged form neonatal intensive care units. *Journal of the American Medical Association* **261:** 1767–72.

— Gortmaker SL, Sobol AM. (1990) Very low birth weight children: behavior problems and school difficulty in a national sample. *Journal of Pediatrics* **117:** 687–93.

McEwen BS. (1992) Steroid hormones: effect on brain development and function. *Hormonal Research* **37** (Suppl 3): 1–10.

Michelsson K, Lindahl E. (1987) School failure in a group of nine-year-old children who neonatally belonged to a high risk group. *Early Child Development and Care* **29:** 61–8.

— — (1993) Relationship between perinatal risk factors and motor development in early and later childhood. In: Kalverboer AF et al., editors. *Longitudinal Approaches.* Cambridge: Cambridge University Press. p 266–85.

— Ylinen A, Donner M. (1981) Neurodevelopmental screening at five years of children who were at risk neonatally. *Developmental Medicine and Child Neurology* **23:** 427–33.

— Lindahl E, Parre M, Helenius M. (1984) Nine-year follow-up of infants weighing 1500 g or less at birth. *Acta Paediatrica Scandinavica* **73:** 835–41.

Mulligan JC, Painter MJ, O'Donoghue PA, et al. (1980) Neonatal asphyxia. II. Neonatal mortality and long term sequelae. *Journal of Pediatrics* **96:** 903–7.

Naye RL, Peters EC. (1987) Antenatal hypoxia and low IQ values. *American Journal of Diseases of Children* **141:** 50–4.

Neligan GA, Kolvin I, Scott D McI, Garside RF. (1976) *Born Too Soon or Born Too Small: A Follow-up Study to Seven Years of Age.* Clinics in Developmental Medicine No. 61. London: Spastics International Medical Publications/William Heinemann Medical Books.

Nelson KB, Ellenberg JH. (1986) Antecedents of cerebral palsy: multivariate analysis of risk. *New England Journal of Medicine* **315:** 81–6.

Nichols PL, Chen TC. (1981) *Minimal Brain Dysfunction: A Prospective Study.* New York: Lawrence Erlbaum.

Nickel RE, Bennett FC, Lamson FN. (1982) School performance of children with birth weights of 1,000 g or less. *American Journal of Diseases of Children* **136:** 105–10.

Nishida H. (1993) Outcome of infants born preterm, with special emphasis on extremely low birthweight infants. *Ballière's Clinical Obstetrics and Gynaecology* **7:** 611–31.

Niswander KR, Gordon M, Drage JS. (1975) The effect of intra-uterine hypoxia on the child surviving to 4 years. *American Journal of Obstetrics and Gynecology* **121**: 892–9.

O'Callaghan MJ, Burns YR, Gray PH, et al. (1996) School performance of ELBW children: a controlled study. *Developmental Medicine and Child Neurology* **38**: 917–26.

Ornstein M, Ohlsson A, Edmonds J, Asztalos E. (1991) Neonatal follow-up of very low birthweight/extremely low birthweight infants to school age: a critical overview. *Acta Paediatrica Scandinavica* **80**: 741–8.

Paneth N, Rudelli R, Monte W, et al. (1990) White matter necrosis in very low birth weight infants: neuropathologic and ultrasonographic findings in infants surviving six days or longer. *Journal of Pediatrics* **116**: 975–84.

— — Kazam E, Monte W. (1994) *Brain Damage in the Preterm Infant.* Clinics in Developmental Medicine No. 131. London: Mac Keith Press.

Parkinson CE, Wallis S, Harvey D. (1981) School achievement and behaviour of children who were small-for-dates at birth. *Developmental Medicine and Child Neurology* **23**: 41–50.

Pasamanick B, Rogers ME, Lilienfeld AM. (1956) Pregnancy experience and the development of behavior disorder in children. *American Journal of Psychiatry* **112**: 613–8.

Polowczyk D, Tejani N, Lauersen N, Siddiq F. (1984) Evaluation of seven-to-nine-year-old children exposed to ritodrine in utero. *Obstetrics and Gynecology* **64**: 485–8.

Prechtl HFR. (1968) Neurological findings in newborn infants after pre- and paranatal complications. In: Jonxis JH, Visser HK, Troelstra JA, editors. *Aspects of Prematurity and Dysmaturity.* Nutricia Symposium Series. Leiden: Stenfert–Kroese. p 303-21.

— Beintema D. (1975) *The Neurological Examination of the Full-Term Newborn Infant.* Clinics in Developmental Medicine No. 12. London: Spastics International Medical Publications/WilliamHeinemann Medical Books.

Reisert I, Pilgrim C. (1991) Sexual differentiation of monoaminergic neurons – genetic or epigenetic? *Trends in Neurosciences* **14**: 468–73.

Rie HE, Rie ED. (1980) *Handbook of Miminal Brain Dysfunctions: A Critical View.* New York: John Wiley and Sons.

Robertson C, Finer N. (1985) Term infants with hypoxic–ischemic encephalopathy: outcome at 3.5 years. *Developmental Medicine and Child Neurology* **27**: 473–84.

— Finer N. (1993) Long-term follow-up of term neonates with perinatal asphyxia. *Clinics in Perinatology* **20**: 483–500.

— Etches PC, Kyle JM. (1990) Eight-year performance and growth of preterm, small for gestational age infants: a comparative study with subjects matched for birthweight or gestational age. *Journal of Pediatrics* **116**: 19–26.

Ross G, Lipper EG, Auld PAM. (1991) Educational status and school-related abilities of very low birth weight premature children. *Pediatrics* **88**: 1125-34.

Roth SC, Baudin J, McCormick DC, et al. (1993) Relation between ultrasound appearance of the brain of very preterm infants and neurodevelopmental impairment at eight years. *Developmental Medicine and Child Neurology* **35**: 755–68.

Rourke BP, Strang JD. (1984) Subtypes of reading and arithmetical disabilities: a neuropsychological analysis. In: Rutter M, editor. *Developmental Neuropsychiatry.* Edinburgh, London, New York: Churchill Livingstone. p 473–88.

Ruoppila I, Röman K, Västi M. (1968). Diagnostic reading test for grades II and III in elementary school. (In Finnish). Institute of Educational Research, Report No. 41. Jyväskylä, Finland: University of Jyväskylä.

— — — (1969). Diagnostic writing test for grades II and III in elementary school. (In Finnish). Institute of Educational Research, Report No. 50. Jyväskylä, Finland: University of Jyväskylä.

Saigal S, Szatmari P, Rosenbaum P, et al. (1991) Cognitive abilities and school performance of extremely low birth weight children and matched term control children at age 8 years: a regional study. *Journal of Pediatrics* **118**: 751–60.

Sameroff AJ, Seifer R, Barocas R, et al. (1987) Intelligence quotient scores of 4-year-old children: social–environmental risk factors. *Pediatrics* **79**: 343–50.

Sampson PD, Streissguth AP, Barr HM, Bookstein FL. (1989) Neurobehavioral effects of prenatal alcohol: Part II. Partial least squares analysis. *Neurotoxicology and Teratology* **11**: 477–91.

Schmand B, Neuvel J, Smolders-De Haas H, et al. (1990) Psychological development of children who were treated antenatally with corticosteroids to prevent respiratory distress syndrome. *Pediatrics* **86**: 58–64.

Seidman DS, Paz I, Laor A, et al. (1991) Apgar scores and cognitive performance at 17 years of age. *Obstetrics and Gynecology* **77**: 875–8.

189

Shankaran S, Woldt E, Koepke T, et al. (1991) Acute neonatal morbidity and long-term central nervous system sequelae of perinatal asphyxia in term infants. *Early Human Development* 25: 135–48.

Sommerfelt K, Ellertsen B, Markestad T. (1995) Parental factors in cognitive outcome of non-handicapped low birthweight infants. *Archives of Disease in Childhood* 73: F135–42.

Soorani-Lunsing RJ, Hadders-Algra M, Olinga AA, et al. (1993a) Is minor neurological dysfunction at 12 years related to behaviour and cognition? *Developmental Medicine and Child Neurology* 35: 321–30.

— — — et al. (1993b) Minor neurological dysfunction after the onset of puberty: association with perinatal events. *Early Human Development* 33: 71–80.

— — Huisjes HJ, Touwen BCL. (1994) Neurobehavioural relationships after the onset of puberty. *Developmental Medicine and Child Neurology* 36: 334–43.

Stott DH, Moyes FA, Henderson SE. (1972) *Test of Motor Impairment.* Guelph, Ontario: Brook Educational Publishing.

Streissguth AP, Bookstein FL, Sampson PD, Barr HM. (1989) Neurobehavioral effects of prenatal alcohol: Part III. Partial least squares analysis of neuropsychologic tests. *Neurotoxicology and Teratology* 11: 493–507.

Swaab DF, Mirmiran M. (1984) Possible mechanisms underlying the teratogenic effects of medicines on the developing brain. In: Yanai J, editor. *Neurobehavioral Teratology.* Amsterdam: Elsevier Science Publ. p 55–71.

Taylor DC. (1981) The influence of sexual differentiation on growth, development and disease. In: Davies JA, Dobbing J, editors. *Scientific Foundations of Pediatrics.* 2nd ed. London: Heinemann Medical Books. p 23–40.

Taylor DJ, Howie PW, Davidson J, et al. (1985) Do pregnancy complications contribute to neurodevelopmental disability? *Lancet* i: 713–6.

Touwen BCL. (1979). *Examination of the Child with Minor Neurological Dysfunction.* 2nd ed. Clinics in Developmental Medicine No. 71. London: Spastics International Medical Publications/William Heinemann Medical Books.

— (1986) Very low birth weight infants. *European Journal of Pediatrics* 145: 460. (Editorial).

— Huisjes HJ. (1984) Obstetrics, neonatal neurology and later outcome. In: Almli CR, Finger S, editors. *Early Brain Damage, Volume 1.* New York: Academic Press. p 169–85.

— — Jurgens-Van der Zee AD, et al. (1980) Obstetrical condition and neonatal neurological morbidity: an analysis with the help of the optimality concept. *Early Human Development* 4: 207–28.

— Lok-Meijer TY, Huisjes HJ, Olinga AA. (1982) The recovery rate of neurologically deviant newborns. *Early Human Development* 7: 131–48.

— Hadders-Algra M, Huisjes HJ. (1988) Hypotonia at six years in prematurely born or small for gestational age children. *Early Human Development* 17: 79–88.

Van der Pol MC, Hadders-Algra M, Huisjes HJ, Touwen BCL. (1991) Antiepileptic medication in pregnancy: late effects on the childrens CNS development. *American Journal of Obstetrics and Gynecology* 164: 121–8.

Verloove-Vanhorick SP, Verwey RA. (1987) Project on preterm and small-for-gestational age infants in the Netherlands 1983 [thesis]. Leiden: University of Leiden, The Netherlands.

Victorian Infant Collaborative Study Group. (1991) Eight-year outcome in infants with birth weights of 500 to 999 grams: continuing regional study of 1979 and 1980 births. *Journal of Pediatrics* 118: 761–7.

Vohr BR, Garcia Coll C, Lobato D, et al. (1991) Neurodevelopmental and medical status of low-birthweight survivors of bronchopulmonary dysplasia at 10 to 12 years of age. *Developmental Medicine and Child Neurology* 33: 690–7.

Volpe JJ. (1991) Cognitive deficits in premature infants. *New England Journal of Medicine* 325: 276–8.

— (1995) *Neurology of the Newborn.* 3rd ed. Philadelphia, London: W B Saunders.

WISC. (1971) *Wechsler Intelligence Scale for Children, Finnish edition.* Helsinki: Psykologien Kustannus.

Werner EE, Smith RS. (1979) An epidemiologic perspective on some antecedents and consequences of childhood mental health problems and learning disabilities: a report from the Kanuai Longitudinal Study. *Journal of the American Academy of Child Psychiatry* 18: 292–306.

Westwood M, Kramer MS, Munz D, et al. (1983) Growth and development of full-term non-asphyxiated small-for-gestational-age newborns: follow-up through adolescence. *Pediatrics* 71: 376–82.

190

9
INSIGHTS FROM INFANTS: TEMPORAL PROCESSING ABILITIES AND GENETICS CONTRIBUTE TO LANGUAGE IMPAIRMENT

April A Benasich and Romy V Spitz

The process of language acquisition is not restricted to the 2- to 6-year period when children actually begin producing words. It can be traced back to roots in the very beginnings of the child's life. These roots can be seen both in the genetic predisposition each of us has for language and also in the child's earliest capabilities and propensities to process language information. The blossoming of language during the first 2 years of life is a universal, cross-cultural phenomenon. From birth, infants are predisposed to attend preferentially to the sounds of language (DeCasper and Fifer 1980, DeCasper and Spence 1986). Even in the first few weeks after birth, infants can discriminate contrasts between phonemes such as /pa/ and /ba/, not only the contrasts existing in their own language but also those in other languages (Eimas et al. 1971, Aslin et al. 1983, Werker and Tees 1984). This early proficiency changes with development, so that by age 10 to 12 months, infants, like adults, only discriminate between the contrasts present in their own language (Werker and Tees 1984, Werker and Lalonde 1988, Kuhl et al. 1992; but see Best 1993). By the end of the first year, children are producing their first words. By the latter half of the second year, they are already beginning to combine these words into short sentences that incorporate many aspects of the syntactic structures present in adult grammar (Bates et al. 1987). Studies of the heritability of language abilities have shown that genetics also plays a significant role in determining language abilities. In fact approximately 50% of the variance in receptive and expressive vocabulary abilities is thought to be due to genetic influences (Scarr and Carter-Saltzman 1983, Plomin et al. 1990). All this evidence leads to the conclusion that infants' propensity to attend to language, early auditory processing competence, and genetic factors are all key determinants of normal language acquisition.

For some children, however, the process of acquiring language is quite protracted and very difficult. They are said to have language impairment (LI), or developmental dysphasia. This classification is applied to children who present with a form of developmental language disorder that cannot be attributed to a known cause such as hearing impairment, mental retardation, childhood schizophrenia, infantile autism, or frank neurological disorder. About 5 to 10% of all children beginning school are estimated to have such language disorders (Robinson 1987, Tomblin 1996). Children with LI may have an increased risk of social and emotional difficulties (Beitchman et al. 1989, Benasich et al. 1993). Moreover the majority of children with LI go on to develop reading problems similar to those seen in individuals with dyslexia (American Psychiatric Association 1987 [DSM-III-R], Tallal 1988). Such data suggest that identification and remediation must begin within the first years of life if early impairments are to be prevented from exerting a cascade of negative effects on language, academic, and social skills. In this chapter we describe findings from studies of early preverbal processing of information and studies of familial aggregation, to show how these two lines of research can provide critical information about the development of language and language impairments.

Preverbal abilities and language acquisition: the case for temporal processing

LI has traditionally been attributed to delays in the learning of semantic and syntactic rules critical to the development of language (Clahsen 1992). At the same time there is strong evidence that children with LI have differences in their basic auditory processing abilities that may be related to their language deficits. This body of research shows that individuals with LI are characterized by deficits on tasks requiring integration of two or more sensory events that enter the nervous system in rapid succession (Tallal et al. 1985a,b). Across laboratories, research investigating sensory processing in individuals with LI suggests that impairment of lower-level auditory temporal processing (that is, the processing of auditory cues in rapid sequence) hinders the development of normal language and reading abilities (Godfrey et al. 1981, Snowling et al. 1986, Werker and Tees 1987, Reed 1989, Stark and Heinz 1996). Children with LI have been shown to have a selectively impaired ability both to perceive and to produce those speech sounds that are characterized by brief or rapidly changing temporal cues; moreover the degree of the language comprehension deficits is highly correlated with the degree of temporal processing deficit (Tallal and Piercy 1973a,b; Tallal et al. 1985a,b). Much of the sensory processing necessary for language comprehension and production occurs within a brief window of time. In order to process speech it is necessary to hear and respond to rapidly occurring, sequential auditory cues that signal what words are being produced. In other words, processing proceeds in a 'bottom-up' manner, with discrimination of basic acoustic properties supporting language acquisition. This information is carried by the elements of the speech sound called 'formants': sound waveforms across time. The rapid transitional cues that facilitate the decoding of language are contained within the consonants, in particular stop consonants such as *p, b, d,* and *g.* These critical transitional cues are short (lasting about 40ms) and must be processed if speech is to be perceived accurately. Vowels, on the other hand, are at steady state across the waveform and thus depend less on temporal processing abilities in the 0-to-50ms range. Many studies of auditory temporal processing in children have provided evidence suggesting that sensory processing in this time range is relevant to language comprehension (see Farmer and Klein 1995 for a review). If such processing deficits could be assessed in infancy or toddlerhood, early identification of children at risk for language delays would be facilitated – a necessary step for early and appropriate intervention.

Given that temporal processing deficits can be used in older children and adults as a behavioral 'marker' of language impairment, our research group predicted that measures of temporal processing would be useful in early (infant) screening for language delays, and indeed we have found that differences in auditory temporal processing thresholds in infancy are related to later language development, both in control infants (Benasich and Tallal 1994, Benasich et al. 1995, Benasich and Spitz 1996) and in infants born into families with a history of language-based learning impairments (Benasich and Tallal 1996, Spitz et al. 1997).

HYPOTHESIZED MECHANISMS FOR A TEMPORAL PROCESSING DISORDER

A number of explanations have been suggested for why children with LI might have slower temporal processing. One hypothesis is that processing speed, like language, has a genetic component (Tallal et al. 1989a,b; Tallal et al. 1991).

Another hypothesis is that such problems could be inherited or acquired as a result of slower sensory processing due to abnormalities of the magnocellular neuronal system (Merzenich et al. 1993). Magnocellular neurons fire preferentially in response to rapid, transient (on/off) stimuli, whereas the smaller, parvocellular, neurons in the same subcortical regions are adapted to respond to steady-state and sustained stimuli. Neurons of both types are located in subcortical sensory areas, specifically visual (lateral geniculate) and perhaps auditory (medial geniculate) subdivisions of the thalamus, and transmit incoming sensory signals to the appropriate cortical areas. Postmorten studies have shown that people diagnosed as dyslexic have smaller and fewer magnocellular neurons than normal in visual subcortical regions (Livingstone et al. 1991, Galaburda and Livingstone 1993, Galaburda et al. 1994). A similar deficit of auditory magnocellular neurons in animal models of dyslexia has been suggested as a plausible explanation for poor discrimination of rapidly presented auditory stimuli (Fitch et al. 1994), although no such deficit has been reported in people with dyslexia. The most common interpretation of such findings is that because of abnormalities in the magnocellular system these neurons may be slower to fire in response to very brief stimuli, thus impeding the encoding of such stimuli. From that point a cascade of processing problems can be hypothesized (see Benasich and Read forthcoming).

A third possible explanation for the slower temporal processing in individuals with LI rests on differences in the structure of the brain itself. These accounts include abnormal asymmetries in the planum temporale, errors in neuronal migration (i.e. ectopias), and the effect of tiny brain abnormalities such as microgyric lesions (Galaburda and Kemper 1979, Galaburda et al. 1985, Humphreys et al. 1990, Plante et al. 1996). Brain imaging studies showing differences in regional brain volumes and in hemispheric asymmetries in the brains of school-age and adult individuals with LI also suggest that the relevant neuropathology probably occurs early in life (Tallal et al. 1990, Hagman et al. 1992, Cowell et al. 1995). Such research, though sparse, also suggests that morphological abnormalities in the caudate nucleus may play a part in temporal processing deficits (Jernigan et al. 1991, Tallal et al. 1994). Further evidence of a physiological basis for slowed temporal processing comes from studies using induced cortical ectopias in rats. In an operant-conditioning paradigm similar to the procedure described below for infants, rats with experimental lesions have shown poorer auditory temporal processing of tone sequences with varying interstimulus intervals (ISIs) (Fitch et al. 1994).

Overall, the findings of these studies support the hypothesis that temporal processing thresholds in individuals with LI could very well be abnormal quite early in life. If so, these thresholds would provide an opportunity for early screening for future LI. Temporal processing thresholds have not previously been studied during the first year of life, however, as assessment tasks have been available only for older children (from age 4 years) and adults. Furthermore, it is critical that such assessments be done prospectively, in order to identify which emerges first, timing problems or language delay – an area of much dispute in the field.

Therefore several prospective longitudinal studies were undertaken to investigate general information processing (as measured by standard habituation/recognition-memory tasks), auditory temporal processing, and cognitive and language outcomes. At 6 and 9 months of age each infant was given an infant-controlled habituation task, a recognition-memory task, and an auditory temporal processing task; cognitive performance was assessed using the Mental Scale of the Bayley Scales of Infant Development (Bayley MDI) (Bayley 1993). Information about the infants' emerging language at 12 and 16 months of age was collected using the MacArthur Communicative Development Inventory (Fenson et al. 1993) and the Preschool Language Scale–3 (Zimmerman et al. 1992). Sociodemographic data and information about infant and maternal health, obstetric history, and familial language-based learning disorders were collected using a parental questionnaire.

MEASURING INFANT AUDITORY TEMPORAL PROCESSING

To assess auditory temporal processing (ATP) in infants, we used operant-conditioning techniques modeled on the Tallal Repetition Test (Tallal and Piercy 1973a), a test of ATP for use with individuals aged 4 years or more. The test accurately discriminates language-impaired from normally developing children, and it predicts language outcomes in preschool and school-age children (Tallal et al. 1993). We developed a paradigm for operant conditioning of infants, designed to have the same parameters as this test (Benasich and Tallal 1993). The methodology (also referred to as visually reinforced conditioned head-turning) allows us to obtain individual ATP thresholds (see Kuhl 1985 and Morrongiello 1990 for reviews). Two operant-conditioning paradigms were used to investigate infant ATP abilities: a two-alternative forced-choice (2AFC) head-turn task and a go/no-go operant head-turn procedure.

During the 2AFC head-turn task, infants learned to discriminate between two auditory tone sequences (the 'stimuli') and to associate each stimulus with a visual reward. The stimuli were two 75ms complex tones combined into two different sequences, with an interstimulus interval (ISI) interposed between the two tones. Infants were first trained to turn their heads to the right for one tone sequence (e.g. 100Hz followed by 300Hz) and to the left for a second sequence (e.g. 100Hz followed by 100Hz) by using as reinforcers two toys (one in either direction) that lit up and moved. When the infants had learned the contingency, they could anticipate from the tone sequence which of the two toys would be activated and would make a head-turn in the correct direction. The initial training was with an ISI of 500ms between the two tones. When the infants had correctly learned which way to turn their head, the ISI between tone pairs was shortened to 300ms and then was gradually decreased, in an

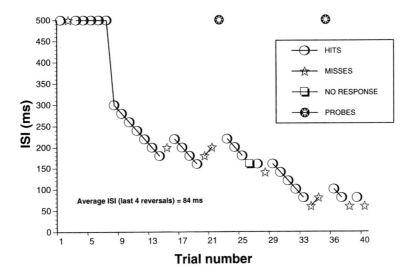

Fig. 9.1. Trial-by-trial record of the test phase of the auditory temporal processing (ATP) task for a normal 26-week-old infant.

Infants were required to score 6 of 7 correct responses at 500ms interstimulus interval (ISI) before proceeding to the test phase. The infant's ATP threshold is 84ms.

up-and-down adaptive procedure, until the interval at which the infants could no longer discriminate between the two tone sequences was identified (an infant's ATP threshold) (see Benasich and Tallal 1996 for further procedural details). Figure 9.1 illustrates a typical infant's trial-by-trial performance on the variable ISI test phase of this task.

Habituation and recognition-memory tasks were also used to evaluate each infant's learning acquisition curve, speed of encoding, and recognition memory (see Bornstein 1985, Benasich and Bejar 1992). During the testing session, each infant received a standard infant-controlled visual habituation and a test of recognition memory, using faces as stimuli (see Bornstein and Benasich 1986).[1]

In one study using the 2AFC head-turn task, ATP thresholds were examined in two groups of infants from 6 to 10 months of age: control infants (called 'FH−') from families with no known history of LI, and infants ('FH+') from families with a history of LI (Benasich and Tallal 1996). Thirty-two FH− infants and eleven FH+ infants were included. All were healthy and had been born at term. The mean ATP threshold for all completed test sessions

---

[1]The mean duration of the infant's first two looks constituted a baseline, considered to be 100%. The same stimuli were presented until the infant reached a habituation criterion of two consecutive looks each 50% of the baseline or less. Immediately after habituation the infant was tested with the habituation stimulus and a novel stimulus, in a 'preferential looking' design. Each pair of stimuli was presented twice, for 10s each, with right/left positions reversed for the second 10s presentation. As infants prefer novelty, the amount of looking at the novel as compared with the familiarized stimulus was computed.

195

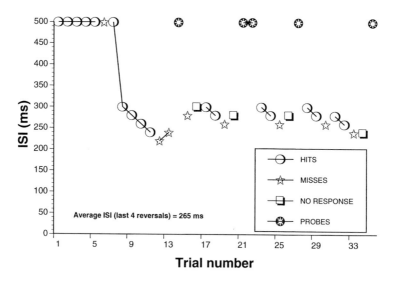

Fig. 9.2. Trial-by-trial record of the test phase of the ATP threshold task for a 26-week-old infant with a family history of language-based learning disability.

At 500ms ISI this infant had no difficulty discriminating one tone sequence from another, but once the ISI dropped below 250ms discrimination dropped to chance levels. The infant's ATP threshold is 265ms.

for the FH– control infants was 70.6ms (SD=25.1) across the last four 'reversals' (switches from a correct response to an incorrect one) in the variable ISI testing phase. However, for the FH+ infants, the mean ATP threshold for all completed test sessions was 148.2ms (SD=77.2) across the last four reversals. Mean thresholds were significantly different in these two samples ($t(41) = -5.04$, $P<0.0001$) with the FH+ group achieving significantly higher mean thresholds than FH– control infants. (Lower temporal processing thresholds correspond to better performance.) Moreover the shapes of the distributions of the ATP threshold scores for these two groups were significantly different ($\chi^2(2)=10.57$, $P<0.01$). Examination of the trial-by-trial plots for a FH+ infant completing the ATP Variable ISI test phase illustrates the longer ISIs necessary for some of these infants to discriminate the two-tone patterns (Fig. 9.2). Five of the 11 FH+ infants tested showed this response pattern and six showed patterns similar to that in Figure 9.1. The pattern of results for the FH+ infants with high ATP thresholds looks very much like the curves found by Tallal et al. (1993) for a sample of children 4 to 8 years of age with LI (Fig. 9.3). Recall that the infants in our study were preverbal and had no present indicators of cognitive delay. In this way we established the normative range of ATP thresholds of 6- to 10-month-old infants using a 2AFC operant-conditioning paradigm.

Differences in general information processing, as indexed by habituation and recognition memory, suggested that these measures of information processing are tapping a similar mechanism, perhaps speed of processing, and that more 'efficient' processing provides an

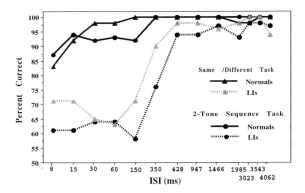

Fig. 9.3. Percentage correct responses on the Tallal repetition task for normal and language-impaired(LI) children with various ISIs.

The 'same/different' task is similar to the auditory temporal processing tasks given to the infants in our study. (From Tallal P, Miller S, Fitch RH. (1993) Neurobiological basis of speech: a case for the pre-eminence of temporal processing. In: Tallal P, Galaburda AM, Llinás RR, von Euler C, editors, *Temporal Information Processing in the Nervous System: Special Reference to Dyslexia and Dysphasia. Annals of the New York Academy of Sciences, Volume 682.* New York: New York Academy of Sciences, p 27–47. Copyright © New York Academy of Sciences 1993. Reprinted by permission.)

advantage in both groups of infants. Measures of habituation, recognition memory, and temporal processing all make independent contributions to prediction of later language abilities both in healthy, control infants and in infants with a family history of language impairments (Benasich et al. 1995, Benasich and Spitz 1996, Benasich and Tallal 1996). Specifically, infants who are better temporal processors (i.e. those with lower ATP thresholds) also habituate more efficiently (i.e. they require fewer trials to achieve the criterion and exhibit steeper habituation slopes). These infants also discriminate better (i.e. they have higher scores on tests of visual recognition memory) and score higher in language tests at 12 and 16 months of age than infants with poorer ATP thresholds.

When the infants from this study were followed longitudinally, it was found that differences in ATP thresholds were related to later language development (Benasich and Tallal 1994). ATP thresholds obtained at a mean age of 7.5 months strongly and significantly predicted language comprehension on the MacArthur Communicative Development Inventory at 16 months (R^2=0.638, $P<0.0001$) and language comprehension and production on the Preschool Language Scale at 24 months (see Figure 9.4).

In sum, these data lend strong support to the notion that the ability to perform fine acoustic discriminations in early infancy is critically important to later language development. This appears to be the case even when specific predictors such as a family history for LI or prematurity are not present. In addition our findings extend research that has shown differences between children with and children without LI to infants at risk of LI because of a family history of language-based learning impairment. Although on individual plots of performance (and of ATP thresholds) just over half of FH+ infants showed functions indistinguishable from those of control infants, the group of FH+ infants as a whole had significantly poorer (higher) ATP thresholds than control infants.

197

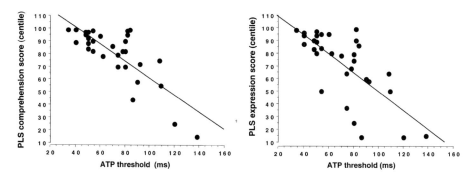

Fig. 9.4. Relation between ATP thresholds (after four 'reversals'; see text) of 32 normal control infants (mean age, 7.5 months) and their later language performance at 24 months on the Preschool Language Scale (PLS), as measured by standardized centile scores for language comprehension *(left)* and language production *(right)*.

A second study examined ATP in infants using a shorter, less-demanding variant of the ATP task: the go/no-go operant head-turn procedure. Using this procedure we were able to replicate our previous findings of a distribution of temporal processing abilities in a sample of 44 normal control infants. The infants were operantly conditioned to turn the head 60° to the left in response to a target tone sequence embedded within a standard repeating sequence, e.g. high–low, high–low, *low–high,* high–low. The training stimuli were paired complex tones (100 and 200Hz; 200 and 100Hz) lasting 75ms and separated by a 500ms ISI. The criterion of successful training was four consecutive correct anticipatory head-turns towards the location of the reward for the target tone sequence. During the test phase, 20 trials were presented (10 'change' trials, 10 'no-change'), each trial consisting of a block of four sequences separated by the same ISI (300, 180, 70, or 10ms for both standard and target sequences). The dependent variable was D′ (the difference between the distributions of 'hits' and false alarms) for detection of the target tone sequence at ISI 70ms (see Benasich et al. 1995 for further procedural details). Systematic correlations were still seen between concurrent ATP, habituation, and recognition memory, suggesting that these three measures are tapping similar processes.

These infants also were given an auditory–visual habituation task that evaluated the ability to discriminate consonant–vowel pairs (i.e. /ba/ and /da/ with normal 40ms transitions). Infants were habituated to an abstract visual pattern paired with one speech stimulus. Then they were given four test trials: two involving the now-familiar auditory–visual pairing, and two involving a novel auditory–visual pairing in which the second speech stimulus was now paired with the unchanged visual stimulus. As infants of this age prefer novelty, our dependent measure was the percentage of looking towards the novel pairing during the recognition-memory test. Because nothing changed in the test but the auditory stimulus, the infants should have preferred to look at (and listen to) the novel pairing if and only if they could detect the change of consonant.

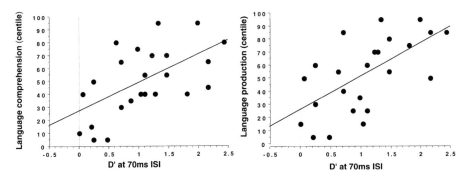

Fig. 9.5. Relation between ATP thresholds as measured by D′ (difference between distribution of 'hits' and false alarms) of 24 normal infants at 9 months and performance on the MacArthur Communicative Development Inventory (CDI) at 16 months, expressed as standardized centile scores for language comprehension *(left)* and language production *(right)*.

The R^2 between D′ and language comprehension was 0.64 ($P<0.0001$) and for language production, 0.51 ($P<0.0001$).

Performance on this task of discriminating consonant–vowel pairs was highly correlated with D′ scores (at 70ms ISI) on the ATP tasks at both 6 months ($r=0.78$, $P<0.001$) and 9 months ($r=0.58$, $P<0.001$). Thus, processing of rapidly changing auditory temporal cues in speech and that in non-speech sounds are related during early infancy. Moreover these differences in ATP abilities in infancy were again related to later language (Benasich et al. 1995; Benasich and Spitz 1996). Figure 9.5 shows the relation in our normal control infants between ATP thresholds at 9 months of age (as measured by D′) and standardized scores of language comprehension and production at 16 months of age.

Using the go/no-go head-turn procedure we also replicated our previous finding of differential performance on ATP tasks according to family history of LI. Twenty-two infants born into families with such a history (FH+ infants) were assessed between 6 and 7 months of age using both the go/no-go head-turn procedure (tones with brief ISIs) and the auditory–visual habituation task (/ba/ versus /da/) described above. In addition a visual-habituation/recognition-memory task that did not require processing of brief temporal cues was given. A control sample of infants with no reported family history of LI (FH–) was selected from our subject pool and matched to the FH+ infants for age at test, gestational age, socioeconomic status, and sex. Differential performance was seen on tasks requiring infants to use their ATP abilities. FH+ infants had significantly higher temporal processing thresholds (i.e. lower D′ scores and poorer discrimination at faster ISIs) on the head-turn task than the control infants (Fig. 9.6). In addition, 12 (54%) of the FH+ infants had non-significant D′ at 70ms ISI. This finding suggests that a subset of these FH+ infants were not discriminating the target tone sequence at an ISI longer than that necessary for discrimination of critical consonant–vowel transitions in language. This implies difficulty in completing a task using actual consonant–vowel syllables. Our next set of results supports that premise. In the visual-habituation/recognition-memory task, novelty preference

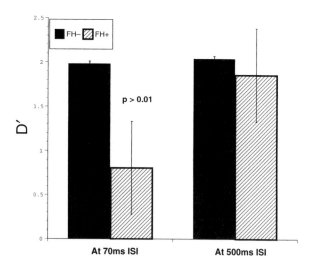

Fig. 9.6. Comparison of ATP thresholds (as measured by D′) of 22 infants with a family history of language-based learning impairments (FH+) and of 22 age-matched normal control infants (FH−).

ATP was assessed from the infant's ability to discriminate between two tone sequences, separated by varying ISIs, on a go/no-go head-turn task, and showed that FH+ infants did less well at 70ms ISI but performed equivalently to FH− infants at 500ms ISI.

(discrimination) scores did not differ between FH+ infants and controls (Fig. 9.7). However, when brief temporal cues were necessary for discrimination of /ba/ from /da/ in the auditory–visual habituation task, the FH+ infants performed significantly worse than the control infants. Furthermore the mean novelty preference scores of the FH+ infants were not significantly different from chance (see Fig. 9.7). Thus temporal processing thresholds in early infancy have been found to differ according to the infants' family history of learning-based language impairments in two studies to date. Taken together the results from these studies provide support for an autosomal dominant pattern of genetic transmission previously documented in older LI individuals (Tallal et al. 1989a, Tomblin 1989).

SUMMING UP: TEMPORAL PROCESSING AND LANGUAGE ACQUISITION
The research discussed so far suggests that even in normal, term infants with no family history of language-based learning disorders, there is a relation between temporal processing efficiency and language in the second year. We have found that 'speed of processing' is also much slower in infants who are later found to have language delay. Processing speed is slower both in the rapid auditory temporal domain (i.e. tens of milliseconds) and for overall acquisition of information (i.e., time in seconds needed for habituation). Thus we have identified – before the onset of verbal language – infants who are going to have language delay. Studies in our laboratory also suggest that ATP thresholds differ in infants with a family history of language-based learning disorders. Specifically, a subset of FH+ infants are poor temporal processors and also have lower achievement in language during the

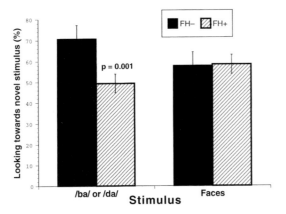

Fig. 9.7. Comparison of discrimination of consonant–vowel syllables (/ba/ versus /da/) *(left)* with discrimination of faces *(right)* in 22 infants with a family history of learning impairment (FH+) and 22 age-matched normal control infants (FH–).

Discrimination was assessed from the infant's differential response to a novel stimulus as compared with the response to a stimulus with which the infant had been familiarized (i.e. after habituation). The two groups did equally well on the visual discrimination task *(right)*, but the FH+ group did significantly less well than the controls on the auditory discrimination task, which required discrimination of brief temporal cues *(left)*.

toddler years. As there have been reports suggesting a genetic component to language-based learning disorders and reports of poorer temporal processing among first-degree relatives of individuals with LI (Tallal et al. 1989a, 1991; Tomblin 1989), the examination of familiality and patterns of genetic transmission becomes an important priority in this previously unexplored population.

Genetic contributions to language
Because of the growing interest in genes and the knowledge gained from studies of the human genome, the past decade has seen a boom in the number of studies examining genetic contributions to language (Hurst et al. 1990, Bishop et al. 1995, Lahey and Edwards 1995, Bishop and Bishop 1998, Fisher et al. 1998, Tomblin and Buckwalter 1998, Rice et al. forthcoming). It is now possible to examine how a particular trait is transmitted – for example, whether a gene is transmitted in an additive or a non-additive (e.g. dominant or recessive fashion and whether or not a particular trait is sex-linked (Brzustowicz 1996; also see Gilger 1995 for a review).

Most studies examining familial aggregation, or patterns of affected individuals within families, have used the developmental history as reported by subjects or their parents to classify family members as affected or unaffected. Typically this is accomplished by sending a questionnaire to the parents, asking if each member of the family has had a history of speech, language, or learning difficulties. Using such a questionnaire Rice et al. (forthcoming) studied the familial aggregation of such difficulties both in first-degree relatives and in members of the extended family. In agreement with the hypothesis that LI is a heritable disorder, the authors found a higher overall prevalence of affected members of the nuclear family (26%), who share more genetic material, than in members of the extended family (16%). Looking at first-degree relatives, Tallal et al. (1989a) reported that children with LI were significantly more likely to have at least one affected first-degree relative than children without LI (77% versus 46%). The proportion of parents reporting a past history of LI for themselves in this study was 61%, and the proportion of those reporting LI in their siblings or the siblings of the proband was 37% (41% of brothers and 26% of sisters). The higher reported prevalence in male than in female family members is consistent with the fact that males are more likely to receive a diagnosis of LI, either because of an increased prevalence of LI in males or, more probably, because of an ascertainment bias (Tomblin et al. 1997). A somewhat lower percentage of overall aggregation of cases in families of affected children (51%) was found by Tomblin (1989); however, a higher percentage was reported for brothers (40%) than for sisters (17%) of children with LI.

Studies using retrospective approaches have also indicated that the prevalence of LI may differ depending on the phenotype, or on how the language disorder is expressed in the proband. For example Lahey and Edwards (1995) found that children with purely expressive delay were more likely to have a family member reported as affected (85%) than were children with receptive–expressive delay (55%). A similar study in our laboratories examined familiality within phenotypes in a sample of 20 children 2 to 3 years old diagnosed as having either mixed receptive–expressive delay ($n=13$) or delayed expressive language and normal receptive language ($n=8$). The children with affected family members in both of these groups were compared with 20 age-matched controls whose language performance was within normal limits. In contrast to Lahey and Edwards' findings, we found that while both groups with delay were more likely to have affected family members than the age-matched controls (76% versus 18%), the children with mixed receptive–expressive delays were more likely to have affected first-degree relatives (82%) than were the children with expressive delay (67%). The overall proportion of members affected in these families was 28%, which is similar to previously reported rates (Neils and Aram 1986, Tomblin 1989, Tomblin 1996) and considerably higher than the 8% of affected family members found for the age-matched controls.

Studies using family-history questionnaires have been shown to underestimate the number of family members classified as affected (Plante et al. 1996). One way to overcome this difficulty is to use current performance rather than the reports of patients or their parents (Tomblin 1996, Spitz et al. 1997). In this method, family members are tested to determine if they meet some criteria for a diagnosis of language impairment. For example Tomblin (1996) identified 44 children with specific language impairment and then tested the language abilities of all their first-degree relatives. Even though he looked only for specific language impairments rather than for a broader range of language disorders, the findings were quite similar to those of previous studies using the family histories given by patients and their parents. In 53% of the families the only affected member was the proband. In the other 47% of the families, however, 42% of the probands' first-degree relatives also had specific language impairment. Such findings suggest that several etiologies may be involved, only some of them showing a strong genetic effect. That study and studies examining familiality in children with LI due to non-genetic causes (such as children born preterm or children who are at risk because of early neonatal health difficulties: Rice et al. 1996) emphasize the need to control strictly the LI phenotype under study.

Instead of using the traditional retrospective approach to studying the familiality of language impairment, we studied familial aggregation prospectively. After identifying a set of proband children, we examined the language and cognitive developmental trajectories of their younger siblings (Spitz et al. 1997). This approach has three main strengths. First, the sample was limited to families with a well-defined classification for language impairment. In order to be classified as having language impairment, the family member had to demonstrate a current non-verbal intelligence score of 80 or above and a language score at least 1 SD below the mean for that age.[2] Thus the younger siblings who participated in the prospective study had at least one family member with a confirmed diagnosis of LI. Second, in most cases the children were inducted into the study between the ages of 6 and 8 months, well before the production of their first word, and were followed at 6, 9, 12, 16, 20, and 24 months, with language testing beginning at 12 months of age. Third, in our sample the classification of a toddler as 'affected' or 'unaffected' was based on current performance on standardized language measures at 16 to 26 months of age rather than on a global impression of previous abilities.

Language acquisition was followed using two measures, the MacArthur Communicative Development Inventory (Fenson et al. 1993) and the Preschool Language Scale–3 (Zimmerman et al. 1992). General cognition was assessed at each visit using the Bayley MDI (Bayley 1993). In addition to using the standardized MDI score, we also examined performance on two subsets of items, one consisting of all the verbal items in each item set and the other, of the remaining (non-verbal) items. Two groups of children were included in the study, one (FH+) consisting of children with a family history of language impairment (i.e. the siblings of the probands, $n=10$) and the other (FH–), of age- and sex-matched controls with a family history that was negative for impairments of speech, language, and learning.

The findings were quite surprising given the youth of the subjects. Most importantly, the results showed that children born into families with a history of LI are at most risk for delays in language acquisition. The receptive and expressive language scores of the FH+ group were far below those of the matched controls (Fig. 9.8). Five of the 10 children in the FH+ group had language scores which fell at least 1.5 SD below the mean (Fig. 9.9). The 50% prevalence of language delay found in this sample is consistent with an autosomal dominant mode of transmission. This mode of transmission is consistent with rates of impairment found in previous studies (Tallal et al. 1989a,b; Hurst et al. 1990; van der Lely and Stollwerck 1996). For most of the children with language delay, scores for both receptive and expressive language were in the range indicating delay. Previous studies have shown that children with receptive–expressive delay are at much greater risk for language problems which persist to school age, unlike children with purely expressive delay, who frequently

---

[2]This study was conducted as part of larger projects on familiality and intervention in children with specific language impairment by P Tallal and S Miller, who were responsible for the identification of probands.

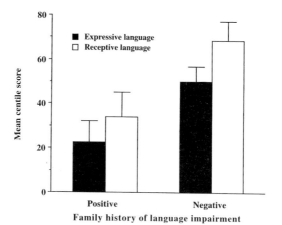

Fig. 9.8. Centile scores for children's receptive and expressive language according to family history of language impairment.
Error bars represent 1 SEM. *$P<0.05$, unadjusted.

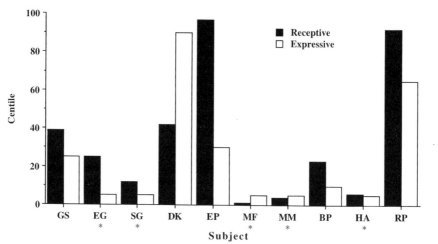

Fig. 9.9. Centile scores for children with a family history of language impairment.
*Children scoring at least 1.5 SD below the mean for their age.

catch up (Rescorla 1993, Whitehurst and Fischel 1994). Thus the results from language testing indicate a high incidence of problems in language acquisition for children with a family history of LI. Because of the limited sample size, sex differences were not analyzed; however, only one of the three girls had language delay, compared with four of the seven boys. Thus here, too, sisters were less often affected than brothers.

The second important finding from this study was that in general the lower language scores of these children could not be explained by delays in general cognition. The mean Bayley MDI for the group of FH+ children was within the normal range. However, when

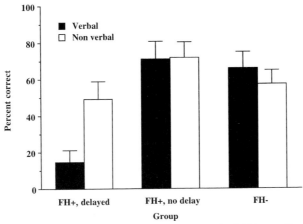

Fig. 9.10. Performance on verbal and non-verbal items of the Bayley MDI according to family history of language impairment and presence or absence of language delay.

The groups' performances differed only on the verbal items.

Error bars represent 1 SEM. *$P<0.05$, unadjusted.

performance on verbal tasks was compared with that on non-verbal tasks, it became clear that the difference in performance was due to poorer performance on the verbal items of the Bayley MDI for the children in the FH+ group who had language delay (Figure 9.10).

Thus there is evidence in this study for the familiality not only of language impairment but also of specific language impairment (i.e. LI not accompanied by cognitive delay). In sum, these results are consistent with models hypothesizing a genetic/familial component of language impairments and indicate that a family history of LI should be regarded as a risk factor for delays in language acquisition.

SUMMMING UP: GENETICS AND LANGUAGE ACQUISITION

Because of the increased interest and knowledge gained from studies of the human genome, the past decade has seen a dramatic rise in the number of studies examining genetic contributions to language impairment. The findings from these studies show good agreement and provide the following information. 1) LI can and does aggregate in families. Its familiality has been proven both retrospectively and prospectively. 2) The prevalence of LI can vary across studies because of differences in proband genotype or population, method of study, and the criteria used to define who is affected. Despite these differences some general findings have emerged. The overall reported incidence of language and learning problems in families with a family history of LI ranges from 20 to 28%. The incidence of language and learning problems tends to be higher in brothers (26 to 41%) and fathers (19 to 43%) than in sisters (17 to 29%) or mothers (16 to 37%). In summary, studies in our laboratories and in others' provide good evidence of a genetic component to some types of LI. Careful studies will be needed to i) more clearly define the phenotypes under study; ii) study familiality using performance-based criteria in multiple generations to allow pedigree analysis; and iii) apply segregation and linkage analyses to determine the possible set of loci involved in the familial transmission of language impairments.

Direction of future research, and conclusions

We have shown that we can identify, very early, those infants who are poor at processing rapid temporal cues in the auditory domain. They appear to be the same infants who are at an increased risk of language delay as toddlers. The studies described here clarify issues pertaining to precedence of ATP versus phonological processing deficits in children with LI. Quite clearly the temporal processing deficits are there preverbally and are predictive of subsequent language delay. Moreover, evidence for familial transmission of LI seen in our laboratories strongly suggests a genetic component in at least a subset of infants who are poor temporal processors. Might it, then, be possible to remedy language-based learning problems before they are even expressed – that is, before the onset of language? During early infancy the critical foundations of phonemic perception and later language are being laid down, and the potential for altering later outcome may be greater in the first 2 years of life than later.

In the future, infants at high risk for language delay may benefit greatly from new interventions modeled on those currently described in the literature. Two recent studies reported the development of a set of learning exercises designed to improve temporal processing abilities in children with LI (Merzenich et al. 1996, Tallal et al. 1996). The intervention was constructed based on research by Tallal and Piercy (1975) showing that stretching of the critical consonant–vowel transition resulted in an increase in the number of children with LI who could then discriminate the phonemes (e.g. /ba/, /pa/, /ta/) and on previous animal studies showing that neuronal reorganization underlies practice-based improvements in temporal segmentation and discrimination (Merzenich et al. 1993, Recanzone et al. 1993). The methods used included an auditory temporal training program (an adaptive shaping procedure) with massed training given using computer games and acoustically modified processed speech that stretched out the troublesome consonant–vowel transitions over a longer period than normal and amplified them. These techniques take advantage of bottom-up processing of sound and were designed to force temporal processing thresholds down (that is, make processing faster). Over a period of 4 weeks, very significant improvements in speech discrimination and language outcomes were shown in two independent groups of 5- to 10-year-old children with LI (Merzenich et al. 1996; Tallal et al. 1996). Such studies provide a potential model for even earlier intervention during the critical period of language acquisition.

Would such techniques work for infants at risk for language impairment? Within a high-risk population (a population showing evidence of familial language impairment or of prematurity), could those individuals most likely to have poor outcomes be identified by early screening and then progress to a closely targeted intervention that could alter basic processing before language is established? Only future research will answer such questions. Further delineation of genetic phenotypes and of patterns of familiality will facilitate early identification of infants at an increased risk for language impairments. Establishing the normative range of ATP across the first 2 years and further elucidating the links among temporal processing and later language is another key priority. Hopefully our knowledge will soon be more comprehensive and language impairments will be identified and remedied before cascading negative effects on language, academic, and social skills have a chance to take hold.

Acknowledgements

The research summarized in this chapter was supported by NICHD grant R01-HD29419 to AAB with additional funding from the Charles A Dana Foundation. A grant supplement to NIDCD grant R01-DC01854 and a grant from the James S McDonnel Foundation (nr JSMF93-25) to RVS provided additional support. RVS's production of this chapter was made possible by support from NIDCD grant T32DC00052 to the University of Kansas.

We thank P Tallal, S Miller, and J Flax for assistance in subject recruitment, and M Gibbons, C Hayes, W Ramel, and J Thomas for assistance with data collection and manuscript preparation. In particular, we are grateful to J Flax for her professional support and guidance. We especially thank the children studied and their parents for their participation and cooperation in these longitudinal studies.

REFERENCES

American Psychiatric Association. (1987) *Diagnostic and Statistical Manual of Mental Disorders.* 3rd ed, revised (DSM-III-R). Washington, DC: American Psychiatric Association.

Aslin RN, Pisoni DB, Juczyk PW. (1983) Auditory development and speech perception in infancy. In: Haith MM, Campos JJ, editors. *Handbook of Child Psychology. Volume 2, Infancy and Developmental Psychobiology.* 4th ed. Mussen PH, series editor. New York: Wiley. p 573–688.

Bates E, O'Connell B, Shore C. (1987) Language and communication in infancy. In: Osofsky J, editor. *Handbook of Infant Development.* 2nd ed. New York: Wiley. p 149–203.

Bayley NB. (1993) *Bayley Scales of Infant Development.* 2nd ed. San Antonio, TX: Psychological Corporation.

Beitchman JH, Hood J, Rochon J, Peterson M. (1989) Empirical classification of speech/language impairment in children: II. Behavioral characteristics. *Journal of the American Academy of Child and Adolescent Psychiatry* **28**: 118–23.

Benasich AA, Bejar II. (1992) The Fagan Test of Infant Intelligence: a critical review. *Journal of Applied Developmental Psychology* **13**: 153–71.

— Read H. (Forthcoming) Representation: picture or process? In: Sigel IE, editor. *Theoretical Perspectives in the Development of Representational (Symbolic) Thought.* Mahwah, NJ: Lawrence Erlbaum Associates.

— Spitz RV. (1996) Relationships among early auditory temporal processing abilities and later language and non-linguistic correlates of early language. Paper presented at the Annual Meeting of the Cognitive Neuroscience Society, San Francisco, California.

— Tallal P. (1993) An operant conditioning paradigm for assessing auditory temporal processing in 6- to 9-month-old infants. In: Tallal P, Galaburda AM, Llinás RR, von Euler C, editors. *Temporal Information Processing in the Nervous System: Special Reference to Dyslexia and Dysphasia. Annals of the New York Academy of Sciences, Volume 682.* New York: New York Academy of Sciences. p 312–4.

— — (1994) Relationships among infant auditory temporal processing thresholds, perceptual-cognitive abilities and language development in the first two years. Paper presented at the meetings of the International Conference on Infancy Studies, Paris, France.

— — (1996) Auditory temporal processing thresholds, habituation, and recognition memory over the first year. *Infant Behavior and Development* **19**: 339–57.

— Curtiss S, Tallal P. (1993) Language, learning, and behavioral disturbances in childhood: a longitudinal perspective. *Journal of the American Academy of Child and Adolescent Psychiatry* **32**: 585–94.

— Spitz RV, Tallal P. (1995) Relationships among infant auditory temporal processing, perceptual–cognitive abilities and early language development. Paper presented at the Annual Meeting of the Cognitive Neuroscience Society, San Francisco, California.

Best CT. (1993) Emergence of language-specific constraints in perception of non-native speech: a window on early phonological development. In: de Boysson-Bardies B, de Schonen S, Jusczyk P, MacNeilage P, Morton J, editors. *Developmental Neurocognition: Speech and Face Processing in the First Year of Life.* Dordrecht, The Netherlands: Kluwer Academic Publishers.

Bishop DVM, Bishop SJ. (1998) 'Twin language': a risk factor for language impairment. *Journal of Speech, Language, and Hearing Research* **41:** 150–60.

— North T, Donlan C. (1995) Genetic basis of specific language impairment: Evidence from a twin study. *Developmental Medicine and Child Neurology* **37:** 56–71.

Bornstein MH. (1985) Habituation of attention as a measure of visual information processing in human infants: summary, systematization, and synthesis. In: Gottlieb G, Krasnegor NA, editors. *Measurement of Audition and Vision in the First Year of Postnatal Life: A Methodological Overview.* Norwood, NJ: Ablex Publishing Company. p 253–301.

— Benasich AA. (1986) Infant habituation: Assessments of individual differences and short-term reliability at 5 months. *Child Development* **57:** 87–99.

Brzustowicz LM. (1996) Looking for language genes: lessons from complex disease studies. In: Rice M, editor. *Towards a Genetics of Language Impairment.* Hillsdale, NJ: Lawrence Erlbaum Associates. p 3–25.

Clahsen H. (1992) The grammatical characterization of developmental dysphasia. *Linguistics* **27:** 897–920.

Cowell PE, Jernigan TL, Denenberg VH, Tallal P (1995) Language and learning impairment and prenatal risk: an MRI study of the corpus callosum and cerebral volume. *Journal of Medical Speech-Language Pathology* **3:** 1–13.

DeCasper AJ, Fifer WP. (1980) Of human bonding: newborns prefer their mothers' voices. *Science* **208:** 1174–6.

— Spence MJ. (1986) Prenatal maternal speech influences newborns' perception of speech sounds. *Infant Behavior and Development* **9:** 133–50.

Eimas PD, Siqueland E, Jusczyk P, Vigorito J. (1971) Speech perception in infants. *Science* **171:** 303–6.

Farmer ME, Klein R. (1995) The evidence for a temporal processing deficit linked to dyslexia: a review. *Psychonomic Bulletin Review* **2:** 460–93.

Fenson L, Dale PS, Reznick JS, et al. (1993) *Technical Manual for the MacArthur Communicative Development Inventory.* San Diego: Singular Press.

Fisher SE, Varga-Khadem F, Watkins K, et al. (1998) Localisation of a gene implicated in a severe speech and language disorder. *Nature Genetics* **18:** 168–70.

Fitch RH, Tallal P, Brown CP, et al. (1994) Induced microgyria and auditory temporal processing in rats: a model for language impairment? *Cerebral Cortex* **4:** 260–70.

Galaburda AM, Kemper TL. (1979) Cytoarchitectonic abnormalities in developmental dyslexia; a case study. *Annals of Neurology* **6:** 94–100.

— Livingstone M. (1993) Evidence for a magnocellular defect in developmental dyslexia. In: Tallal P, Galaburda AM, Llinás RR, von Euler C, editors. *Temporal Information Processing in the Nervous System: Special Reference to Dyslexia and Dysphasia. Annals of the New York Academy of Sciences, Volume 682.* New York: New York Academy of Sciences. p 70–82.

— Sherman GF, Rosen GD, et al. (1985) Developmental dyslexia: four consecutive cases with cortical anomalies. *Annals of Neurology* **18:** 222–33.

— Menard MT, Rosen GD. (1994) Evidence for aberrant auditory anatomy in developmental dyslexia. *Proceedings of the National Academy of Sciences, USA* **91:** 8010–3.

Gilger JW. (1995) Behavioral genetics: Concepts for research and practice in language development and disorders. *Journal of Speech and Hearing Research* **38:** 1126–42.

Godfrey JJ, Syrdal-Lasky AK, Millay KK, Knox CM. (1981) Performance of dyslexic children on speech perception tests. *Journal of Experimental Child Psychology* **32:** 401–24.

Hagman J, Wood F, Buchsbaum M, et al. (1992) Cerebral brain metabolism in adult dyslexics assessed with positron emission tomography during performance of an auditory task. *Archives of Neurology* **49:** 734–39.

Humphreys P, Kaufmann WE, Galaburda AM. (1990) Developmental dyslexia in women: neuropathological findings in three cases. *Annals of Neuroscience* **28:** 727–38.

Hurst JA, Baraitser M, Auger E, et al. (1990) An extended family with a dominantly inherited speech disorder. *Developmental Medicine and Child Neurology* **32:** 352–5.

Jernigan T, Hesselink JR, Sowell E, Tallal P. (1991) Cerebral structure on magnetic resonance imaging in language- and learning-impaired children. *Archives of Neurology* **48:** 539–45.

Kuhl P. (1985) Methods in the study of infant speech perception. In: Gottlieb G, Krasnegor NA, editors. *Measurement of Audition and Vision in the First Year of Postnatal Life: A Methodological Overview.* Norwood, NJ: Ablex Publishing Company. p 233–51.

— Williams KA, Lacerda F, et al. (1992) Linguistic experience alters phonetic perception in infants by 6 months of age. *Science* **255:** 606–8.

Lahey M, Edwards J. (1995) Specific language impairment: Preliminary investigation of factors associated with family history and with patterns of language performance. *Journal of Speech and Hearing Research* **38**: 643–57.

Livingstone MS, Rosen GD, Drislane FW, Galaburda AM. (1991) Physiological and anatomical evidence for a magnocellular defect in developmental dyslexia. *Proceedings of the National Academy of Sciences USA*: 88, 7943–7.

Merzenich MM, Schreiner CE, Jenkins WM, Wang X. (1993) Neural mechanisms underlying temporal integration, segmentation, and input sequence representation: some implications for the origin of learning disabilities. In: Tallal P, Galaburda AM, Llinás RR, von Euler C, editors. *Temporal Information Processing in the Nervous System: Special Reference to Dyslexia and Dysphasia. Annals of the New York Academy of Sciences, Volume 682*. New York: New York Academy of Sciences. p 1–22.

— Jenkins WM, Johnston P, et al. (1996) Temporal processing deficits of language-learning impaired children ameliorated by training. *Science* **271**: 77–81.

Morrongiello BA. (1990) The study of individual differences in infants: auditory processing measures. In: Colombo J, Fagen J, editors. *Individual Differences in Infancy: Reliability, Stability, Prediction*. Hillsdale, NJ: Lawrence Erlbaum Associates. p 271–320.

Neils J, Aram D. (1986) Family history of children with developmental language disorders. *Perceptual and Motor Skills* **63**: 655–8.

Plante E, Shenkman K, Clark MM. (1996) Classification of adults for family studies of developmental language disorders. *Journal of Speech and Hearing Research* **39**: 661–7.

Plomin R, DeFries JC, McClearn GE. (1990) Behavioral Genetics: A Primer. 2nd ed. New York: Cambridge University Press.

Recanzone GH, Schreiner CE, Merzenich MM. (1993) Plasticity in the frequency representation of primary auditory cortex following discrimination training in adult owl monkeys. *Journal of Neuroscience* **13**: 87–104.

Reed MA. (1989) Speech perception and the discrimination of brief auditory cues in reading disabled children. *Journal of Experimental Child Psychology* **48**: 270–92.

Rescorla L. (1993) Outcome of toddlers with specific expressive delay (SELD) at ages 3, 4, 5, 6, 7, and 8. *Society for Research in Child Development Abstracts* **9**: 566.

Rice ML, Spitz RV, O'Brien M. (1996) Familiality and language impairment in NICU survivors: implications for genetic studies. Paper presented at University of Kansas.

— Haney KJ, Wexler K. (Forthcoming) Family histories of children with SLI who show optional infinitives. *Journal of Speech, Language, and Hearing Research*.

Robinson RJ. (1987). Introduction and overview. In: *Proceedings of the First International Symposium on Specific Speech and Language Disorders in Children*. London: AFASIC.

Scarr S, Carter-Saltzman L. (1983) Genetics and intelligence. In: Fuller J, Simmel E, editors. *Behavioral Genetics: Principles and Applications*. Hillsdale, NJ: Lawrence Erlbaum and Associates.

Snowling M, Goulandris N, Bowlby M, Howell P. (1986) Segmentation and speech perception in relation to reading skill: a developmental analysis. *Journal of Experimental Child Psychology* **41**: 489–507.

Spitz RV, Tallal P, Flax J, Benasich AA. (1997) Look who's talking: a prospective study of familial transmission of language impairments. *Journal of Speech and Language Research* **40**: 990–1001.

Stark RE, Heinz JM. (1996) Perception of stop consonants in children with expressive and receptive–expressive language impairments. *Journal of Speech and Hearing Research* **39**: 676–86.

Tallal P. (1988) Developmental language disorders. In: Kavanagh J, Tarkton TT, editors. *Proceedings of the National Conference on Learning Disabilities*. Parkton, MD: York Press. p 181–272.

— Piercy M. (1973a) Defects of non-verbal auditory perception in children with developmental aphasia. *Nature* **241**: 468–9.

—— (1973b) Developmental aphasia: impaired rate of nonverbal processing as a function of sensory modality. *Neuropsychologia* **11**: 389–98.

— — (1975) Developmental aphasia: the perception of brief vowels and extended stop consonants. *Neuropsychologia* **13**: 69–74.

— Stark R, Mellits D. (1985a) Identification of language impaired children on the basis of rapid perception and production skills. *Brain and Language* **25**: 314–22.

—— (1985b) Relationship between auditory temporal analysis and receptive language development: evidence from studies of developmental language disorders. *Neuropsychologia* **23**: 527–36.

— Ross R, Curtiss S. (1989a) Familial aggregation in specific language impairment. *Journal of Speech and Hearing Disorders* **54**: 167–73.

209

——— (1989b) Unexpected sex-ratios in families of language/learning-impaired children. *Neuropsychologia* **27:** 987–98.

— Wood F, Buchsbaum M, et al. (1990) Decoupling of PET measured left caudate and cortical metabolism in adult dyslexics. *Society for Neuroscience Abstracts* **16:** 1241.

— Townsend J, Curtiss J, Wulfeck B. (1991) Phenotypic profiles of language impaired children based on genetic/family history. *Brain and Language* **41:** 81–95.

— Miller S, Fitch RH. (1993) Neurobiological basis of speech: a case for the preeminence of temporal processing. In: Tallal P, Galaburda AM, Llinás RR, von Euler C, editors. *Temporal Information Processing in the Nervous System: Special Reference to Dyslexia and Dysphasia. Annals of the New York Academy of Sciences, Volume 682.* New York: New York Academy of Sciences. p 27–47.

— Jernigan T, Trauner D. (1994) Developmental bilateral damage to the head of the caudate nuclei: implications for speech–language pathology. *Journal of Medical Speech Language Pathology* **2:** 23–8.

— Miller S, Bedi G, et al. (1996) Language comprehension in language-learning impaired children improved with acoustically modified speech. *Science* **271:** 81–4.

Tomblin JB. (1989) Familial concentration of developmental language impairment. *Journal of Speech and Hearing Disorders* **54:** 287–95.

— (1996) Genetic and environmental contributions to the risk for specific language impairment. In: Rice ML, editor. *Toward a Genetics of Language.* New York: Lawrence Erlbaum Associates.

— Buckwalter PR. (1998) Heritability of poor language achievement among twins. *Journal of Speech, Language, and Hearing Research* **41:** 188–99.

— Records NL, Buckwalter P, et al. (1997) Prevalence of specific language impairment in kindergarten children. *Journal of Speech, Language, and Hearing Research* **40:** 1245–60.

van der Lely HKJ, Stollwerck L. (1996) A grammatical specific language impairment in children: an autosomal dominant inheritance? *Brain and Language* **52:** 484–504.

Werker JF, Lalonde CE. (1988) Cross-language speech perception: initial capabilities and developmental change. *Developmental Psychology* **24:** 672–83.

— Tees RC. (1984) Cross-language speech perception: evidence for perceptual reorganization during the first year of life. *Infant Behavior and Development* **7:** 49–63.

— — (1987) Speech perception in severely disabled and average reading children. *Canadian Journal of Psychology* **41:** 48–61.

Whitehurst GJ, Fischel JE. (1994) Practitioner review: Early developmental language delay: What, if anything, should the clinician do about it. *Journal of Child Psychology and Psychiatry* **35:** 613–48.

Zimmerman IL, Steiner VG, Pond RE. (1992) *Preschool Language Scale–3.* New York: Psychological Corporation.

10
PSYCHOSOCIAL FACTORS IN THE AETIOLOGY AND COURSE OF SPECIFIC LEARNING DISABILITIES

Thomas G O'Connor and Robert C Pianta

Our understanding of the aetiology and course of learning disabilities and of how to assess, diagnose, and treat them has progressed greatly in recent years (Maughan and Yule 1994). In this chapter on aetiological factors we focus on several sets of key findings regarding the environmental influences associated with such disabilities in general, with special reference to *specific* learning disabilities. In addition we draw attention to the difficulties of interpreting research findings and suggest directions forward for further studies.

Four major themes are addressed. First, we review what is known about the epidemiology of specific learning disorders and highlight the variations in prevalence rates across ethnic, geographic, and demographic settings. The variability in prevalences of specific learning disorders and of general cognitive impairment across socioeconomic status is consistent with the notion that the aetiology of learning problems may be linked to psychosocial factors, and raises many questions about which environmental influences might be important and by which mechanisms they exert their influence.

Second, using the model of research on the environmental influences – broadly defined – on intellectual development (e.g. Detterman 1996), we identify some of the lessons and challenges for research into links between psychosocial influences and learning disorders, whether specific or global. There are numerous parallels between research on general intellectual functioning and research on learning disorders: in both cases there is a need to integrate genetic and psychosocial factors, to assess any correlations with and between psychosocial risk factors, and to address the extent to which specific learning disorders are aetiologically distinct from individual differences in cognitive skills within the normal range.

Third, we examine how environmental influences may indirectly contribute to the development and course of learning disabilities in children through their influence on co-occurring behavioural and emotional disorders. It has been known for some time that the population of children with learning problems has an elevated prevalence rate of psychopathology; recent findings suggest that environmental factors may be most aetiologically salient through their influence on the likelihood of a child's developing behavioural problems.

Finally, we examine what clues interventions provide regarding the environmental aetiology of specific learning disorders. To be sure, interventions may alleviate learning problems through mechanisms unrelated to those that caused the disorder. Nonetheless, research into intervention may provide clues to the psychosocial correlates of learning disorders and to the most effective primary prevention strategies. Throughout this chapter we pay close attention to the distinction between broadly defined and specific learning disabilities. The distinction is important in a chapter covering a range of topics, as not all research distinguishes between the two, and, to complicate matters further, much more is known about some specific learning disorders than others.

The role of epidemiological findings in identifying psychosocial risk factors

Epidemiological studies are critical to an understanding of a disorder in at least two ways. First, epidemiological data provide an estimate of the prevalence, which makes it possible to estimate the need to address the problem and the cost of doing so. Second, and more central to this chapter, by revealing the social correlates of a disorder as well as trends over time and across regions, epidemiological data can provide clues to the underlying causes of the disorder (Rutter and Smith 1995). Although there are important limitations to inferring causal mechanisms from epidemiological data (Taubes 1995), gathering such data is nevertheless a critical first step in understanding a disorder. In this section we briefly examine three risk indicators – socioeconomic differences, sociocultural differences, and sex differences – that epidemiological research has shown to be associated with learning problems. A fourth finding, regarding the overlap of learning and behavioural problems, is considered in the penultimate section.

In the study of specific learning disorders, several issues regarding epidemiological findings should be noted. There is a clear consensus that individuals with learning disorders form a heterogeneous group, even when children with a specific type of learning disorder (e.g. reading disability) are examined (Rourke 1983). Thus, underlying each prevalence rate and variation in base prevalence rates is a complex mix of individuals who vary with respect to, among other dimensions, co-occurring learning problems, co-occurring behavioural problems, genetic risk, response to interventions, age-based changes in the profile of difficulties, and putative underlying cognitive and processing difficulties. In addition, studies vary in how they define learning problems. Some studies have assessed distinct subtypes of learning disorder, most notably the distinction between specific reading disorder and general reading backwardness (see Maughan and Yule 1994), whereas other studies have not made such a distinction. Also, certain problems of definition plague research on learning difficulties from country to country, and even from region to region within the same country (Hallahan and Kauffman 1991, Chapman 1992). Moreover – as further evidence of the definitional problems in the field – even experts have difficulty in differentiating individuals with learning disorder from low-achieving individuals (Shinn et al. 1986, Algozzine and Ysseldyke 1988).

Furthermore, large-scale studies of learning problems cannot include the detailed assessments that are the hallmark of small-scale and clinical studies. Consequently, large-scale studies cannot identify specific deficit profiles and thus cannot assess heterogeneity in much detail. Large-scale studies also cannot examine processes such as qualities of parent–child interactions, which have been implicated in the development of learning problems (Pianta and McCoy, forthcoming).

Thus there are several reasons to expect variability in estimated prevalences of specific learning disorders. To the extent that such variability reflects methodological rather than substantive influences, it will inevitably obscure some of the clues to causation that epidemiological data could otherwise provide.

There have been several epidemiological studies of general learning problems, but few of specific learning disorders, and it is quite rare for studies to assess each learning disorder independently (e.g. each of those listed in DSM IV [American Psychiatric Association 1994] or ICD–10 [World Health Organization 1993]). Consequently, little is known about geographic and demographic variations in rates of these specific disorders. Thus we limit our discussion of what connections there may be between variation in prevalences of learning problems and psychosocial aetiology to reading problems. It remains to be seen whether the lessons learned from research on reading problems provide a more general model of research on specific learning disabilities.

Some of the initial and now best-known epidemiological data on reading disorders were derived from an epidemiological study of 10-year-olds on the Isle of Wight in the UK (Rutter et al. 1970). The finding that approximately 4% of the children were affected has been replicated in other normal-risk studies, and most estimates range from 4 to 10%. Cross-cultural prevalences of learning problems are relatively consistent with this range (e.g. Silva et al. 1985).

The base prevalence of specific learning problems in very deprived (e.g. developing) countries has not been reported and may not be obtainable given the need for established schools and validated and culturally sensitive assessment measures. Accordingly, little can be concluded at present regarding the variation between cultural economic deprivation and relative prevalences of diagnosed learning problems *across* cultures. Nonetheless there has been an increase in the number of studies examining the cognitive and social development of children in very poor countries. Among the important findings that have emerged is that nutrition, physical health, and the extent to which basic needs are met are clearly linked both to general cognitive development and to specific learning abilities (Wachs et al. 1993, Gorman and Pollitt 1996). Thus, although it may not be possible to ascertain the prevalences of specific learning problems in diverse cultures, it is fairly clear that risk exposure varies significantly across cultures.

SOCIOECONOMIC STATUS
The link between socioeconomic well-being and the prevalences of specific learning problems can be explored by examining the variation in prevalences across socioeconomic status and demographic groups *within* a culture. Studies of low-income and urban populations have reported prevalences of learning problems much higher than 4 to 10% – often double or triple in magnitude (Eisenberg 1966, Berger et al. 1975). These findings provide some of the most compelling evidence for risk factors relating to social class, but leave unanswered the question of which psychosocial factors associated with socioeconomic conditions might be most important, and by what mechanisms these factors operate.

The mechanisms underlying the link between the level of socioeconomic disadvantage and the prevalence of learning problems need to be examined in the context of the many risks correlated with economic adversity. That is, low socioeconomic status indexes a wide range of causally more proximal influences. Among those factors associated with low socioeconomic status *and* with cognitive development are birth complications, very low birth weight, poor prenatal nutrition, and exposure to environmental toxins such as lead (Sameroff et al. 1987, Fergusson et al. 1993, Wachs et al. 1993). In low socioeconomic groups, there are not only elevated medical 'environmental' risks but also elevated risks relating to environmental stimulation at home and at school.

SOCIOCULTURAL FACTORS

It is very difficult to isolate the 'effects' of one risk factor from another. Although it is certainly possible to examine statistically the independent effects of correlated risk factors (see Fergusson et al. 1992), such an approach may have little meaning outside a research context; that is, they may have little ecological validity. Similar difficulties arise in understanding the significance of the variation in prevalences of learning problems and poor school performance across ethnic groups *within* cultures, because minority status is correlated with many of the risk factors already mentioned. When environmental and medical risks are accounted for, sociocultural and ethnic differences in prevalences of learning problems are eliminated or substantially reduced (Fergusson et al. 1991; see also Brooks-Gunn et al. 1996). The difficulties that correlated risk factors create for understanding *how* psychosocial factors influence the aetiology and course of (specific) learning disabilities are examined in more detail in the next section.

SEX

The disproportionate numbers of boys diagnosed with learning disorders is a replicated epidemiological finding that might have implications for psychosocial aetiology. The difference between the base prevalences of learning problems is not disputed: most studies find that boys are anywhere between 2 and 5 times more likely than girls to receive a diagnosis of reading disorder. This finding parallels the reported sex differences in verbal ability within the normal range in children and adults (Hyde and Linn 1988).

Some authors have suggested that the sex ratio of diagnosed learning problems in boys to those in girls may be inflated because of referral biases that stem from associated disruptive behaviour. That is, boys may be more likely to be identified as having learning disabilities not because of the disability per se but rather because of the higher prevalences of the associated behavioural problems (notably, poor conduct and hyperactivity/inattention) that prompt the referral. Some support for this hypothesis is found in the report by Sanson and colleagues (1996), who used different cut-off scores for boys and girls to define the presence or absence of behavioural problems comorbid with learning problems in order to identify a group of boys and girls large enough for statistical analyses. Another piece of evidence supporting the hypothesis of a referral bias in children is that in adults the prevalences of specific learning disorders in the two sexes are roughly equal (see Maughan and Yule 1994).

However, assuming that boys do outnumber girls in the actual prevalence of learning problems, it is not clear what psychosocial implications this imbalance may have for understanding the aetiology of learning disorders. Both psychosocial and genetic or other biological explanations have been proposed to explain the sex difference within the normal and clinical range. Boys may be more vulnerable to learning disorders, but it is not clear whether sex is a 'main effect' or modifies key environmental risks (Morisset et al. 1995). We address this question in the next section.

At the very least these findings highlight the severe limitations of relying on clinic samples and the continuing need to include psychiatric and specific and global learning disorders in epidemiological research on children and adults. The usefulness of future epidemiological research in identifying directions for detailed experimental and clinical investigations in this field will depend on how far it goes beyond assessing risk indicators such as social class and economic resources, and cultural and sex differences, to assess the risk factors associated with these indicators, and the putative processes by which these factor operate.

Assessing psychosocial influences on learning disorders
Much is known about the ontogeny of specific language skills and disorders, how they can be assessed, the presumed underlying cognitive structures, and the rate of development (Bradley and Bryant 1979, Bishop 1992, Goswami 1994, Wagner et al. 1994). Fewer studies focus on the social context associated with learning difficulties and the development of related learning skills or on the relation between individual differences in specific learning abilities and psychosocial experiences. Before discussing some recent and key findings, we examine the current debates and controversies regarding the mechanisms by which psychosocial influences operate – that is, how they increase the risk of learning disorders and how they shape the developmental paths of the affected individuals. We then examine three issues that are central to interpreting the available findings, in particular those from research in developmental psychology: the aetiological distinction between individual differences within the normal range and severe or clinical disorders, the need to integrate environmental and genetic models of development and disorder, and the power of longitudinal follow-up studies for sorting out risk processes.

MODELS OF PSYCHOSOCIAL INFLUENCE
If the role of psychosocial risks in learning disorders is to be understood, the mechanisms by which these risks may operate must be explained. Research relating psychosocial influences to individual differences in learning abilities has adopted one of two general models. The most straightforward model assumes 'direct effects', whereby psychosocial influences have a direct impact on the emergence and course of learning skills and disabilities. For example, lack of support for learning and reading in the family, which may especially characterize families with low socioeconomic status, has been linked to a long-term trajectory of academic failure (Walker et al. 1994). This finding, which has been replicated in many studies, underlies the 'cultural/familial' model of mental retardation. The assumption underlying these studies is that the cause of the delay is the child's poor social environment.

Factors other than those directly involved with socioeconomic status have also been cited as playing a direct role in the development of learning problems or, as is more often assessed, academic failure, including stressful life events, family type, and behavioural problems. An issue that often goes unrecognized in these studies is that a model that assumes direct effects is compelling only if the mechanism of action (rather than just the risk factor) is also specified. Unfortunately, research has tended to focus more on identifying risks than on specifying the mechanisms.

In the other model, psychosocial factors are assumed to act indirectly. Risks such as those associated with lower socioeconomic status may exacerbate existing biological and medical risks but not lead to learning problems in the absence of other risks. Evidence is accumulating that this process may hold for babies with low birthweight, as low-birthweight babies who show poor cognitive and academic adjustment in childhood are disproportionately from families with low socioeconomic status. Similarly, studies are increasingly adopting a model positing cumulative effects (Sameroff et al. 1987), in which the accumulation of risk factors, rather than a particular factor or combination of factors, is linked to learning difficulties. In these studies, the risk processes are assumed to be multiplicative, not additive (e.g. Pungello et al. 1996).

Understanding the mechanisms by which psychosocial factors operate is critical to understanding their role in learning disorders. General models proposed by, for example, Bronfenbrenner (1986), and many others, assume a bidirectional, multiplicative, and hierarchical arrangement of psychosocial influences in normal and abnormal development, and the conceptual advantages of such inclusive models are widely acknowledged. There is, however, considerable confusion about how such models can be reified and empirically tested. Although attempts have been made to operationalize some of the implications of these models in the context of cognitive development (Super and Harkness 1986, Pianta and O'Connor 1996), progress in the field of learning disabilities lags behind, especially in integrating research on genetic and psychosocial risks. Despite the absence of an accepted general and empirical model for understanding psychosocial influences on learning development (and development generally), it is clear that a 'main effects' model has fallen out of favour. Researchers are playing closer attention to the factors that moderate and mediate the connection between specific risk factors and learning skills, and it is this research into the covariation among risk factors that has made the most important contributions to our understanding of learning disorders and individual differences in learning abilities.

A critical theme in recent discussions of the nature of psychosocial influences is the question of whether there are correlations between social factors and cognitive development. Similarly, medical and psychosocial risks for learning disorders are correlated with one another, such that birth complications and poor prenatal care and a poor learning environment in the home and school are all more common among families with low socioeconomic status. Recent findings in research on the psychosocial factors associated with intellectual development further underscore the correlated nature of genetic and psychosocial influences, as those environmental factors associated with academic success and intellectual development are more common among intellectually more able parents (Pianta and O'Connor 1996). These

216

findings underscore the complexity of documenting the specific ways in which psychosocial factors operate and simultaneously emphasize the need for a multidisciplinary perspective in research designs.

Natural experiments are often very helpful in distinguishing the correlated social and biological influences in the development of specific learning abilities – and perhaps disorders. A recent study by Morrison et al. (1995) provides a good example. The authors made use of the fact that whether a child is enrolled in first grade or in kindergarten depends on an arbitrary cut-off date – the child's fifth birthday. By comparing children who were just old enough to enter first grade with those who were not, those authors could compare the development of cognitive skills as a function of maturation and of the more 'academic' environment of first grade. After the first year, the children who had attended first grade had much better memory skills than those who had attended kindergarten, but this gap disappeared after the second group of children had attended first grade for a year. The design also allowed the authors to conclude that advances in phonological skills that are critical for reading (such as segmentation of sounds) are related to exposure to formal reading instruction in first grade rather than to maturational changes (Morrison et al. 1995).

CATEGORIES AND DIMENSIONS

Many studies report psychosocial correlates of learning problems, but few report whether these risks are associated with learning disorders, that is, what percentage of the children in the sample have diagnosed problems, as distinct from, for example, underachievement. Of course many intervention studies focus on policy implications of psychosocial interventions, and these reports make explicit an estimate of the number of children whose learning problems may have been prevented (Campbell and Ramey 1994, Seitz and Apfel 1994). However, the majority of studies examining psychosocial factors associated with learning abilities and school success adopt a dimensional view of learning abilities and pay little attention to learning disorders as distinct from comparatively lower ability. Consequently it is difficult to interpret findings that link qualities of maternal interaction, extent of reading and of exposure to academic materials in the home, quality of school (and day-care) environments, exposure to school, the extent to which numeracy is practised, and many other factors (e.g. see Morisset et al. 1995), to the aetiology of learning disorders. Virtually all of the studies that have examined the above factors have examined them in relation to individual differences in learning abilities and not in relation to the presence or absence of disorder. An important general lesson from psychiatric research is that the aetiology of the extremes (i.e. of a disorder) is often not different from the aetiology of individual differences, though there may be exceptions. Using research on intelligence as an example, it is clear that the aetiology of extreme mental retardation is qualitatively different from the aetiology of mild mental retardation and of individual differences within the normal range.

THE NEED TO INTEGRATE PSYCHOSOCIAL AND GENETIC INFLUENCES

Research into the aetiology of learning disabilities has been changed dramatically by recent findings regarding the important role of genetic influences (Lewitter et al. 1980). Much of quantitative genetic and molecular genetic research on learning disorders has focused specifically on reading disorders. The degree of genetic influence found has differed, but most studies now suggest that in reading disorders approximately one-third of the variance in individual differences can be attributed to genetic factors (Stevenson 1991, and Chapter 7 in this book). While questions remain about the nature of genetic influences and the mechanisms by which they act (Bishop et al. 1995), it is clear that future studies on the aetiology of specific learning disorders must take into account the role of genetic and familial factors.

What are the implications of these findings for psychosocial studies of specific learning disorders? As several authors have pointed out (Plomin 1994), behavioural genetic studies provide some of the most critical support for environmental influences in development and pathology, by examining the role of environmental factors while controlling for genetic influences. This is certainly true in the context of specific learning disorders: if genetic influences account for one-third of the variance in individual differences in learning disorders, then non-genetic factors account for the remainder. There are, of course, many pitfalls in estimating the relative contributions of genetic and non-genetic factors on the basis of analyses that partition the relative influences in quantitative models, but it is significant that behavioural genetic analyses ascribe an important role to psychosocial and other non-genetic influences.

At the very least these findings highlight the need to incorporate both genetic and environmental hypotheses in research designs. To date, relatively few studies hypothesizing that parent–child interactions and related proximal processes explain individual differences in children's learning abilities have included controls to take parental cognitive abilities into account (Pianta and O'Connor 1996). Pianta and McCoy (forthcoming) found, for example, that the quality of child–mother interactions was predictive for learning problems even after maternal education had been taken into account. Similarly, in a different sample of children Pianta and Egeland (forthcoming) found that changes in children's intellectual abilities in the early school years were significantly associated with the quality of parent–child interactions even after the effects of maternal cognitive ability had been taken into account. This approach needs to be extended to research on children with specific learning disabilities.

The genetic evidence also suggests that these findings on the variation in prevalences of learning disorders across social class do not unambiguously suggest psychosocial risks. Adults with learning disorders are reported to be more likely to drop out of school and less likely to obtain educational qualifications than their peers without learning (and especially reading) disorders. Consequently it is hardly surprising that these adults have lower wages and lower-skill occupations as adults (Maughan 1995). Thus the finding that children and adolescents in low social classes have relatively high prevalences of learning problems may be partly influenced by a higher prevalence of learning problems in their parents – that is, the risk arises from genetic factors rather than from social class per se. Similarly, the finding that children from lower social classes experience a less positive reading environment (for example are read to less often, or have fewer books availability) may be a function of the disinterest and difficulty their parents have in reading. In this way a correlation exists between environmental risk and genetic risk, and social class is accordingly an ambiguous variable from the perspective of aetiology.

An additional lesson learned from recent studies is that genetic influences may act not on the phenotype per se but rather on the central component processes underlying the disorder. Thus the genetic influence on reading disorders appears to operate through phonological processing (rather than through orthographic coding; Stevenson 1991). There is a need to take a similar approach in linking psychosocial influences to learning disorders. The implication is that social class and related factors (including, for example, birth complications, nutrition, school quality) may influence reading abilities via their connection with phonological processing or other related skills rather than directly. Although few studies have examined the association between psychosocial factors and phonological processing, available data do not support a link (MacLean et al. 1987). Differences in phonological processing between able and poor readers and between disadvantaged and advantaged children appear only after the children have started school and have been exposed to formal reading instruction (Goswami 1994; cf. Morrison et al. 1995). These null findings may help to narrow the focus in further research on specific psychosocial influences and specific components of learning disorders.

FOLLOW-UP STUDIES
Follow-up studies are reviewed in more detail in the next section. Suffice it to note here that longitudinal research has significantly shaped the emerging models of psychosocial influence in learning disabilities. For example, research findings indicate that the negative long-term effects of learning problems appear to bear most heavily on lower socioeconomic groups; the eventual educational and occupational attainment of better-off individuals appear unaffected, or at least less affected (O'Connor and Spreen 1988, Maughan 1995). As already noted, the many factors indexed by social class may play a central role in the developmental course of learning problems, but here again the available studies do not allow firm conclusions. This matter is revisited in the last section, on intervention.

The role of social factors in learning disorders: links with behavioural problems
Research from more than two decades has identified behavioural problems, usually defined as inattentiveness, overactivity, and problems of conduct, as a frequent correlate of learning problems in children. For example, Sanson et al. (1996) reported that 36% of children with behavioural problems have reading problems, and 69% of children with reading problems have behavioural problems. The mechanisms underlying this association are unclear. The disorders may share a common biological or genetic cause, or the overlap may be entirely psychosocially mediated. Many researchers have used longitudinal designs to test the temporal association between learning problems and behavioural problems (Rutter and Yule 1970, Sanson et al. 1996). The findings offer clear evidence that behavioural problems, especially inattention and conduct problems, lead to later reading problems and underachievement (Horn and Packard 1985), and evidence also suggests that reading problems exacerbate behaviour problems (McGee et al. 1986). Thus the effects are reciprocal.

Several studies have examined whether comorbid reading and behavioural problems are aetiologically different from problems solely of reading or of behaviour. In a longitudinal cohort investigation spanning nearly 8 years and including a range of temperamental problems, behavioural problems, and social class variables, Sanson and colleagues (1996) found that among children as young as 3 to 4 years of age who later were found to have a reading disorder, those who turned out to have co-occurring behavioural problems could be distinguished from those without behavioural problems; in contrast there was a striking absence of distinguishing characteristics of children who later had reading problems only and those who later had no reading or behavioural problems. Those findings are consistent with other reports (cf. Pennington et al. 1993) suggesting that single disorders have a different causal pathway from comorbid disorders. Equally importantly, the overlap of learning and behavioural problems at such an early age suggests that, at least for a subset of children with co-occurring learning and behavioural problems, feelings of frustration and failure in school cannot explain comorbidity. However, very few studies, including that of Sanson et al. (1996), have examined the differential patterns of social and demographic risk associated with single and comorbid groups of children.

In a subset of studies focusing on the link between learning and behavioural problems, the problem of inattention and overactivity has been distinguished from problems of conduct. The evidence from these studies suggests that antisocial behaviour or conduct problems arise primarily through their association with inattention and overactivity rather than through a direct link with reading problems (Frick et al. 1991, Maughan et al. 1996). These findings underscore the need to study the patterns of comorbidity among the behavioural problems as well as in relation to learning problems, and to anticipate the problems that will arise if the subtle but critical distinctions among the disruptive behaviour disorders are ignored.

Finally, age-based change in the patterns of learning and behavioural disorders may offer important insights into aetiology. In particular, long-term follow-up studies suggest that learning problems per se are stable and continue into adulthood, but that the patterns of co-occurring behavioural and emotional problems may be limited to adolescence (Maughan et al. 1996). Implications of the above findings for aetiology and intervention are examined in the next section.

Lessons from interventions and follow-up studies

In this final section some lessons for understanding the aetiology of learning disorders are drawn from intervention and follow-up studies. An important distinction is that between aetiology and course. Factors that maintain or shape the course of a disorder may be very different from those that initiate the disorder. To date, much more is known about the psychosocial influences on the course of learning problems than on their aetiology.

The research findings on the influence of social class on the aetiology and course of learning problems are relatively consistent. Children from the middle and upper classes are not only less likely to be diagnosed with learning problems, but also more likely to have a positive prognosis in terms of educational and occupational attainment if they do have a learning problem. Rawson's (1968) follow-up of children with learning problems in childhood suggested that the adjustment in young adulthood was relatively favourable in terms of college attendance and occupational status. However, the vast majority of the children were from very privileged backgrounds and had relatively high intelligence. Thus it is not clear what can be concluded from these findings except that social class may carry significant protective effects. It is also not clear what processes associated with higher socioeconomic status afford the protection; some of the more likely explanations would be access to remedial care, prevention of the development of co-occurring behavioural and emotional problems, and promotion of academic attainment outside the range of the particular learning disability. Alongside these findings it is important to note that an increasing number of intervention studies report that interventions based at home, school, or day-care centre have beneficial effects only, or at least mainly, for children considered to be at risk (for socioeconomic or related reasons) and not for children in normal or low-risk categories (e.g. Caughy et al. 1994).

As noted above, several early-intervention studies that included a day-care-based or school-based component appeared to prevent the development of learning problems, and some family-based intervention approaches showed that the decrease in learning and school-related problems applied not only to the targeted children but also to their siblings born after the intervention had ended (Seitz and Apfel 1994). Unfortunately, few specific conclusions regarding the mechanisms of influence of social factors on learning problems can be drawn from the extant intervention and prevention studies because they vary widely in their treatment focus, with some being very clearly focused on learning and school-related success (Campbell and Ramey 1994) and others being focused on more general family social and economic needs and paying more attention to social and emotional than to cognitive development (Seitz and Apfel 1994). Specifying the mechanisms of treatment is the next step for intervention research. Intervention studies are also positioned to assess both direct and, perhaps more importantly, indirect mechanisms of influence. For example, interventions originally designed to treat learning difficulties may reduce their severity across time or prevent their emergence by treating behavioural problems, promoting sensitive parent–child interactions, increasing family support, or other processes.

An additional caveat is required in interpreting the intervention research. Many intervention studies do not define the type of learning problems, so it remains to be seen whether they are concerned more with underachievement than with specific learning problems in reading, mathematics, and other areas. Nonetheless, extant studies provide ample evidence of a link between individual differences in experiences at home and school, and learning competence and learning difficulties.

Case studies in learning disabilities and psychosocial factors

THE CASE OF U *(all initials have been changed)*

U is a 9-year-old boy who attends an elementary school in the suburban USA. He is the oldest of three children of highly educated parents. His appearance is somewhat odd, though not remarkable for any specific features or patterns. He is healthy and growing normally and his size is above the 50th centile for his age.

From the time he started school U appeared somewhat socially odd. He was highly verbal; most of his interactions were (and still are) with adults. In kindergarten he was identified as a precocious reader, yet his focus was mostly on 'scary' books. His quantitative and spatial skills were weak and his handwriting and gross motor skills were poor. Specifically, he had difficulty with early mathematic concepts and skills and required considerable help to perform skills the other children in the kindergarten mastered more easily. His fine motor coordination was poor (his handwriting was illegible) and so was his gross motor coordination (he was clumsy). Although he played soccer on a local team of children his age and was mildly interested in the game, he rarely participated on the field. When he attempted to charge the ball and kick, he would usually miss. Socially, U was an outsider. He appeared to not know the 'rules of engagement' with peers, even in fairly structured situations in which there was an adult present to mediate his peer interactions. In less structured situations he stayed apart from the group and the vast majority of his interactions were with adults. Despite these concerns, no referrals were made for special education or other concerns for U throughout his first 4 years of school (kindergarten to grade 3), although he did receive some tutoring with a volunteer in math. U was not bothered by children, who mostly ignored him. Adults viewed him as somewhat odd.

When U was in the second grade (age 7 years) his parents, concerned about his poor mathematics, asked for an assessment by the school's special-education team. He scored in the 'mildly retarded' range on an IQ test. His performance on an achievement test was high in reading and language and was low for age, but not for IQ, in mathematics. The parents were quite upset at the IQ score, believing it did not adequately reflect his verbal abilities. At that time the team did not identify a need for him to have special-education services. In the fourth grade U became increasingly withdrawn and appeared stressed and generally depressed. He often cried himself to sleep. His parents grew increasingly distressed. In interactions with his peers, U rarely if ever sought out age-mates and instead interacted only (and rarely) with younger children. Interactions were almost exclusively with adults and were repetitive, focusing on the same idea over several instances of interaction, and increasingly were narrowed and rigid. He clearly had little or no age-appropriate interaction or social skills. In the classroom he was quiet and isolated, but worked hard.

The parents consulted an independent psychologist (outside the school) for an evaluation, which indicated that U's scores were widely scattered. His verbal scores were at the 98th centile while nonverbal reasoning, spatial processing, and attention were in the 10th to 15th centile range. At that time U was viewed as having a severe learning disability. An independent consultant worked with the school, which now provided tutoring for U. At the end of the fourth grade, U's parents enrolled him in a summer programme at a private school for learning-disabled children. The director of that programme noted that U had one of the most serious learning disabilities she had seen; she also emphasized his social problems.

The case illustrates several issues raised in the discussion of the research. First, it illustrates how thorny diagnostic issues make epidemiological and other types of research difficult in practice. U's learning disability is neither clearly specific (for example to quantitative or spatial skills) nor clearly global (for example he has above-average verbal ability). Moreover, although there is clearly evidence of a learning disability it is also clear that U has impairments in a range of other cognitive areas, notably social cognition and the ability to process social information. Impairments in these areas are often not assessed directly, but they may nonetheless be a source of considerable disability and distress. In fact U shows some mild signs of pervasive developmental disorder. Second, the case highlights the complex ways in which learning and behavioural problems coexist. It is difficult to know for sure, but it seems most likely that U's behavioural and emotional problems were secondary to his learning difficulties and problems of social cognition. It also seems that his learning problems led to emotional difficulties and frustrations and had ever-increasing social impact on his standing in the class and his self-esteem. The case also illustrates how development modifies the relations among behavioural and learning problems. U's apparent lack of interest in interacting with others initially may have led to underestimation of his difficulties and of the range of abilities affected, thus delaying intervention that might have prevented further problems. Third, the case illustrates the difficulties of matching intervention to the types of U's needs. Although tutoring and other academic interventions may help, it is clear that U also needs an intervention for his social problems, which are presumed to derive from difficulties of social cognitive processing. School programmes for these types of complex problems are essentially non-existent.

THE CASE OF B

An underachiever who has no apparent emotional or social problems, B was given special education from grade 2 (he is now in grade 6, age 11 years). An amiable, social boy with friends throughout the school, he performs at an average level on cognitive tests. His performance indicates little scatter, but his verbal IQ is somewhat lower than his nonverbal IQ. B's achievement is significantly lower, at the 25th centile.

Although his early school performance was generally positive, by the second grade (age 7) – when academic expectations rise – B had a hard time keeping up with his classmates. His achievement plummeted that year after the death of his parents in a car accident. B was adopted by an aunt and uncle. Late in the school year he was referred for special education because of his very poor academic 'behaviour' in school. The test scores, noted above, indicated that he performed in the normal range in cognitive abilities but had lowered achievement. No behavioural problems were reported by the school, which in general made no attempt to understand his emotional development and concerns regarding his parents' deaths. He was identified as having a learning disability and received resource-room help (20 hours per week). The label 'learning disability' was applied because of the discrepancy between achievement and IQ.

B flourished in the resource environment for 2 years. He worked very hard and formed a close attachment to teachers in that environment (with whom he remained for 3 years of middle school). By the end of the sixth grade (age 11 years) he was achieving at near-grade-level expectations.

The case of B raises a number of additional issues. First, as with the case of U, there are inevitable diagnostic issues. In practice the school primarily saw B as having a 'learning disability'; little effort was put into understanding the nature of the problem (i.e. which skills were affected) or what the possible causes were (i.e. the role of the traumatic loss). Thus the label 'learning disability' was what the school was interested in. Second, regarding the intervention, was B 'cured' of his learning disability, or had his problem been misdiagnosed (specifically on the basis of discrepancies between IQ and achievement)? Children may underachieve for many reasons, only some of which pertain to issues concerning learning disabilities. How sensitive and specific is the IQ–achievement discrepancy commonly applied in schools? This diagnostic practice has received relatively little close empirical scrutiny. Third, what aspect of the intervention may have had the greatest impact on B's 'recovery': his increased contact with a teacher, his relationship with a teacher, or some other aspect? How might an intervention be specifically designed for B given the school's resources and expertise? Fourth, in this case it seems likely that the learning disability was secondary to the emotional trauma of his parents' death. Nonetheless it is striking that the school recorded no behavioural or emotional problems in B; therefore from the perspective of traditional research methods he would probably not seen as having a learning disability secondary to behavioural or emotional problems.

These cases highlight the complex ways in which a) questions raised in research programmes may seem unrealistically clear-cut in contrast to the complex realities of school systems, b) precise diagnosis sometimes plays a remarkably minor role in the intervention applied by schools, and c) behavioural and emotional problems may lead to, exacerbate, or result from learning disabilities. The cases also illustrate that the relation between learning disabilities and behavioural and emotional problems changes as the child develops.

Conclusion

In this chapter we reviewed some of the current debates and findings regarding the psychosocial influences on the aetiology and course of specific learning problems. Epidemiological data suggest an important role of social and cultural influences on the aetiology of learning disorders, and intervention and follow-up studies are equally convincing that social factors play a critical role in the course of these individuals. In the absence of research focused on risk mechanisms, no firm conclusions can yet be drawn about specific factors or the manner in which they operate. Directions for further clinical and epidemiological research are highlighted with a particular emphasis on the types of challenges clinical and developmental research must address.

REFERENCES

Algozzine B, Ysseldyke JE. (1988) Questioning discrepancies: Retaking the first step 20 years later. *Learning Disabilities Quarterly* **11**: 307–18.

American Psychiatric Association. (1994) *Diagnostic and Statistical Manual of Mental Disorders.* 4th ed. (DSM IV). Washington, DC: American Psychiatric Association.

Berger M, Yule W, Rutter M. (1975) Attainment and adjustment in two geographic areas – II. The prevalence of specific reading retardation. *British Journal of Psychiatry* **126**: 510–9.

Bishop D. (1992) The underlying nature of specific language impairment. *Journal of Child Psychology and Psychiatry* **33**: 3–67.

— North T, Donlan C. (1995) Genetic basis of specific language impairment: Evidence from a twin study. *Developmental Medicine and Child Neurology* **37**: 56–71.

Bradley L, Bryant PE. (1979) The independence of reading and spelling in backward and normal readers. *Developmental Medicine and Child Neurology* **21**: 504–14.

Bronfenbrenner U. (1986) Ecology of the family as a context for human development. *Developmental Psychology* **22**: 723–42.

Brooks-Gunn J, Klebanov PK Duncan, GJ. (1996) Ethnic differences in children's intelligence test scores: role of economic deprivation, home environment and maternal characteristics. *Child Development* **67**: 396–408.

Campbell FA, Ramey CT. (1994) Effects of a early intervention on intellectual and academic achievement: a follow-up study of children from low-income families. *Child Development* **65:** 684–98.

Caughy MO'B, DiPietro JA, Strobino DM. (1994) Day-care participation as a protective factor in the cognitive development of low-income children. *Child Development* **65:** 457–471.

Chapman JW. (1992) Learning disabilities in New Zealand: Why Kiwis and kids with learning disorders can't fly. *Journal of Learning Disorders* **25:** 362–70.

Detterman D. (1996) *Current Topics in Human Intelligence. Volume 5, The Environment.* Norwood, NJ: Ablex.

Eisenberg L. (1966) Reading retardation: I. Psychiatric and sociologic aspects. *Pediatrics* **37:** 352–65.

Fergusson DM: Horwood LJ, Lynskey MT. (1992) Family change, parental discord and early offending. *Journal of Child Psychology and Psychiatry* **33:** 1059–75.

— — — (1993) Early dentine lead levels and subsequent cognitive and behavioural development. *Journal of Child Psychology and Psychiatry* **34:** 215–227.

— Lloyd M, Horwood LJ. (1991) Family ethnicity, social background and scholastic achievement: An eleven year longitudinal study. *New Zealand Journal of Educational Studies* **26:** 49–63.

Frick PJ, Schmidt MH, Lahey BB, et al. (1991) Academic underachievement and the disruptive behavior disorders. *Journal of Consulting and Clinical Psychology* **59:** 289–94.

Gorman KS, Pollitt E. (1996) Does schooling buffer the effects of early risk? *Child Development* **67:** 314–26.

Goswami, U. (1994) Development of reading and spelling skills. In: Rutter M, Hay D, editors. *Development through Life: A Handbook for Clinicians.* Oxford: Blackwell Scientific. p 284–302.

Hallahan DP: Kauffman JM. (1991) *Exceptional children.* 5th ed. Englewood Cliffs, NJ: Prentice-Hall.

Horn WF, Packard T. (1985) Early identification of learning problems: a meta-analysis. *Journal of Educational Psychology* **77:** 597–607.

Hyde JS, Linn MC. (1988) Gender differences in verbal ability: A meta-analysis. *Psychological Bulletin* **104:** 53–69.

Lewitter FI, DeFries JC, Elston RC. (1980) Genetic models of reading disability. *Behavior Genetics* **10:** 9–30.

MacLean M, Bryant, PE, Bradley L. (1987) Rhymes, nursery rhymes and reading in early childhood. *Merrill-Palmer Quarterly* **33:** 255–82.

Maughan B. (1995) Annotation: Long-term outcomes of developmental reading problems. *Journal of Child Psychology and Psychiatry* 36: 357–71.

— Yule M. (1994) Reading and other learning disabilities. In: Rutter M, Taylor E, Hersov L, editors. *Child and Adolescent Psychiatry.* 3rd ed. Oxford: Blackwell Scientific. p 647–65.

— Pickles A, Hagell A, et al. (1996) Reading problems and antisocial behaviour: developmental trends in comorbidity. *Journal of Child Psychology and Psychiatry* **37:** 405–18.

McGee R, Williams S, Share DL, et al. (1986) The relationships between specific learning retardation, general reading backwardness and behavioural problems in a large sample of Dunedin boys. *Journal of Child Psychology and Psychiatry* **27:** 597–610.

Morisset CE, Barnard KE, Booth CL. (1995) Toddlers' language development: sex differences within social risk. *Developmental Psychology* **31:** 851–65.

Morrison FJ, Smith L, Dow-Ehrensberger M. (1995) Education and cognitive development: a natural experiment. *Developmental Psychology* **31:** 789–99.

O'Connor S, Spreen O. (1988) The relationship between parents' socioeconomic status and education level and adult occupational and educational achievement of children with learning disabilities. *Journal of Learning Disabilities* **21:** 148–53.

Pennington BF, Groisser D, Welsh MC. (1993) Contrasting cognitive deficits in attention deficit hyperactivity disorder versus reading disability. *Developmental Psychology* **29:** 511–23.

Pianta RC, Egeland B. Predictors of instability of children's mental test performance at 24, 48, and 96 months. *Intelligence.* Forthcoming.

— McCoy S. The first day of school: the predictive utility of a kindergarten screening battery. *Journal of Applied Developmental Psychology.* Forthcoming.

— O'Connor TG. (1996) Developmental challenges to the study of specific environmental effects: an argument for niche-level influences. In: Detterman D, editor. *Current Topics in Human Intelligence. Volume 5, The Environment.* Norwood, NJ: Ablex. p 45–58.

Plomin R. (1994) *Genes and Experience: The Interplay between Nature and Nurture.* Thousand Oaks, CA: Sage.

Pungello EP, Kupersmidt JB, Burchinal MR, Patterson CJ. (1996) Environmental risk factors and children's achievement from middle childhood to early adolescence. *Developmental Psychology* **32:** 755–67.

Rawson M. (1968) *Developmental Language Disability: Adult Accomplishments of Dyslexic Boys.* Baltimore: Johns Hopkins University Press.

Rourke BP. (1983) Outstanding issues in research on learning disabilities. In: Rutter M, editor. *Developmental Neuropsychiatry.* New York: Guilford. p 564–76.

Rutter M, Tizard J, Whitmore K. (1970) *Education, Health and Behaviour.* London: Longmans.

— Yule W. (1970) Reading retardation and antisocial behaviour – the nature of the association. In Rutter M, Tizard J, Whitmore K., editors. *Education, Health and Behaviour.* London: Longmans. p. 240–55.

— Smith DJ, editors. (1995) *Psychosocial Disorders in Young People: Time Trends and Their Causes.* Chichester, England: Wiley.

Sameroff AJ, Seifer R, Barocas R, et al. (1987) Intelligence quotient scores of 4-year-old children: social environment risk factors. *Pediatrics* **79:** 343–50.

Sanson A, Prior M, Smart D. (1996) Reading disabilities with and without behaviour problems at 7–8 years: prediction from longitudinal data from infancy to 6 years. *Journal of Child Psychology and Psychiatry* **37:** 529–41.

Seitz V, Apfel NH. (1994) Parent-focused intervention: diffusion effects on siblings. *Child Development* **65:** 677–83.

Shinn MR, Ysseldyke JE, Deno SL, Tindal GA. (1986) A comparison of differences between students labeled learning disabled and low achieving on measures of classroom performance. *Journal of Learning Disabilities* **9:** 545–52.

Silva PA, McGee R, Williams S. (1985) Some characteristics of 9-year-old boys with general reading backwardness or specific reading retardation. *Journal of Child Psychology and Psychiatry* **26:** 407–21.

Stevenson J. (1991) Which aspects of processing text mediate genetic effects? *Reading and Writing: An Interdisciplinary Journal* **3:** 249–69.

Super CM, Harkness S. (1986) The developmental niche: a conceptualization at the interface of child and culture. *International Journal of Behavioral Development* **9:** 545–69.

Taubes G. (1995) Epidemiology faces its limits. *Science* **269:** 164–9.

Wachs TD, Moussa W, Bishry Z, et al. (1993) Relation between nutrition and cognitive performance. *Intelligence* **17:** 151–72.

Wagner RK, Torgesen JK, Rashotte CA. (1994) Development of reading-related phonological processing abilities: new evidence of bidirectional causality from a latent variable longitudinal study. *Developmental Psychology* **30:** 73–87.

Walker D, Greenwood C, Hart B, Carta J. (1994) Prediction of school outcomes based on early language production and socioeconomic factors. *Child Development* **65:** 606–21.

World Health Organization. (1993) *The ICD–10 Classification of Mental and Behavioural Disorders: Diagnostic Criteria for Research.* Geneva: World Health Organization.

11
IDENTIFICATION OF SPECIFIC LEARNING DISORDER AT THE AGE OF 5 YEARS

Guy Willems and Philippe Evrard

There are two routine circumstances in which a clinician seeing a child will conclude that the child may have a specific learning (neurodevelopmental) disorder. One is when the examination is requested because the child's teachers or parents think that the child, after a year or two of school, has unusual difficulty in learning the '3 Rs' – reading, writing, and arithmetic – or in socializing reasonably. They particularly want to know from the paediatric assessment whether there may be a biological cause for the difficulty and, if the problem in socializing is greater than the delay in learning the 3 Rs, whether it is an intrinsic feature of a learning disorder or only a consequence of the delay. The paediatric opinion might significantly influence planning for the child's education. Such a paediatric contribution to diagnosis is discussed more fully in Chapter 15.

The second routine opportunity to identify specific learning disorder is when the clinician carries out routine physical and neurodevelopmental examination of indiviual children when they begin formal, compulsory education in school. The object of such examination is to be sure that the child's health is satisfactory and that the child has no unrecognized physical, sensory, or neurological disorder that might appreciably interrupt learning or attendance at school. This objective is discussed in this chapter with particular reference to the early identification of specific learning disorders, although there is considerable overlap in the clinical tests used in the two situations.

History of school-entrant health examinations

In Europe health examinations for school entrants were introduced at the beginning of the century, soon after the provision of free milk in school and when education became compulsory. Both the examinations and the milk were aimed at reducing the malnutrition, ill health, and disability that so often compromised children's education in school. The doctors' and nurses' examinations understandably focused on the assessment of physical health by methods that are essentially the same today. The school health services that evolved around these examinations often took on a therapeutic role until primary health-care services, as they are now called, became available. Comparable services for preschool children were also preceded by measures for countering malnutrition, in the form of free milk depots. Initially, at the turn of the century, these were run by health visitors, who soon started offering advice to mothers on infant care. The health visitors were the forerunners of child-welfare clinics, where doctors undertook immunizations and periodically checked on young children's physical growth and development.

After the Great Depression that overtook the economies of the United States and European countries in the late 1920s, the nutrition and health of children of all ages improved measurably and attention turned to more subtle indicators of functional maturity than motor development. The paediatricians Gesell and Amatruda laid the foundation for what we now call neurodevelopmental assessment. After studying the early signs of mental deficiency in children, Gesell and his colleagues (Gesell et al. 1930) launched an unprecedented study of the normal infant and young child (Gesell and Amatruda 1941), from which they drew the following conclusions:

- The developmental status of a child can be gauged from their reactions – the way they behave.
- All behaviour patterns, whether prenatal or postnatal, reflex or learned, are simply defined responses of the neuromotor system to specific situations, more advanced patterns reflecting an increasing maturity of the nervous system, i.e. developmental status.
- The human organism is a complicated action system that is the summation of four principal kinds of behaviour: motor, adaptive, language, and personal–social.

At the same time Gesell and Amatruda (1941) published the first brief manual describing the techniques (test procedures and materials) for clinical use that 'constituted controlled devices for eliciting patterns of behaviour indicative of [the] developmental status' of children up to the age of $3^{1}/2$ years, including developmental norms for the population of children they examined. Assessment of developmental status soon became widely incorporated into periodic health assessments of preschool children.

For many years children missed out on developmental assessment once they entered school. The emphasis of medical inspection continued to be on their physical state rather than their behaviour, and when problems in either learning or personal–social behaviour arose, it was the children's response to tests of their intelligence that were thought to be relevant. However, the concept of minimal brain damage (MBD) heralded an important change in clinical practice. Gesell and Amatruda (1941) reported that this concept was 'gradually forced upon us by our clinical experience with atypical infants'. The concept received considerable support when Strauss and Lehtinen (1947) described what was later to be known as the Strauss syndrome. This was regarded as a unitary syndrome due to minor brain damage of nonspecific origin, consisting in abnormal distractibility, hyperactivity, clumsiness, and motor–perceptual difficulties. Bender (1947) unwittingly popularized the term 'soft signs' as a description of the responses to neurological examination of a group of children with schizophrenia, because it was then used for similar responses of children 'diagnosed' as having MBD. It continued to be used when the concept of MBD gave way to that of minimal cerebral dysfunction (MCD) and the latter became a generic aetiological classification of specific learning disorders, e.g. dyslexia, which were presumed to have a neurological basis (Gaddes and Edgell 1993). It is historically interesting that as long ago as 1934 Gesell and Thompson wondered whether some infants and young children had 'specific lags or accelerations among components of their behaviour', and in 1941 Bender and Yarnell suggested that the reading disability of children in whom the findings on classical neurological examination were normal might be due to developmental or maturational lag.

Years of debate on both topics ensued and certainly in respect of soft signs it can hardly be said that there is a clear consensus (Touwen 1979, Shaffer et al. 1983, Denckla 1985, Silver and Hagin 1990). What has become clear is that whatever word one chooses to describe the responses of young children to tests of their development, similar tests are no less important in their first term in school than in their infant and toddler years. Their purpose is still an initial assessment of the functional maturity of the child's central nervous system as a first step in the early identification of neurological dysfunction. Only if signs of dysfunction are found does the question arise: what do they signify? Are they inappropriate for the age of the child, i.e. developmental, or are they abnormal for any age, i.e. pathological? Some signs such as clumsiness, motor impersistence, or associated movements are said to be common to both immaturity and abnormality (Spreen et al. 1995). Which of these is the most likely will be a matter of clinical judgement and experience that may govern a decision to refer the child for specialist assessment; paediatricians are uniquely and crucially able to adopt a holistic perspective in such decisions, mindful of the interests of the child as a whole in summing up the results of physical and behavioural examination.

The only difference between the developmental testing of toddlers and of pupils is less reliance on tests of motor behaviour for the older children and the inclusion of suitable tests of the more extensive and complex functional repertoire (perceptual–motor performance) of 5- to 6-year-old children that follows advancing sensory and motor organization and integration. This is the common ground between paediatric neurology and neuropsychology, involving the use of tests that focus more exactly than for toddlers on specific aspects of adaptive and language behaviour, particularly finesse in executing intentional or exploratory neuromotor behaviour and the quality and effectiveness of verbal communication, including reading and writing.

Comprehensive health and neurodevelopmental assessment of school entrants

Bax and Whitmore were among the first to investigate the practicability and value of including a short battery of neurodevelopmental tests in a school-entrant medical examination. Their first study was of the entire population of children who entered ordinary schools in the Isle of Wight at the age of 5 years (Bax and Whitmore 1973). The study included a 3-year follow-up examination and tests on the reliability and validity of the neurodevelopmental subtests, the latter by comparison with the results of examination by educational psychologists using a battery particularly devised to identify children likely to have reading difficulties.

Their study showed that it was certainly feasible to include a number of neurodevelopmental tests in an entrant medical examination lasting 15 to 20 minutes. More importantly, they found that there was a significant (and therefore encouraging) high correlation between the children who did worst on the psychological battery and those who had a high neurodevelopmental test score (that is, a score indicating neurodevelopmental problems). This exploratory study did not include the full, detailed diagnostic examination that such children should have, but Bax and Whitmore noted that over half of the children with high scores at age 5 had by age 9 been independently referred by their schools to the educational psychologist on account of learning or behavioural difficulties.

Bax and Whitmore carried out a more refined study of the neurodevelopmental assessment of entrants to schools in the Paddington district of London (Whitmore and Bax 1986, Bax and Whitmore 1987), in which the children were followed up for learning or behavioural difficulties at the ages of 7 and 10 years. The revised tests that contributed to a full neurodevelopmental score (NDS) were subgrouped to provide separate neurological, motor, visual-perception, speech-and-language, and ability scores (Table 11.1). The results were as follows:

1   The children with a high neurodevelopmental score (NDS) at entrance to school were very vulnerable and had significantly higher rates of learning difficulty at the age of 10 years.
2   A high NDS at entrance to school correlated well with poor academic achievement at age 7 years and was a good predictor of the likelihood of referral to a psychologist during infant-school years (ages 5 to 7); such referral was in turn a predictor of learning difficulties persisting or arising in the junior school (ages 7 to 11).
3   The NDS was a more effective predictor of learning difficulties at 10 years than a simple assessment of intelligence (ability score), probably because it reflects a wide range of developing functions of the central nervous system and a child with a high NDS is one with a neurological disadvantage that is not manifest solely as limited intellectual ability.
4   Children with a reading quotient of 80 or less usually did not have a high NDS, but they quite often did have a poor visual perception score. They seldom had both.
5   Children with high motor scores (indicating clumsiness) had significantly more learning difficulties at the age of 10 than children with normal motor scores.
6   Impaired hearing or problems with speech and language at the age of 5 years were significantly associated with a high NDS.
7   The school doctor's clinical judgement based on the complete entrant examination gave a better prediction of learning disorder and of behaviour difficulties at the age of 10 than did the NDS score alone.

The search for more discriminating tests for specific learning disorders

Many paediatricians will no doubt be familiar with manuals of so-called soft neurological tests for learning disorders in general in young children (Touwen 1979, Denckla 1985). In the Groningen Perinatal Project Touwen and his colleagues (Huisjes et al. 1980) used a neurological examination to detect the presence of minor signs of neurological dysfunction. The signs were arranged according to subsystems of the nervous system: posture in various positions, hypotonia of the sensorimotor system (reflexes and responses), coordination, fine manipulation, and the presence or absence of choreiform dyskinesia. The children were examined at age of 4 and again at 6, 9, and 12 years and at puberty by the same group of authors (Hadders-Algra et al. 1986, 1988).

TABLE 11.1
Tests contributing to the neurodevelopmental score at the age of 5 years

Neurological score	*Visual perception score*
Head circumference	Squint
Bergès-Lézine	Visual acuity
Finger–nose	Building with bricks
Motor symmetry	Drawing shapes
Motor persistence	Bergès-Lézine
Tongue movements	*Speech and language score*
Nystagmus	Picture vocabulary
Cranial nerves	Definitions
Squint	Articulation (words and sentences)
Reflexes	Renfrew Action Pictures (information)
Motor score	*Ability score*
Motor precision (quality of drawing skills)	Picture vocabulary
Pencil grip	Definitions
Hand patting	Materials
Finger–nose	Sentence repetition
Gait	Practical reasoning items
Heel–toe walk	Renfrew Action Pictures (information)
Hopping	Building with bricks
	Drawing shapes

(From The school entry medical examination, Whitmore K, Bax MCO, 1986, *Archives of Disease in Childhood* **61:** 807–17, with permission from the BMJ Publishing Group.)

At 9 years of age undesirable behaviour and learning problems were found in excess among children with MND compared with the control group (Hadders-Algra et al. 1988). MND was also found to be more closely related to learning difficulties than to behavioural problems (Hadders-Algra and Touwen 1992).

Learning disorders have now been more precisely differentiated, for instance language disorders (Rapin and Segalowitz 1992), subtypes of reading disorder (Cantwell and Baker 1991, Kaplan et al. 1995, Lyon 1995, Stanovich et al. 1997), mathematics disorders (Badian 1983, O'Hare et al. 1991), verbal and non-verbal disabilities (Rourke 1993), and motor learning disorders (Henderson 1987, Cratty 1994).

Finger succession has been studied by Denckla (1973, 1974) and Wolff et al. (1983) with the intention of identifying children who are at risk of severe writing disabilities (handwriting, spelling, composition) later in their development. This examination (a test of planning, programming, and execution of fine motor movements) was also studied by Berninger and Rutberg in 1992.

Finger recognition and finger agnosia, on a verbal task, were studied in relation to later reading achievement (Fletcher et al. 1982).

Finger discrimination and finger localization, on a non-verbal task, were studied by Kinsbourne and Warrington (1963), and the presence of finger localization errors in children of preschool age seems to be an indicator of high risk for learning disabilities in general and reading retardation in particular (Satz et al. 1974). Lindgren (1975) also proposed the finger localization examination as a predictor of reading and arithmetic disabilities. Levine et al. (1981) found that half their sample had finger agnosia (elicited by imitative finger movement and finger differentiation); all those with finger agnosia also had fine motor problems (e.g. using a pencil or putting things together), and 72% of the ones with fine motor problems also displayed finger agnosia. The speed of verbal naming is impaired in the verbal naming of pictures (picture naming) and also in the verbal naming of fingers (finger agnosia). The verbal-fluency deficit is highly correlated with the naming task, and the verbal-sequencing deficit present in finger agnosia may affect the speed and accuracy of reading (see Wolf et al. 1986, Denckla 1985).

Balancing on one leg. Powell and Bishop (1992) reported signs of clumsiness at the age of 6 in children with specific language impairment. Poor performance on motor tasks (balancing on one foot) in combination with imperfect visual-perceptual performance (comparing the length of two lines) was effective in discriminating between the language-impaired and the control children.

Judgements of length (visual discrimination, visual perception). Hulme et al. (1982) found that clumsy children were poor at making visual judgements of length. Lord and Hulme (1987) found consistently poorer performance by clumsy children in processing visuospatial information unrelated to variance of visual acuity. Powell and Bishop (1992) found that 6-year-olds with language impairment also had problems of perception and clumsiness.

However, from neuropsychological studies there have been glimpses of the processes (mechanisms) that may explain the chain of cerebral activities between sensory arousal and intentional motor response. Such processes are still largely hypothetical and the aetiology of their dysfunction is far from certain. However, a review of the literature suggests that there are some worthwhile tests that might be incorporated into a comprehensive neurodevelopmental assessment of children on entry to school.

Jorn et al. (1986) carried out a study with 453 Australian children with an average age of 5 years 4 months. This 3-year study was intended to identify the weaknesses of future poor readers and to see if any differences emerged in the patterns of deficiency between readers with global retardation (indicated by a Neale reading test score below that predicted on the basis of age alone) and those with a specific retardation (indicated by a Neale reading test score 1.5 standard deviations below that predicted on the basis of age and IQ). Of 453 children, 14 exhibited general reading retardation, 25 had a specific reading retardation, and 414 could read normally.

In the third year of kindergarten, the poor readers with specific problems had difficulties with letter naming, recognition and discrimination between letters and numbers, remembering rhyming and non-rhyming phrases, speed of identifying the names of pictures and colours, phoneme segmentation, finger discrimination, and finger agnosia.

In a longitudinal predictive study, Ellis and Large (1987) identified the precise area of the inability of poor readers. The authors monitored 40 children between the ages of 5 and 8 years. Forty-four tests were administered every year to evaluate their intellectual level; level of reading and spelling; short-term visual and auditory memory; visual, auditory, and visuoauditory perception; and knowledge of syntax, vocabulary, and organization of time (days in the week, low numbers). After 3 years, three groups of five subjects each were created: a group of readers with global retardation (signalled by low IQ and low reading level), a group of children with reading disorders (signalled by average IQ and low reading level), and a group of good readers (signalled by average IQ and good reading level). The three groups of readers were matched on the basis of chronological age and sociocultural environment. The only tests in which the interaction between group and age was significant were the reading and spelling tests and, at the age of 5, the auditory-number or word-span test, the letter-identification test, the WISC coding test, the phoneme-segmentation test, the ability to recognize or create rhymes, and the ability to recognize a dictated word among five written words.

Mann and Liberman (1984) and Lecocq (1988) have studied the relations between short-term memory measured at the age of 5 years and the reading scores measured at age 7. Most of the tests used for the 5-year-olds by these authors consisted of the repetition of lists of phonetically different words, phrases with no phonetic similarity, and rhyming words; the repetition of ever longer phrases or of phonetically similar or dissimilar phrases with the same syntactic structure (e.g., respectively, *Mike – likes – bikes* or *Dave – likes – cars*); and the repetition of lists of numbers backwards or forwards.

Wolf et al. (1986) examined 86 5-year-old children and reviewed their reading level at the age of 8. The study concluded that at the age of 5 the children with reading disorders were significantly slower than the eventually good readers in the colour-, object-, number-, and letter-naming tests. Unlike the good readers, they made little progress in these tests between the ages of 5 and 8 years.

Clearly tests of short-term memory are important, but solely with respect to the linguistic material – e.g. verbal short-term memory, repetition of phonologically coded words, phrases (rhymes) – when it is presented in a certain order (verbal-sequential memory), or with respect to the ability to segment words or syllables. In reality some of the other tests used at the age of 5 are not purely memory tests, but also measure the attention span in continuous performance tasks, such as quickly naming colours or objects, or repeating numbers. The repetitive tasks measuring the verbal short-term memory span are also related to the speed of articulation (dependent on the articulatory loop), which can be examined in children by considering their buccolinguofacial gestures, pronunciation of syllables or rhymes, and speed of subvocal pronunciation. It may be possible for children to use these systems to develop an information-processing strategy (articulatory memory) enabling information to be stored in longer-term memory.

Of course, short-term memory is important in learning to read, but the situation is complex, since those children who can learn to read will develop short-term memory in parallel with their reading ability, whereas children with reading disorders will probably not have this option.

One important prerequisite of normal reading acquisition seems to be the capacity for rapid lexical retrieval, as examined by confrontation naming tasks (Denckla and Rudel 1976, Wolf 1986, Wolf and Goodglass 1986). Difficulty in naming colours (Denckla and Rudel 1976) indicates and measures a specific slowness in the retrieval of symbolic material from long-term memory, i.e. finding phonological information in the long-term memory.

Equally important in testing for specific reading disorders are tests of phonological awareness processing. There is mounting evidence that children with dyslexia have difficulty with tasks relying on phonological awareness. Frith (1997) has summarized the impairments: slowness in automatic naming, poor verbal learning and memory, poor non-word repetition and phoneme awareness, difficulties in segmenting phonemes, and difficulties in naming objects.

The question of which aspects of language deficiency may result in late reading and spelling has also been addressed in some studies, all of which have focused on a specific component of language. Some of the data show a rather striking similarity between the deficits in children with language disorders at age 5 to 6 years and in future poor readers. Children with language disorder took longer than children in the control group to name pictures of objects or animals: in other words they took longer to retrieve phonological information from long-term memory. Kamhi and Catts (1986) monitored from age 6 to 9 years a group of children who had language disorder leading to reading disorder. At age 6 the best tests of oral language capacity, which most successfully predicted reading success, were the tests of word segmentation, rhyming, sound blending, and elision.

In some children disorders of oral language are diagnosed much later, when they are learning to read. Knowledge about language acquisition remains very patchy and the knowledge that does exist is shared to differing degrees between doctors and psychologists. Oral language development can also vary greatly between children. It may be developed well enough to allow communication but not well enough for some aspects of learning to read. For example in children with language disorders the understanding of syntactic structures at the age of 5 or 6 years appears to be another good indicator of the chance of reading success (Bowey 1986, Tunmer et al. 1987).

Korkman and Peltomaa (1994) studied 26 boys with language impairment, with the aim of instituting preventive treatment to reduce the risk of reading disorders. These authors found that the boys they studied were affected most by language disorders, but also by attention disorders (seen on tests of sustained concentration and of selective auditory attention), and visuomotor disorders (visuomotor integration) (Beery and Buktenica 1967).

The Brussels study

In the light of such reports we and our colleagues set up the Brussels study (Willems et al. 1984a), with two objectives. The first was to determine which were the best tests for school doctors and community paediatricians to use in a school-entrant examination to identify the children most a risk of having specific learning disorders (the 3-year phase of the study). The second objective was to find out how effective they might be in practice (the 5-year phase). We addressed this task with caution because of the many problems. Apart from problems of the validity and reliability of the tests, there is the complication of the co-occurrence of specific disorders and their clinical diagnosis. A number of authors have found that certain difficulties can co-occur, such as reading, spelling, and mathematics disabilities (Rutter 1978, Satz and Morris 1981, Siegel 1989), and clumsiness, perceptual problems, and language impairment (Stark and Tallal 1981, Noterdaeme et al. 1988, Powell and Bishop 1992).

The term *motor learning disorders* (or *motor learning difficulties*) is being increasingly used (Hulme and Lord 1986, McKinlay 1987) to describe the problems of children who experience perceptual and motor difficulties, whether or not these are associated with learning disorders. It seems that there is considerable overlap between the two kinds of disorder, though the estimates of overlap vary greatly.

Neurodevelopmental difficulties are associated with language difficulties (Johnston et al. 1981, Wolff et al. 1985), with psychiatric problems of the anxiety type (Shaffer 1985), and with signs of problems of attention or hyperactivity (Rasmussen et al. 1983).

However, others consider that some problems are specific, such as reading disorders (Critchley 1970, Boder 1973, Benton and Pearl 1978), developmental clumsiness (Gubbay 1975, Gordon and McKinlay 1980), and language disabilities (Ingram 1969). These problems are presumably independent of one another (for example, some children with dyslexia learn mathematics easily). Pennington (1991) treats reading disorders and attention-deficit disorders as unitary syndromes, an approach that is criticized by Bishop (1992).

For our studies we used the definitional criteria of learning disorders as set out in the law of the USA [Public Law 94-142 (S.6); Nov. 19, 1975. Education for All Handicapped Children Act of 1975]:

Specific learning disability means a disorder in one or more of the basic psychological processes involved in understanding or in using language, spoken or written, which may manifest itself in an imperfect ability to listen, think, speak, read, write, spell, or to do mathematical calculations. The term includes such conditions as perceptual handicaps, brain injury, minimal brain dysfunction, dyslexia, and developmental aphasia. The term does not include children who have learning problems which are primarily the result of visual, hearing, or motor handicaps, of mental retardation, of emotional disturbance, or of environmental, cultural, or economic disadvantage.

This meant that the initial group of children on whom tests would be carried out in the initial, 3-year phase of the study had to be as homogeneous as possible with respect to social, linguistic, cultural, environmental, and educational backgrounds, of normal intelligence, and free from any severe auditory or visual defect. Accordingly from 355 children in 19 different schools of the same area in Brussels who attended school regularly, we selected 281 boys aged $5^1/2$ to $6^1/4$ years, all of whom were of Belgian nationality, monolingual, from families whose socioeconomic status was average to high, and whose IQ (on the WISC) was normal. Boys were chosen because many authors argue that the results of tests for learning disorder for boys and girls must be analysed separately, because the two sexes probably have different hemispheric strategies or specialization at this age (5 to 10 years) and are subject to different environmental and familial factors. Thus results from girls may distort results obtained from boys and vice versa.

From among the tests used by many authors to establish a neurodevelopmental profile (Jansky and de Hirsch 1972, Bax and Whitmore 1973, Satz et al. 1974, Silver and Hagin 1975, Touwen 1979), 45 were used in the full battery given to the 281 boys (Table 11.2). Three years later, when they were in grade 3 (aged $8^1/2$), the children were given standardized academic achievement tests: the 'Poucet' (Simon 1954), a test of expressive reading; the California reading test (Tiegs and Clark 1967), which tests receptive or semantic reading; and a mathematics achievement test (Bonboir 1969). By stepwise discriminant analysis we

TABLE 11.2
The neurodevelopmental examination between 5¹/₂ and 6¹/₄ years of age

Classic neurological examination	*Intelligence*
Head circumference	Performance
Cranial nerves	Picture arrangement
Eye movements	Block design
Squint	Coding
Nystagmus	Verbal
Extrapyramidal involuntary movements	Arithmetic
Choreoathetiform syndrome (Prechtl)	Similarities
Diadochokinesia	Vocabulary
Dysmorphic signs or stigmata	*Short-term memory*
	Digit repetition
Development of praxis (motor learning)	Verbal-sequential memory
Finger praxis (fine coordination)	Sentence memory
Pencil grip	*Sensory integration*
Associated movements (synkinesia)	Crossing midline
Gross motor coordination (equilibrium)	Tactile recognition
Stand on one foot, jump on one foot	Graphiaesthesia
Constructional praxis	Imitation of gestures
Buccolinguofacial praxis	*Sequential organization*
Imitation of gestures	Digit repetition
	Finger discrimination
Gnosis	Finger gnosia
Stereognosis	*Position in space*
Finger gnosis, finger discrimination: simultanagnosia	Lamb chop
	Block design
Visual perception	Spatial discrimination
Embedded figure test	*Laterality*
Visual discrimination	Arm-extension test
Bender gestalt	*Verbal naming*
Constructional praxis	Finger gnosia
Imitation of gestures	Picture naming
Crossing midline	Hearing (before tests)
Visual acuity (before testing)	*Attention*
	Double simultaneous stimuli (simultanagnosia)
Speech and language	Motor impersistence
Buccolinguofacial praxis	Digit span
Phonological awareness	Coding
Auditory discrimination	Arithmetic
Vocabulary	
Sentence memory	

(Based on findings in Willems et al. 1984a, 1986.)

identified which tests from the initial battery correlated with eventual poor performance on the academic achievement tests.

The tests we used gave a correct classification in 85 to 98% of cases, with 89 to 92% specificity (Table 11.3). The tests that correlated most strongly with reading and mathematics disorders are shown in Table 11.4. Surprisingly, among the children who on academic tests given in grade 3 were found to have learning disorder, the largest group was of children with difficulties in more than one area of learning (for example severe reading disorder with moderate or mild problems in mathematics). This observation is important because most studies on learning disorder investigate only reading disorders, which rarely occur alone.

TABLE 11.3
Diagnostic value for outcome in grade 3 of tests given at school entry

Specific learning disabilities diagnosed	Correct classification (%)	Sensitivity (%)	Specificity (%)
3-year study[a]			
Expressive reading disorders (speed, accuracy)	85.4	61	89
Receptive reading disorders (comprehension)	84	58	89
Mathematics disorders	90.5	80	92
Specific learning disorders (overall)	98.6	71	100
5-year study[b]			
Specific learning disorders (overall)	80	59	79

(Based on findings in Willems et al. 1984a.)
[a]Full neurodevelopmental examination; *N*=281 (boys).
[b]Abridged neurodevelopmental examination; *N*=2941 (boys and girls).

WHICH TESTS SHOULD THE SCHOOL DOCTOR OR PAEDIATRICIAN USE FOR 5-YEAR-OLDS?

Tests of speed and accuracy of reading (expressive reading)

To detect disorders in speed and accuracy of reading, a test for finger agnosia seems unquestionably useful. In our examination battery the task assigned required verbal naming (i.e. naming the number corresponding to the finger touched by the tester); this implied retrieving into memory the exact number and also the mental representation (body schema) of the sequence of fingers (sequential memory). A deficit in semantic categorization (measured on the Similarities scale of the WISC) is also found at preschool age in reading disorders and is related to the semantic-processing deficit (Milles and Haslum 1986). Some children who do not know the meaning of a word may formulate semantic paraphasias (e.g. saying *church* for *priest*) in reading, which reduces accuracy. Constructional apraxia (in drawing shapes, assessed on the Bender test) is considered to be a general action-planning deficit involving coordination of the various parts of the drawing and size scaling within the object and between objects. It is considered a visual-perception deficit critical to many academic tasks and is usually impaired before the child learns to read.

The lack of perception of double tactile stimuli (simultanagnosia) seems to be correlated with the level of vigilance and the quality of attention needed to perceive double stimulation in kinaesthetic perception.

Tests for comprehension deficits in reading (receptive reading)

Comprehension deficits seem to be related to the same difficulties in verbal naming as in the children with disorders of speed and accuracy; however, the children with comprehension deficits also have difficulties in placing words in the right position within a long sentence – a task requiring a short-term verbal memory of six items in the test used. A deficit in sequencing from memory and in oral language, especially with a poor vocabulary, may

237

TABLE 11.4
Tests correlating most strongly with specific learning disorders

Function tested	Reading (speed/accuracy)	Reading (comprehension)	Mathematics	SLDs
Speech and language				
Verbal naming	X	X		
Finger gnosis (naming)	X			X
Semantic categorization	X			
Word morphology			X	
Phonological awareness			X	X
Motor learning				
Diadochokinesia		X		
Finger discrimination			X	
Visual perception				
Constructional praxis (drawing shapes)	X			X
Simultanagnosia	X			X
Graphiaesthesia		X		
Stereognosis			X	
Picture arrangement			X	
Sequential memory				
Finger discrimination (non-verbal)		X		
Sentence repetition (verbal)		X		X
Attention				
Sustained concentration	X	X	X	X
Staying with task	X	X	X	X

(Based on findings in Willems et al. 1984a.)

interfere with comprehension in reading. Ordering deficits also appear in finger discrimination, which is a non-verbal sequencing task. A comprehension deficit may be related to both verbal and non-verbal sequencing deficits. The sequence of motor movements is also limited (dysdiadochokinesia), and these children also show a deficit in perceiving a design drawn on the back of the hand (dysgraphiaesthesia), lacking sufficient duration and quality of attention. They seem to lack global or holistic perception. To comprehend a written sentence a child must be able to perceive it as words in sequence and to combine the words to form a whole, but these children cannot do this.

Tests for mathematics disorders
Mathematics disorders at age 9 years 3 months seem to be related to functions of both the left hemisphere (word recognition and phonological awareness) and the right hemisphere (image sequences, spatial orientation). The relation with the two hemispheres has been discussed by Gordon and McKinlay (1980).

What clearly appears is the identification of the Gerstmann syndromes (Kinsbourne and Warrington 1963; Benton 1985) in astereognosis of blocks presenting different heights for each finger (finger localization task), and of non-verbal-sequencing deficit or sequential-memory deficit in finger discrimination or in categorization of sequences of images.

Numeration disorders can appear at the age of $5^1/2$ years as disorders of mental representation (spatial imagery) or as inaccuracy in finger ordering (sequencing deficit), which is needed in finger discrimination and in finger praxis (counting to 5). Deficits in visual perception or spatial organization appear in astereognosis and in deficits of spatial orientation. Preschool children begin with material objects, which they can handle, arranged in space, and later they acquire number facts from visual and manual contact with the objects when they learn to write numbers. This leads to the formation of tabular calculation (e.g. sometimes by using the sequence of fingers) and then automated learning through oral recitation and writing in a particular spatial arrangement. They finally learn to think symbolically with numbers and to reason abstractly (O'Hare et al. 1991, Shalev et al. 1993).

A deficit in word recognition (discriminating whether words are the same or different) and in phonological awareness may be related to some disorders in oral language (Gaddes 1980), or to some disorders of reading of numbers (for example saying '61' when '16' is intended) or of reading the verbal statement of a problem.

Disorders of perceptual–motor and visuospatial skills constitute a risk for low achievement in geometry.

Tests for learning disorders in general
The neurodevelopmental tests in our battery that correlated most strongly with learning disorders in general (both types of reading disorder, and mathematics disorders) are also shown in Table 11.4.

The inability to name fingers in the finger-touch tests underlines the importance of disabilities in three major areas: verbal naming, sequencing, and the internal lexicon of the verbal material needed in reading.

A short-term memory deficit regarding sequential words in sentences indicates that it is mainly again a sequencing deficit that provokes a short-term memory deficit: either the short-term memory deficit itself occurs in the sentence memory or there is a deficit in duration of attention (tested by, e.g., digit repetition) that causes the sequencing deficit.

A deficit in phonological awareness (tested here by the ability to extract the same syllable presented in three different words – for example 'pa' in *repas, papier,* and *pavé* [Chevrie-Muller et al. 1981]) can be used to distinguish between good and poor readers at $5^1/2$ years of age (results not presented here). In the group with learning disorders a phonological-awareness deficit can occur with both reading and mathematics disorders. Few studies have examined such a narrowly defined group. In a study in Florida (Fletcher et al. 1982) some of the pupils met the criteria for both reading and mathematics disability.

The test for constructional apraxia is a basic visuomotor or visual-perceptual task (spatial) involving planning of action when drawing in a non-verbal learning task. Difficulties with planning of actions can be due to disorders in perception or in motor learning, or to a deficit in attention or concentration.

Simultanagnosia, or tactile discrimination of two points, involves spatial perception and elementary somataesthesia, involving the parietal regions (right or left or both). In the absence of any brain lesion it is usually related to the level of vigilance or quality of attention in a discriminative learning task (for a discussion see Rourke 1993). Deficits on tasks requiring motor learning are seen in dysdiadochokinesia, which is a complex deficit of motor planning and of coordination under visual control.

Our study also showed that deficits in attention (its quality and duration) and memory, considered here as neurodevelopmental factors, play a role in information-processing deficits and consequently in learning disorders (for a discussion see Thomas and Willems 1997).

Attention deficits can be seen in finger agnosia and in deficits in coding, digit span, and finger discrimination; and memory deficits can be seen in sentence memory and verbal-sequential memory (Willems et al. 1996).

THE 'ABRIDGED' NEURODEVELOPMENTAL EXAMINATION
From the 45 tests used in the full neurodevelopmental examination (in the 3-year phase of our study), we selected 23 items for inclusion in an abridged version, intended for use by school doctors or paediatricians in Belgium (Table 11.5):

- The non-verbal aspect of sequential organization can be evaluated by the finger-discrimination test, and its verbal aspect, by the tests of finger gnosis and of verbal-sequential memory.

- Short-term verbal memory is involved in the finger-gnosis and sentence-repetition tests, and short-term non-verbal memory is involved in the gesture-sequence (imitation of gestures) and Schilder arm-extension tests.

- The articulatory aspect of speech can be evaluated using the buccolinguofacial-praxis and tongue-protrusion tests, and the syntactic aspect of oral speech itself, using the sentence-repetition test.

- Tests of attention are the simultanagnosia test (for the physiological aspect of attention), the graphiaesthesia test (for its quality and duration), and tests of bimanual coordination such as crossing the midline and gesture imitation (for its gestural aspects).

- Visual perception can be tested using the Bender gestalt test (of constructional praxis) and the gesture-imitation and crossing-the-midline gestural tests.

- Manual laterality can be tested by the pencil-grip, finger-praxis, diadochokinesia, and Schilder arm-extension tests.

- In addition to the results of the conventional neurological examination (i.e. head circumference) the anamnesis should include information on the presence of epilepsy, headache, difficulties in falling asleep, disorders of attention and mental perseveration, and signs of mental fatigue.

- Minor neurological signs, the so-called soft signs, found in children with developmental dyspraxia and developmental clumsiness can be tested using the Prechtl test (Prechtl and Stemmer 1962) (for the choreoathetiform syndrome), finger-praxis test, fine-motor-coordination test, the test for dysdiadochokinesia, the

TABLE 11.5
Abridged neurodevelopmental examination that community paediatricians and school
doctors can give to children aged 5^1/$_2$ to 6^1/$_4$ years

Non-verbal
    Finger discrimination
    Graphiaesthesia (tactile recognition, skin writing, haptic perception)
    Simultanagnosia (two-point discrimination, double tactile stimulation, haptic perception)
    Gestural praxis (praxis + visual gnosia)
    Crossing midline of the body
    Arm-extension test (Schilder)
    Constructional praxis (visuopractic function)

Verbal
    Finger gnosis
    Verbal-sequential memory (sentences memory, syntactic structures, short-term memory (verbal))
    Phonological recognition
    Buccolinguofacial praxis (oromotor praxis)

Praxis
    Finger praxis (manual dexterity)
    Pencil grip

Neurology
    Diadochokinesia
    Head circumference
    Gross motor coordination (jumping on one foot, standing on one foot)
    Dysmorphic signs or stigmata
    Choreathetiform syndrome (Prechtl)

Complaints
    Headache, sleep problems (from the anamnesis)
    Abdominal pain, nausea

Behaviour
    Attention span, signs of mental fatigue, perseveration, slowness, comprehension, impulsivity
    Hyperactivity, hypoactivity, normal activity

Diseases
    Epilepsy, etc. (from the anamnesis)

(Translated and adapted from *Les troubles d'apprentissage scolaire, examen neuropédiatrique des fonctions d'apprentissage de l'enfant en âge préscolaire,* Willems G, Noël A, Evrard P, 1984, Paris, Doin.)

gesture-imitation test, the type of pencil grip, and tests of gross praxis (hopping on one foot) and balance (standing on one foot).

- Behaviour can be observed during the examination (cognitive slowness, presence of hyperactivity or hypoactivity, impulsive cognitive style) and documented by the anamnesis.
- From a paediatric point of view the examiner can look for strabismus, signs of facial dysmorphia, or a particular phenotype. Finally complaints of symptoms such as nausea or abdominal pains, and any diseases, may be recorded.

This version of the examination was evaluated in the 5-year, clinical phase of our study by administering it at the end of kindergarten to 2941 children aged 5^1/$_2$ to 6^1/$_4$ years). Each child was subsequently given academic achievement tests in reading and mathematics either 1, 3, or 5 years later, at the end of grade 1 ($n=1729$), 3 ($n=793$), or 5 ($n=419$); the

TABLE 11.6
Neuropsychological tests proposed by Korkman and Peltomaa for 6- to 7-year-olds

Auditory perception
 Auditory analysis of speech (phonemic awareness)
 Selective auditory attention
Visual perception
 Developmental test of visuomotor integration (visuomotor precision, visual precision, copying-skill)
Motor learning
 Developmental test of visuomotor integration (visuomotor precision, visual precision, copying-skill)
 Tactile finger discrimination
Short-term memory
 Storytelling (remembering of the story)
 Word span (repeat long series of words)
 Delayed recall of names (half an hour after the name-learning test)
Language
 Token test (receptive language functions)
 Naming tokens (name size 'colour and shape')
 Concepts of relativity (such as 'equally', 'many', 'forward')
Attention concentration
 Sustained concentration (stay on task)
 Selective auditory attention
Learning information processing
 Inhibition and control (measure of impulsive cognitive style)

(From Preventive treatment of dyslexia by a preschool training program for children with language impairments, Korkman M, Peltomaa AK, 1994, *Journal of Clinical Child Psychology* **22**: 277–87. Copyright © 1994 Lawrence Erlbaum Associates, Inc.)

TABLE 11.7
Neuropsychological tests proposed by Wilson for 5- to 6-year-olds

Auditory perception
 Auditory discrimination (discriminate like-sounding words in quiet and in noisy surroundings)
 Auditory cognition (ability to decode vocal language)
 Auditory–visual cognition (ability to process in both modalities)
Visual perception
 Visual discrimination (differences and similarities in visual stimuli)
 Visuospatial function (constructional abilities)
 Visual cognition (visual apprehension)
Motor learning
 Fine motor skills (eye–hand coordination, finger dexterity)
 Graphomotor skills (spontaneous or copying from representations)
 Praxis (imitation of a series of movements)
Short-term memory
 Auditory-sequential memory (memory for sentences)
 Short-term auditory memory (retell a story just heard)
 Visual-sequential memory (sequence of visual stimuli)
Attention concentration
 Auditory discrimination
 Effects of distracters on auditory discrimination (discriminate like-sounding words in quiet and in noisy surroundings)
Language
 Organization – formulation of language
 Word retrieval (verbal fluency)

(Based on findings in Wilson 1992.)

results were compared with their performance 1, 3, or 5 years before on the abridged paediatric neurodevelopmental examination. A diagnostic evaluation of this battery showed that it correctly classified 80% of the children who had a specific learning disorder in grade 3, with a specificity of 79% (see Table 11.3). The full neurodevelopmental examination yielded better results than the abridged version mainly because the latter was less extensive (taking 30 minutes rather than 3 hours) and the population studied included both boys and girls, irrespective of their social status. The abridged examination showed disturbance as early as $5^{1}/_{2}$ to $6^{1}/_{4}$ years in the children with learning disorders in comparison with the control group. Preliminary results were published by Loute and Willems (1992) and Willems et al. (1996).

The need for a comprehensive assessment of 5-year-old children

Some children have an unexpected specific difficulty in learning to read, write, or calculate, but we believe that such difficulties should rarely come as a surprise to teachers and parents: they are often preceded by 'markers', the vast majority of which could be identified if all children had a comprehensive paediatric examination at the end of kindergarten or on entry to school. Evidence of some of these can be obtained from the family history (e.g. of dyslexia) and the child's personal medical and developmental history (e.g. epilepsy, or otitis media with effusions) and especially delay in the onset of speech and language (Whitmore and Bax 1986). Evidence of other markers requires testing of certain key neurodevelopmental functions. The minutiae of any test battery may vary, but there is closer agreement as to functions that need testing (see Tables 11.1, 11.2, 11.6, and 11.7). Although by definition learning disorders are not specific if due to environmental factors, social and family circumstances need to be included in any assessment; they may still determine the severity of the difficulties in school (Hunt et al. 1988) and influence the development of compensatory skills.

REFERENCES

Badian NA. (1983) Developmental dysclaculia. In: Mykelbust HR, editor. *Progress in Learning Disabilities.* New York: Grune and Stratton.

Bax M, Whitmore K. (1973) Neurodevelopmental screening in the school entrant medical examination. *Lancet* **2:** 368–70.

—— (1987) The medical examination of children on entry to school. The results and use of neurodevelopmental assessment. *Developmental Medicine and Child Neurology* **29:** 40–55.

Beery DC, Buktenica N. (1967) *Developmental Test of Visual-Motor Integration.* Chicago: Follett.

Bender L. (1947). Childhood schizophrenia: clinical study of 100 schizophrenic children. *American Journal of Orthopsychiatry* **17:** 40.

— Yarnell H. (1941) An observation nursery. *American Journal of Psychiatry* **97:** 1158–72.

Benton A. (1985) Body schema disturbances: finger agnosia and right–left disorientation. In: Heilman KM, Valenstein E, editors. *Clinical Neuropsychology.* New York: Oxford University Press. p 115–23.

— Pearl D. (1978) *Dyslexia: An Appraisal of Current Knowledge.* New York: Oxford University Press.

Berninger VW, Rutberg J. (1992) Relationship of finger function to beginning writing: application to diagnosis of writing disabilities. *Developmental Medicine and Child Neurology* **34:** 198–215.

Bishop D. (1992) *Developmental Medicine and Child Neurology* **34:** 838–9. (Book review).

Boder E. (1973) Developmental dyslexia: a diagnostic approach based on three atypical reading-spelling patterns. *Developmental Medicine and Child Neurology* **15:** 663–87.

Bonboir A. (1969) *Test d'arithmétique. Ecole Primaire.* Commission Consultative Universitaire de Pédagogie. Ministère Belge de l'Education Nationale de la Culture. Louvain, Belgium: Laboratoire de Pédagogie Expérimentale, Université Catholique de Louvain.

Bowey JA. (1986) Syntactic awareness and verbal performance from preschool to fifth grade. *Journal of Psycholinguistic Research* **15**: 285–308.

Cantwell DP, Baker L. (1991) Association between attention deficit–hyperactivity disorders and learning disorders. *Journal of Learning Disabilities* **24**: 88–95.

Chevrie-Muller C, Simon AM, Decante P. (1981) *Epreuves pour l'examen du langage.* Paris: Centre de Psychologie Appliqué.

Cratty BJ. (1994) *Clumsy Child Syndromes: Descriptions, Evaluation and Remediation.* Chur [Switzerland]: Harwood Academic Publishers.

Critchley M. (1970) *The Dyslexic Child.* Springfield [IL]: Charles C Thomas.

Denckla MB. (1973) Development of speed in repetitive and successive finger-movements in normal children. *Developmental Medicine and Child Neurology* **15**: 635–45.

— (1974) Development of motor co-ordination in normal children. *Developmental Medicine and Child Neurology* **16**: 729–41.

— (1985) Revised neurological examination for subtle signs. *Psychopharmacology Bulletin* **4**: 773–800.

— Rudel RG. (1976) Rapid 'automatized' naming: dyslexia differentiated from other learning disabilites. *Neuropsychologia* **14**: 471–9.

Ellis NC, Large B. (1987) The development of reading: as you seek so shall you find. *British Journal of Psychology* **78**: 1–128.

Fletcher J, Taylor HG, Morris R, Satz P. (1982) Finger recognition skills and reading achievement: a develomental neuropsychological analysis. *Developmental Psychology* **18**: 124–32.

Frith U. (1997) Brain, mind and behaviour in dyslexia. In: Hulme C, Snowling M, editors. *Dyslexia, Cognition and Intervention.* London: Whurr Publishers. p 1–19.

Gaddes WH. (1980) *Learning Disabilities and Brain Function: A Neuropsychological Approach.* New York, Heidelberg, Berlin: Springer-Verlag.

— Edgell D. (1993) *Learning Disabilities and Brain Function.* 3rd ed. New York: Springer.

Gesell A, Amatruda CS. (1941) *Developmental Diagnosis.* London: Hoeber.

— Thompson H. (1934) *Infant Behaviour: Its Genesis and Growth.* New York: McGraw–Hill.

— Amatruda CS, Castner BM, Thompson H. (1930) *Biographies of Child Development.* London: Hamish Hamilton.

Gordon N, McKinlay I. (1980) *Helping Clumsy Children.* Edinburgh, London, New York: Churchill Livingstone.

Gubbay SS. (1975) *The Clumsy Child: A Study of Developmental Apraxia and Agnosic Ataxia.* London: Saunders.

Hadders-Algra M, Touwen BCL. (1992) Minor neurological dysfunction is more closely related to learning difficulties than to behavioural problems. *Journal of Learning Disabilities* **25**: 649–57.

— — Huisjes HJ. (1986) Neurologically deviant newborns: neurological and behavioural development at the age of six years. *Developmental Medicine and Child Neurology* **28**: 569–78.

— Huisjes HJ, Touwen BCL. (1988) Perinatal risk factors and minor neurological dysfunction: significance for behaviour and school achievement at nine years. *Developmental Medicine and Child Neurology* **30**: 482–91.

Henderson SE. (1987) The assessment of 'clumsy' children: old and new approaches. *Journal of Child Psychology and Psychiatry* **28**: 511–27.

Huisjes HJ, Touwen BC, Hoekstra J, et al. (1980) Obstetrical-neonatal neurological relationship. A replication study. *European Journal of Obstetrics, Gynaecology and Reproductive Biology* **10**: 247–56.

Hulme C, Lord R. (1986) Clumsy children - A review of recent research. *Child: Care, Health and Development* **12**: 257–69.

— Biggerstaff A, Moran G, McKinlay I. (1982) Visual, kinesthesic and cross-modal judgements of length by normal and clumsy children. *Developmental Medicine and Child Neurology* **24**: 461–71.

Hunt JV, Cooper BAB, Tooley WH. (1988). Very low birth weight infants at 8 and 11 years of age: role of neonatal illness and fmily status. *Pediatrics* **82**: 596–603.

Ingram TTS. (1969) Developmental disorders of speech. In: Vinken PJ, Bruin W, editors. *Handbook of Clinical Neurology, Volume 4.* Amsterdam: North-Holland. p 407.

Jansky J, de Hirsch K. (1972) *Preventing Reading Failure – Prediction, Diagnosis, Intervention.* New York: Harper and Row.

Johnston RB, Stark RE, Mellits ED, Tallal P. (1981) Neurological status of language-impaired and normal children. *Annals of Neurology* **10:** 159–63.

Jorn AF, Share DL, Matthews R, Maclean R. (1986) Behaviour problems in specific reading retarded and general reading backword children: a longitudinal study. *Journal of Child Psychology Psychiatry* **27:** 33–43.

Kamhi A, Catts UW. (1986) Toward an understanding of developmental language and reading disorders. *Journal of Speech and Hearing Disorders* **51:** 337–47.

Kaplan BJ, Wilson BN, Crawford SG. (1995) The genetic basis of clumsiness and its overlap with other disorders. In: Polatajko HP, Fox AM. *Final Report on the Conference: Children and Clumsiness: A Disability in Search of Definition. International Consensus Meeting.* London, Ontario. Not numbered.

Kinsbourne M, Warrington EK. (1963) The developmental Gerstmann syndrome. *Archives of Neurology* **8:** 490–501.

Korkman M, Peltomaa AK. (1994) Preventive treatment of dyslexia by a preschool training program for children with language impairments. *Journal of Clinical Child Psychology* **22:** 277–87.

Lecocq O. (1988) Conscience phonologique, mémoire de travail et acquisition de la lecture. In: *L'Orthophonie, ici... ailleurs... autrement: approches cognitivistes et pragmatiques.* Isbergues: ORTHO Edition. p 356–87.

Levine MD, Oberklaid F, Meltzer L. (1981) Developmental output failure: a study of low productivity in school-aged children. *Pediatrics* **67:** 18–25.

Lindgren SD. (1975) The early identification of children at risk for reading disabilities: finger localization ability, verbal skills, and perceptual-motor performance in kindergarten children. Unpublished master's thesis, University of Iowa.

Lord R, Hulme C. (1987) Perceptual judgements of normal and clumsy children. *Developmental Medicine and Child Neurology* **29:** 250–7.

Loute J, Willems G. (1992) The use of a neurodevelopmental examination at the end of kindergarten. European Meeting on Dyslexia, Louvain, Belgium, 16 October 1992. *Bulletin of School Medicine, University of Louvain*, No. 15, December 1992. p 40–8.

Lyon GR. (1995) Research initiatives in learning disabilities: contributions from scientists supported by the National Institute of Child Health and Human Development. *Journal of Child Neurology* **10:** S120–6.

Mann VA, Liberman IY. (1984) Phonological awareness and verbal short-term memory. *Journal of Learning Disabilities* **17:** 592–8.

McKinlay I. (1987) Children with motor learning difficulties: not so much a syndrome - more a way of life. *Physiotherapy* **73:** 635–8.

Milles TR, Haslum MN. (1986) Dyslexia: anomaly or normal variation. *Annals of Dyslexia* **36:** 103–17.

Noterdaeme H, Amorosa H, Ploog M, Scheimann G. (1988) Quantitative and qualitative aspects of associated movements in children with specific developmental speech and language disorders and in normal pre-school children. *Journal of Human Movement Studies* **15:** 151–69.

O'Hare AE, Brown JK, Aitken K. (1991) Dyscalculia in children. *Developmental Medicine and Child Neurology* **33:** 356–61. (Annotation).

Pennington BF. (1991) *Diagnosing Learning Disorders: A Neuropsychological Framework.* Lawrence Erlbaum, Hove (Eds), London, New York: Guilford Press.

Powell RP, Bishop DVM. (1992) Clumsiness and perceptual problems in children with specific language impairment. *Developmental Medicine and Child Neurology* **34:** 755–65.

Prechtl HRF, Stemmer CJ. (1962) The choreiform syndrome in children. *Developmental Medicine and Child Neurology* **4:** 119–27.

Rapin I, Segalowitz SJ. (1992) *Handbook of Neuropsychology.* Amsterdam: Elsevier.

Rasmussen P, Gillberg C, Waldenström E, Svenson B. (1983) Perceptual, motor and attentional deficits in seven-year-old children: neurological and neurodevelopmental aspects. *Developmental Medicine and Child Neurology* **25:** 315–33.

Rourke BP. (1993) Arithmetic disabilities specific and otherwise: a neuropsychological perspective. *Journal of Leaning Disabilites* **26:** 214–26.

Rutter M. (1978) Prevalence and types of dyslexia. In: Benton AL, Pearl D, editors. *Dyslexia. An Appraisal of Current Knowledge.* London, New York: Oxford University Press. p 3–28.

Satz P, Morris R. (1981) Learning disability subtypes: a review. In: Pirrozolo F, Wittrock J, editors. *Neuropsychological and Cognitive Processes in Reading.* New York: Academic Press.

— Friel J, Rudegeair F. (1974) Differential changes in the acquisition of developmental skills in children who later became dyslexic. In: Stein DG, Rosen JJ, Butters N, editors. *Plasticity and Recovery of Function in the Central Nervous System.* New York: Academic Press. p. 175–202

Shaffer D. (1985) Brain damage. In: Rutter M, Hersov L, editors. *Child and Adolescent Psychiatry: Modern Approaches.* Oxford: Blackwell Scientific. p 123–51.

— O'Connor PA, Shaffer SQ, Prupis S. (1985) Neurological 'soft' signs. In: Rutter M, editor. *Developmental Neuropsychiatry.* New York: Guilford. p 114–64.

Shalev R, Manor O, Amir N, Gross-Tsur V. (1993) The acquisition of arithmetic in normal children: assessment by a cognitive model of dyscalculia. *Developmental Medicine and Child Neurology* 35: 593–601.

Siegel LS. (1989) IQ is irrelevent to the definition of learning disabilities. *Journal of Learning Disabilities* 22: 469–86.

Silver AA, Hagin RA. (1975) *Search: A Scanning Instrument for the Identification of Potential Learning Disability. Experimental Edition.* New York: New York University Medical Center.

— — (1990). *Disorders of Learning in Childhood.* New York: John Wiley and Sons.

Simon J. (1954) *Psychopedagogie de l'orthographe.* Paris: Ed. P.U.F.

Spreen O, Risser AT, Edgell D. (1995) *Developmental Neuropsychology.* Oxford: Oxford University Press.

Stanovich KE, Siegel LS, Gottardo A. (1997) Progress in the search for dyslexia sub-types. In: Hulme C, Snowling M, editors. *Dyslexia: Biology, Cognition and Intervention.* London: Whurr Publishers.

Stark RE, Tallal P. (1981) Perceptual and motor deficits in language impaired children. In: Keith RW, editor. *Central Auditory and Language Disorders in Children.* San Diego: College-Hill Press.

Strauss AA, Lehtinen LE. (1947) *The Psychopathology and Education of the Brain-Injured Child.* Volume 1. New York: Grune and Stratton.

Thomas J, Willems G. (1997) *Troubles de l'attention, impulsivité et hyperactivité chez l'enfant: approche neurocognitive. [Attention Deficit, Impulsivity and Hyperactivity in Children: Neurocognitive Approach.]* Paris: Masson. (In French).

Tiegs EW, Clark WK. (1967) *California Reading Test.* Monterey [CA]: California Test Bureau (Division McGraw-Hill Book Company).

Touwen BCL. (1979) *Examination of the Child with Minor Neurological Dysfunction.* 2nd ed. Clinics in Developmental Medicine No. 71. London: Spastics International Medical Publications / William Heinemann Medical Books; Philadelphia: JB Lippincott Co.

Tunmer WE, Nesdale AR, Wright AD. (1987) Syntactic awareness and reading acquisition. *British Journal of Developmental Psychology* 5: 25–34.

Whitmore K, Bax MCO. (1986) The school entry medical examination. *Archives of Disease in Childhood* 61: 807–17.

Willems G, Berte-Depuydt R, de Leval N, et al. (1984a) A neuropediatric and neuropsychological prospective study of learning disorders: a three-year follow-up. In: Bloomingdale LM, editor. *Attention Deficit Disorder: Diagnostic, Cognitive, and Therapeutic Understanding, Volume 5.* Jamaica [NY]: Spectrum Publications. p. 73–118.

— Noël A, Evrard P. (1984b) *Les troubles d'apprentissage scolaire, examen neuropédiatrique des fonctions d'apprentissage de l'enfant en âge préscolaire. [Learning Disabilities: Neuropediatric examination of the Learning Functions of Preschool-aged Children.]* Paris: Doin. (In French).

— — — et al. (1986) Models of neuropediatric prediction of learning disability: neuropediatric and neuropsychological prospective study of learning disorders. In: *Child Development and Learning Behaviour.* Stuttgart, New York: Gustav Fischer Verlag. p 191–201.

— de Leval N, Bouckaert A, et al. (1996) Persistency of neurodevelopmental problems (attention and memory deficits) in children with high risk for learning disorders (a six year follow-up study). In: *Neuropsychology of Children with Learning Disorders.* Anae. Paris: PDG Communication. 37: 54–61.

Wilson BC. (1992) The neuropsychological assessment of the preschool child: a branching model. In: Rapin I, Segalowitz SJ, editors. *Handbook of Neuropsychology. Volume 6, Child Neuropsychology.* Amsterdam: Elsevier. p. 377–99.

Wolf M. (1986) Rapid alternating stimulus naming in the developmental dyslexias. *Brain and Language* 27: 360–79.

— Goodglass H. (1986) Dyslexia, dysnomia and lexical retrieval: a longitudinal investigation. *Brain and Language* 28: 154–68.

— Bally H, Morris R. (1986) Automaticity, retrieval processes and reading: in average and impaired readers. *Child Development* 57: 988–1000.

Wolff PH, Gunnoe CE, Cohen C. (1983) Associated movements as a measure of developmental age. *Developmental Medicine and Child Neurology* 25: 417–29.

— — — (1985) Neuromotor maturation and psychological performance: a developmental study. *Developmental Medicine and Child Neurology* 27: 344–54.

12
IMAGING IN LEARNING DISORDERS

Peter Born and Hans C Lou

Little is known about the aetiology and pathogenesis of learning disorders in childhood. A variety of sophisticated, recently developed imaging techniques are helping to elucidate these by shedding new light on brain physiology and pathology. With regard to learning disorders these techniques are at present used only in the context of research, where some of the insights gained may have implications for patient management.

This chapter provides a brief introduction to the main imaging techniques that have been used to study learning disorders in children and summarizes the findings so far.

The techniques
SINGLE PHOTON EMISSION COMPUTED TOMOGRAPHY
Single photon emission computed tomography (SPECT), in use since the late 1970s, utilizes the detection of single photons emitted from tracers such as ^{133}Xe and ^{99m}Tc hexamethyl-propyleneamineoxime (HMPAO) by scintillation detectors surrounding the head. SPECT is a comparatively inexpensive tomographic imaging technique. The half-life of the tracers used is long enough to obviate the need for a nearby cyclotron. SPECT allows the absolute, three-dimensional, quantitative determination of regional cerebral blood flow (rCBF) by inhalation of ^{133}Xe. The method is convenient for use in children, because it is non-invasive and repeated measurements can be taken in one session. The radiation dose is relatively small: when administered at 10mCi/l for one minute of rebreathing, lung doses of 0.001 to 0.002Gy and total body doses of the order of 0.0001Gy may be expected (Goddard and Ackery 1975). One drawback of the ^{133}Xe technique is the relatively poor spatial resolution, approximately 12mm.

^{99m}Tc HMPAO gives better spatial resolution (approximately 9mm) but usually does not allow repeated measurements in one session, gives only relative values of rCBF, and requires venipuncture. This tracer gets trapped in the brain after injection, and imaging can be performed as the tracer decays. This means that it can be injected in an awake child, who is later sedated for imaging or during a clinical event such as a seizure.

SPECT is also potentially very useful for neuroreceptor studies, using, for example, ^{123}I-labelled epidepride, a tracer with affinity for dopaminergic receptors.

POSITRON EMISSION TOMOGRAPHY
Positron emission tomography (PET), like SPECT, has also been used in humans since the late 1970s. In PET, substances labelled with a positron-emitting isotope are introduced into the body by intravenous injection or inhalation, and the signal is then collected by external

detectors. The commonly used isotopes are ^{11}C, ^{13}N, ^{15}O, and ^{18}F. Because these isotopes have short half-lives (for example 2 minutes for ^{15}O-labelled water), a cyclotron is usually needed at the PET site to generate the labelled molecules. One of the most widely used PET techniques is the determination of the local cerebral metabolic rate for glucose with ^{18}F-labelled deoxyglucose (Sokoloff et al. 1977). This technique has been used to elucidate the functional development of the brain in infants and young children (Chugani et al. 1987). Because among these commonly used isotopes ^{18}F has a relatively long half-life (109 min), studies of activation related to particular tasks are difficult to perform with this method, and most studies of the local cerebral metabolic rate for glucose are of the resting rate. PET has provided task-related measurements of absolute and relative cerebral blood flow by use of the tracer $H_2^{15}O$ (Fox et al. 1988). This tracer makes it possible to acquire 8 to 12 scans, under various conditions, in one session; subsequent statistical analysis makes it possible to depict the task-related brain activation. The technique has recently been used to study a wide variety of neurological and neuropsychological problems. PET gives somewhat better spatial resolution than SPECT and, like SPECT, makes it possible to perform receptor studies. For these, labelled ligands binding to, for example, opiates, benzodiazepine, serotonin, and dopamine have been produced. A wide variety of molecules, such as neurotransmitters or pharmacological agents, can be labelled, and the possible applications are numerous. Only radionuclide techniques can detect the minute concentrations of labelled ligands bound to receptors. PET and SPECT have a promising future in this field.

Drawbacks of PET include the high cost of tracers and equipment and the relatively high radiation exposure (e.g. 0.003 Gy for measurement of the local cerebral metabolic rate for glucose [Chugani et al. 1987]), which has limited its use in children and young adults.

MAGNETIC RESONANCE IMAGING

The first successful nuclear magnetic resonance (NMR) experiment was performed in 1946, and over the next three decades the technique was used in chemical spectroscopy. In the 1970s the discovery that NMR signals could be rendered spatially dependent made it possible to generate images, and since then magnetic resonance has undergone a stunning development. With NMR it is now possible not only to create high-resolution images of tissue, but also to assess a variety of physiological parameters.

For an MR experiment the tissue of interest is placed in a static magnetic field. In clinical whole-body scanners this field is typically of the magnitude of 0.5 to 1.5 tesla. In such a magnetic field, the nuclei will perform a precessing movement, whose frequency depends on the type of the nucleus and the strength of the magnetic field. The NMR of various nuclei, such as those of ^{31}P, ^{23}Na, ^{13}C, and ^{1}H, can be measured. Because ^{1}H, being present in water, is numerically preponderant in biological systems, it is currently the only nucleus used for MRI in clinical settings. For the magnetic resonance experiment the nuclei in the magnetic field have to be excited at their specific precession frequency, also called the Larmor frequency, by a radiofrequency (RF) pulse of precisely this frequency. On return to the resting state the nuclei emit the absorbed energy: the returned energy depends strongly on the surrounding tissue. The RF pulse is transmitted and received by coils, which should be close to the part of the body that is being examined. In neuroimaging, the coil is usually helmet-shaped and surrounds the head. Images can be created by periodically superimposing the field gradient, which can be rapidly altered. This field gradient causes the nuclei to precess at slightly different frequencies, depending on their position. Imaging is performed using a series of RF pulses and field gradient changes; these series are called sequences and can give different types of contrast, depending on the tissue of interest.

If performed according to the existing guidelines, NMR imaging (or 'MRI') is free of known adverse biological effects. Consequently, healthy individuals can also be examined, making MRI especially attractive as a tool for examining a population of developing individuals. Children are sometimes frightened by the narrow, deep bore of the magnet, and by the considerable noise generated during some imaging sequences. Therefore children less than about 5 to 7 years of age usually require sedation during the examination. Claustrophobic reactions can be avoided by the use of wide-bore or open scanners, which are now commercially available. Scanner noise will probably be reduced considerably in future generations of scanners.

Morphometric MRI

Since MRI now makes it possible to obtain anatomical information that could previously be obtained only by autopsy, a new interest has arisen in measuring the sizes of various brain regions in normal and abnormal development. With the technical development of MRI, the possibilities for morphometric acquisitions have been refined. While earlier studies used time-consuming and relatively coarse conventional two-dimensional acquisitions, a complete three-dimensional data set of the brain with a voxel size of $1\,mm^3$ can now be obtained in less than 15 minutes. Automatic and semi-automatic procedures have been developed for segmenting the brain into different regions and tissue classes. As described below, a number of studies have been performed on populations with learning disorders, with sometimes conflicting results. The many different methodological approaches used make direct comparison of studies difficult. Filipek (1996) has published an excellent review of the application of morphometric MRI to the study of learning disorders.

Functional MRI

The blood-oxygen-level-dependent (BOLD) change in the magnetic properties of haemoglobin was first described by Ogawa et al. (1990). This effect was exploited to provide an MRI method of demonstrating brain activation (Kwong et al. 1992). This method, functional MRI (fMRI), has developed rapidly. As in PET, the basis for signal generation is the physiological uncoupling of cerebral blood flow (CBF) and metabolism during brain activation (Fox and Raichle 1986). During brain activation CBF increases, with a concomitant decrease of the overall concentration of deoxyhaemoglobin per voxel (Kwong 1995). The result is that in an MRI system using, say, 1.5T the MRI signal rises by about 4 to 6% during brain activation on visual stimulation with, for example, an alternating chequerboard pattern. A change in the BOLD signal depends not only on CBF, but also on several other parameters, such as oxygen consumption, cerebral blood volume, and haematocrit. The exact nature of the change in the BOLD signal is at present still subject to intense research, but comparisons of findings from

PET and fMRI show good agreement between the two methods (Ramsey et al. 1996, Small et al. 1996). Although attempts are under way to quantify CBF in fMRI (Kim 1995, Kwong et al. 1995), most fMRI experiments at present are performed using *relative* signal change. As the relative BOLD signal change is similar to the noise level, to improve statistical significance several cycles of rest and activation are usually performed while images are being continuously obtained. Whereas early fMRI studies performed measurements on only a few selected slices, modern MRI systems equipped with spiral or echoplanar imaging capability can acquire images covering the whole brain in 3 to 4 seconds. Temporal resolution in fMRI is limited by the haemodynamic response, which is maximal after 4 to 8 seconds.

Only a few fMRI studies in children have been performed, and there are a number of questions to be answered before the full potential of the technique can be exploited. A more diffuse activation pattern seen in 9- to 11-year-old children than in adults during a language task (Hertz-Pannier et al. 1995) was attributed to ongoing synaptic pruning in the children. In infants under the age of 3 years diffuse light stimulation causes a *decrease* of the BOLD signal, in contrast to the increase usually seen in adults (Born et al. 1996).

ELECTROPHYSIOLOGICAL IMAGING

The general purpose of brain imaging is threefold: (1) to gain insight into normal neurophysiological functions, including states such as sleep and wakefulness and tasks such as cognitive functions, (2) to explore the plasticity of the central nervous system, for example changes with age or changes after injury, and (3) to understand the pathophysiology of diseases afflicting the central nervous system.

For each of these purposes EEG, the oldest of the imaging modalities treated in this chapter, has a distinct advantage over the newer ones such as SPECT, PET, and fMRI, in that it registers neuronal events in real time at a resolution of 10^{-4} seconds. Other advantages are its much lower cost, the fact that EEG can be performed on ambulatory subjects in a natural setting, and its non-invasive nature.

EEG has, however, two major drawbacks: (1) the spatial resolution, although often underestimated, is comparatively poor, being of the order of a few centimetres, and (2) EEG does not offer true three-dimensional analysis of brain physiology, being essentially limited to the neocortex.

The origin of the EEG signal recorded at the scalp is largely the graded postsynaptic potentials of the cell bodies and large dendrites of vertically oriented pyramidal cells in cortical layers III to V. These postsynaptic potentials are of lower voltage than action potentials, but they last much longer and involve a large area of the cellular membranes, facilitating their conductance to the scalp. At the scalp level most of the recordable signals originate from the vicinity of the electrode, although in exceptional cases large signals originating from a distance may affect the recording. The amplitude usually is a few microvolts to about 75, and the frequency varies from a few hertz to 20 or 30, increasing with the degree of the individual's wakefulness and alertness. The EEG is conventionally described as patterns of activity in four frequency bands, delta (<4Hz), theta (4 to 8Hz), alpha (8 to 12Hz), and beta (>12Hz). The postsynaptic potentials, and hence the EEG, are thought to be synchronized by rhythmic discharges from the thalami.

Normative developmental equations have been calculated within the above frequency bands. Mapping with colour scales has improved visual identification of abnormalities, allowing, for instance, mild cognitive impairment to be ascertained by an increasing presence of theta activity (John et al. 1988). A word of caution has been raised by Duffy (1989), who stressed the need for solid normative databases, the existence of marked intrapersonal variations with time, and the susceptibility to artifacts. In his opinion, and ours, the qualitative electrophysiological methods can never be diagnostic. At most they may be indices of 'organicity'. However, this indication in itself may be helpful in the management of learning disabilities.

The spatial resolution is, as mentioned, poorer than that of the newer imaging methods based upon emission tomography. However, attempts at improving the spatial resolution have been fruitful. One way is to increase the number of electrodes from the usual 16 to 64 or even more, especially for experimental purposes, with the aim of sequencing mental operations. For instance Posner and coworkers at the University of Oregon used a geodesic sensor net of 64 electrodes to examine event-related potentials recorded from the scalp while the subjects looked at words or consonant strings (Posner and Raichle 1994). Event-related potentials, that is, potentials elicited by a stimulus, can be seen by averaging multiple stimulation experiments, so that the spontaneous EEG signals disappear, leaving the event-related signals intact. Posner and Raichle found pronounced asymmetry 100ms after a visual stimulus, with large potentials in the posterior right hemisphere. This finding is consistent with findings in PET experiments demonstrating activation in the right occipital lobe by visual features. The timing of the EEG measurements suggested that the PET image consistent with such activation appears about 100ms after the stimulus. Fifty milliseconds later (150ms after the stimulus), focal EEG activation was detected over the posterior sites in the *left* hemisphere – but only if the stimulus was interpretable as a word: if it was a nonsense string of consonants, no left hemisphere activation was seen on the EEG. Again the EEG signal in this area corresponded to a PET focus of increased activity. It was therefore evident that the two foci of activity seen in PET, one in the right occipital lobe and the other in the anterior left occipital lobe near the midline, appeared not simultaneously, but rather in a sequence, in the right focus at 100ms after the stimulus for visual detection, and in the left focus at 150ms for word operation. This experiment illustrates how the spatial resolution of PET can be fruitfully combined with the temporal resolution of the EEG. An example of an integration of PET and EEG during a word-generation task in adults is given in Figure 12.1.

Even when many electrodes are used, one problem is inherent in the spatial resolution of the EEG: the heterogeneous electrical conduction in the widely heterogeneous tissues of the skull and scalp. One way of circumventing this heterogeneity is to use magnetoencephalography (MEG) to measure the magnetic field associated with the brain's electrical activity; this field is uniformly circular around the dipole. However, there are major problems with this approach. One is the high cost and sensitivity to external noise. Another is the fact that MEG is primarily sensitive to dipoles oriented tangentially to the surface of the brain, whereas most cortical dipoles are radially organized because of

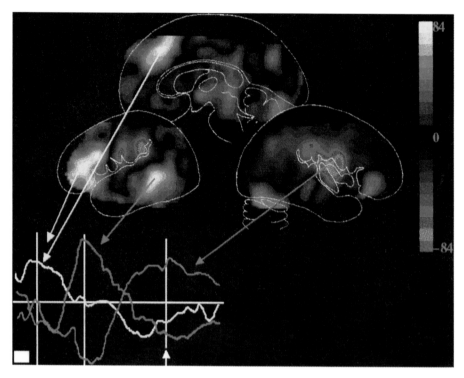

Fig. 12.1. Example of a combination of PET and event-related potential (ERP).

Both PET and ERP data sets represent response differences between reading aloud a visually presented noun (reading-aloud task) and saying aloud an appropriate use for the same nouns (use-generation task). PET images show cortical areas of blood flow changes depicted by subtracting the ERP for the reading-aloud task from that for the use-generation task. The colour coding represents positive (yellow/red) and negative (blue/green) flow changes. The upper image was obtained 1mm from the midline, and the lower left and lower right images were obtained from the left and right hemispheres, respectively. There is a prominent flow increase in the anterior cingulate and frontal and temporal cortex of the left hemisphere and a bilateral flow decrease in the sylvian–insular region. ERP wave recordings from the nearest electrodes for these regions are presented, showing the difference in response patterns.

(From Snyder AZ, Abdullaev YG, Posner MI, Raichle ME, 1995, Scalp electrical potentials reflect regional cerebral blood flow responses during processing of written words. *Proceedings of the National Academy of Sciences of the USA* **92**: 1689–93. Copyright 1995 National Academy of Sciences, USA.)

the columnar organization of cortical neurons. It therefore remains to be seen how useful MEG will prove to be. In the meantime, improvement in the mathematical models of EEG signal processing is a realistic expectation.

Imaging in specific learning disorders
ATTENTION-DEFICIT/HYPERACTIVITY DISORDER (ADHD)

Findings from the available imaging studies suggest that the striatum plays a key role in the pathogenesis of ADHD. Such findings can be interpreted as expressions of a dysfunctional frontostriatal loop. In a ^{133}Xe SPECT study of a group of children with ADHD alone or with ADHD plus dysphasia, the striatal region was found to be hypoperfused (see also Fig. 12.2), whereas the primary sensory and sensorimotor areas were relatively hyperperfused (Lou et al. 1989). The central, low-flow area was found to be larger in the children who had ADHD plus dysphasia. Methylphenidate, a central stimulant used for treatment of ADHD, increased flow in the central regions and less conspicuously decreased flow in the cortical areas.

A number of morphometric MRI studies have been performed in populations with ADHD. Of all global indices, the volume of the right hemispheric white matter was found to be reduced (Semrud Clikeman et al. 1994). The asymmetry (left>right) of the caudate nucleus in control subjects has been found to be reversed in individuals with ADHD (Hynd et al. 1993), while other workers have report symmetrical caudate volumes in patients with ADHD but the same asymmetry just mentioned (left>right) in controls (Castellanos et al. 1994). While the total callosal volume seems to be normal in ADHD, various workers have reported anomalies of various areas of the corpus callosum: genu and splenium (Hynd et al. 1991), rostrum and rostral body (Giedd et al. 1994), and splenium (Semrud Clikeman et al. 1994). Semrud Clikeman and colleagues found the smallest callosal size in patients whose condition did not respond to stimulants. These studies are difficult to compare, as different methodologies were used to measure the callosal area.

The demonstration of striatal dysfunction in ADHD as the prime pathophysiological fact has, in retrospect, provided a breakthrough in the understanding of a number of behavioural aberrations: obsessive–compulsive disorder, Tourette syndrome, and even Parkinson's disease, Huntington's chorea, and schizophrenia. These conditions are all examples of behavioural disturbances of frontostriatothalamic circuits, or loops. However, the exact delineation of one condition from another is not yet possible.

AUTISM

A number of PET studies using ^{18}F-labelled deoxyglucose in subjects with autism have shown either no significant differences from control subjects (De Volder et al. 1987, Herold et al. 1988, Heh et al. 1989) or regional abnormalities of glucose metabolism in the subjects with autism (Buchsbaum et al. 1992). Regional abnormalites of flow distribution in temporal and parietal lobes were noted in a SPECT study using [99m]TC HMPAO (Mountz et al. 1995). Horwitz et al. (1988) found a lower positive correlation of the local cerebral metabolic rate for glucose between different brain regions in subjects with autism than in a control group in a PET study. These authors hypothesized that there was a functionally impaired interaction between frontal and parietal regions, and between neostriatum and thalamus.

A number of morphometric MRI studies point towards cerebellar anomaly in autism, but reports about the involved cerebellar structures vary. There is some evidence for involvement of the cerebellar vermis (for a review see Filipek 1995a), and somewhat less evidence for involvement of the cerebellar hemispheres (Gaffney et al. 1987) and the brainstem (Hashimoto et al. 1995).

In early morphometric studies using CT, a reversal of the normal asymmetry of the parietooccipital region was reported (Hier et al. 1979). Later studies have not confirmed this finding and have been inconclusive about the involvement of the cerebral hemispheres and hemispheric substructures.

DYSLEXIA

Neurophysiological abnormalities in both hemispheres of patients with dyslexia were first detected by a combination of EEG and evoked potentials (Duffy et al. 1980). In adults with dyslexia, metabolic activity in the inferior occipital (lingual) regions during reading was found to be higher than that in controls (Duara et al. 1991). Asymmetry of the inferior occipital regions was leftward (i.e. left>right) in controls but rightward in patients with dyslexia. During reading of single words, abnormalities of function of areas of visual association and of frontal association were found. This finding was supported by an fMRI study in which adults with dyslexia showed abnormal function of motion processing (Eden et al. 1996). Conflicting results were reported in a ^{133}Xe SPECT study of adults with developmental dyslexia, in which an increased hemispheric asymmetry (left>right) was found (Rumsey et al. 1987). In both studies, frontal lobe activity was found to be deficient. Involvement of the insular lobe in adults with dyslexia was confirmed by the finding of an increased local cerebral metabolic rate for glucose in a PET study of reading (Gross Glenn et al. 1991); the increase could be due to a reduction in the size of the insular lobe (Hynd et al. 1990).

The perisylvian regions, particularly on the left, have been in focus in much of the earlier pathoanatomical studies of dyslexia. Recently such studies have been carried out using imaging techniques. Rumsey et al. (1992) found that individuals with dyslexia fail to activate the left temporoparietal cortex during a rhyming task, and Paulesu et al. (1996) found evidence from PET studies that Broca's area and the left temporoparietal cortex do not operate in concert in such individuals and suggested that developmental dyslexia is a disconnection syndrome (see also Chapter 3).

Various morphometric MRI studies have shown that the posterior perisylvian region is in some way abnormal in patients with dyslexia (Jernigan et al. 1991, Plante et al. 1991) and their parents and siblings (Plante 1991). The size of the corpus callosum has been measured as an indicator for interhemispheric connection (Duara et al. 1991). There have been varying reports about the involvement of the planum temporale: studies have differed in methodology and are difficult to compare (Filipek 1995b).

DYSPHASIA

Using ^{133}Xe SPECT, four groups of children (aged 7 to 15 years) plus controls were studied (Lou et al. 1990) (Fig. 12.2): children with phonologic–syntactic dysphasia plus ADHD, or with pure ADHD, or with verbal auditory agnosia, or (not shown in the figure) with phonologic–syntactic dysphasia alone. In the children with phonologic–syntactic dysphasia (either alone or with ADHD as well), flow to the left prefrontal region was lower than that to the right (not shown in the figure). In the children with pure ADHD, flow to the two prefrontal regions was symmetrical. In the children with verbal auditory agnosia, flow was lower in the left central perisylvian region than in the right. Similar observations of reduced

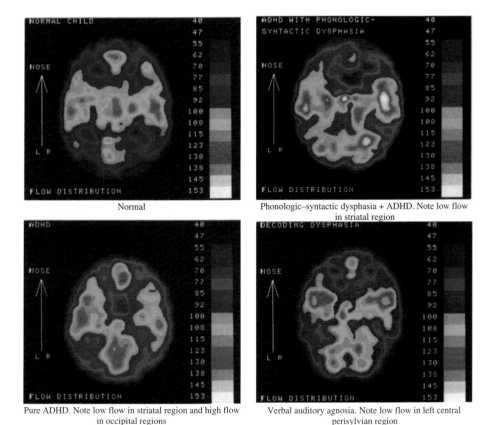

Fig. 12.2. Regional cerebral blood flow seen in SPECT.

Images from (left to right, top to bottom) a normal 12-year-old boy, a boy with ADHD and phonologic–syntactic deficit, a girl with ADHD, and a boy with verbal auditory agnosia.

(From Lou HC, Henriksen L, Bruhn P, 1990, Focal cerebral dysfunction in developmental learning disabilities. *Lancet* **335** (Jan 6 1990): 8–11. © by The Lancet Ltd. 1990.)

activation in the left hemisphere were made in another ^{133}Xe SPECT study of children with dysphasia, using a simple auditory task (Tzourio et al. 1994). The notion of disturbed interhemispheric collaboration in dysphasia is also supported by the finding of a thicker corpus callosum in children with familial dysphasia or dyslexia by morphometric MRI (Filipek 1995b), possibly as a result of faulty axonal elimination. In another morphometric study on children with various language impairments (Jernigan et al. 1991), reduction of volume in the left posterior perisylvian region, right diencephalon, and caudate nucleus was found.

GILLES DE LA TOURETTE SYNDROME

A number of imaging studies have been performed in patients with this condition. In an ^{18}F-labelled deoxyglucose PET study in 18 drug-free adult patients, increased metabolic activity was found in orbitofrontal cortices, related to associated behavioural features. A similar finding, though less robust, was made regarding the insula and putamen (Braun et al. 1995).

Conclusion

As advanced imaging techniques have become more accessible and more suitable for the study of populations of individuals as they develop, imaging studies to shed new light on the pathophysiology of learning disorders are increasingly being undertaken. In this chapter we concentrate on the techniques that at present are most used and most useful for this purpose.

Learning disorders can arise from a variety of generalized conditions (e.g. neurofibromatosis, lead poisoning) or from localized conditions (e.g. intracerebral haemorrhage, hypoxic–ischaemic encephalopathy) in the central nervous system. MRI alone can detect a variety of organic causes of learning disorders. The therapist evaluating a patient who presents with a learning disorder faces the challenge of rapidly diagnosing any underlying condition. This diagnosis can provide clues important for patient management and, maybe more importantly, prognostic information for the individual patient.

In recent years NMR scanners have become more accessible, and MRI even in young children has become routine in many centres. We think that all patients presenting with a learning disorder serious enough to disrupt everyday functioning should be referred for a cerebral structural MRI examination, particularly if the history or general physical examination gives clues of a generalized or localized neurological condition. The MRI examination should be combined with a full EEG to detect any subclinical seizure activity. At present other imaging studies are indicated only rarely. For example if epileptic foci are suspected on the EEG, SPECT can be used to detect areas of interictal hypoperfusion. It is, however, to be foreseen that in the future, functional imaging methods may be used to identify inter- and intraindividual variability.

Most of the other techniques mentioned in this chapter cannot yet provide useful information about the individual patient, but as new knowledge arises from ongoing research the role of imaging may well evolve, and the more advanced techniques discussed here may become an integral part of patient management.

REFERENCES

Born P, Rostrup E, Leth H, et al. (1996) Change of visually induced cortical activation patterns during development. *Lancet* **347**: 543. (Letter).

Braun AR, Randolph C, Stoetter B, et al. (1995) The functional neuroanatomy of Tourette's syndrome: an FDG-PET Study. II: Relationships between regional cerebral metabolism and associated behavioral and cognitive features of the illness. *Neuropsychopharmacology* **13**: 151–68.

Buchsbaum MS, Siegel BV Jr, Wu JC, et al. (1992) Brief report: attention performance in autism and regional brain metabolic rate assessed by positron emission tomography. *Journal of Autism and Developmental Disorders* **22**: 115–25.

Castellanos FX, Giedd JN, Eckburg P, et al. (1994) Quantitative morphology of the caudate nucleus in attention deficit hyperactivity disorder. *American Journal of Psychiatry* **151**: 1791–6.

Chugani HT, Phelps ME, Mazziotta JC. (1987) Positron emission tomography study of human brain functional development. *Annals of Neurology* **22**: 487–97.

De Volder A, Bol A, Michel C, et al. (1987) Brain glucose metabolism in children with the autistic syndrome: positron tomography analysis. *Brain and Development* **9**: 581–7.

Duara R, Kushch A, Gross Glenn K, et al. (1991) Neuroanatomic differences between dyslexic and normal readers on magnetic resonance imaging scans. *Archives of Neurololgy* **48**: 410–6.

Duffy FH. (1989) Clinical value of topographic mapping and quantified neurophysiology. *Archives of Neurology* **46**: 1133–4.

— Denckla MB, Bartels PH, et al. (1980) Dyslexia: automated diagnosis by computerized classification of brain electrical acticity. *Annals of Neurology* **7**: 421–8.

Eden GF, VanMeter JW, Rumsey JM, et al. (1996) Abnormal processing of visual motion in dyslexia revealed by functional brain imaging. *Nature* **382**: 66–9.

Filipek PA. (1995a) Quantitative magnetic resonance imaging in autism: the cerebellar vermis. *Current Opinion in Neurology* **8**: 134–8.

— (1995b) Neurobiologic correlates of developmental dyslexia: how do dyslexics' brains differ from normal readers? *Journal of Child Neurology* **10** (Suppl 1): S62–9.

— (1996) Structural variations in measures in the developmental disorders. In: Thatcher RW, Reid Lyon G, Rumsey JM, Krasnegor N, editors. *Developmental Neuroimaging.* San Diego, London: Academic Press.

Fox PT, Raichle ME. (1986) Focal physiological uncoupling of cerebral blood flow and oxidative metabolism during somatosensory stimulation in human subjects. *Proceedings of the National Acadademy of Sciences of the USA* **83**: 1140–4.

— Mintun MA, Reiman EM, Raichle ME. (1988) Enhanced detection of focal brain responses using inter-subject averaging and change-distribution analysis of subtracted PET images. *Journal of Cerebral Blood Flow and Metabolism* **8**: 642–53.

Gaffney GR, Tsai LY, Kuperman S, Minchin S. (1987) Cerebellar structure in autism. *American Journal of Diseases in Childhood* **141**: 1330–2.

Giedd JN, Castellanos FX, Casey BJ, et al. (1994) Quantitative morphology of the corpus callosum in attention deficit hyperactivity disorder. *American Journal of Psychiatry* **151**: 665–9.

Goddard BA, Ackery DM. (1975) Xenon-133, ^{127}Xe, and ^{125}Xe for lung function investigations: a dosimetric comparison. *Journal of Nuclear Medicine* **16**: 780–6.

Gross Glenn K, Duara R, Barker WW, et al. (1991) Positron emission tomographic studies during serial word-reading by normal and dyslexic adults. *Journal of Clinical and Experimental Neuropsychology* **13**: 531–44.

Hashimoto T, Tayama M, Murakawa K, et al. (1995) Development of the brainstem and cerebellum in autistic patients. *Journal of Autism and Developmental Disorders* **25**: 1–18.

Heh CW, Smith R, Wu J, et al. (1989) Positron emission tomography of the cerebellum in autism. *American Journal of Psychiatry* **146**: 242–5.

Herold S, Frackowiak RS, Le Couteur A, et al. (1988) Cerebral blood flow and metabolism of oxygen and glucose in young autistic adults. *Psychol Med* **18**: 823–31.

Hertz-Pannier L, Gaillard WD, Mott S, et al. (1995) Functional MRI of language tasks: frontal diffuse activation pattern in children. *Human Brain Mapping* (Suppl 1): 231. (Abstract).

Hier DB, LeMay M, Rosenberger PB. (1979) Autism and unfavorable left–right asymmetries of the brain. *Journal of Autism and Developmental Disorders* **9**: 153–9.

Horwitz B, Rumsey JM, Grady CL, Rapoport SI. (1988) The cerebral metabolic landscape in autism. Intercorrelations of regional glucose utilization. *Archives of Neurology* **45**: 749–55.

Hynd GW, Semrud Clikeman M, Lorys AR, et al. (1990) Brain morphology in developmental dyslexia and attention deficit disorder/hyperactivity. *Archives of Neurology* **47**: 919–26.

— — — et al. (1991) Corpus callosum morphology in attention deficit–hyperactivity disorder: morphometric analysis of MRI. *Journal of Learning Disabilities* **24**: 141–6.

— Hern KL, Novey ES, et al. (1993) Attention deficit–hyperactivity disorder and asymmetry of the caudate nucleus. *Journal of Child Neurology* **8**: 339–47.

Jernigan TL, Hesselink JR, Sowell E, Tallal PA. (1991) Cerebral structure on magnetic resonance imaging in language- and learning-impaired children. *Archives of Neurology* **48**: 539–45.

John ER, Prichep LS, Fridman J, Easton P. (1988) Neurometrics: computer-assisted differential diagnosis of brain dysfunctions. *Science* **239**: 162–9.

Kim SG. (1995) Quantification of relative cerebral blood flow change by flow-sensitive alternating inversion recovery (FAIR) technique: application to functional mapping. *Magnetic Resonance in Medicine* **34**: 293–301.

257

Kwong KK. (1995) Functional magnetic resonance imaging with echo planar imaging. *Magnetic Resonance Quarterly* **11:** 1–20.

— Belliveau JW, Chesler DA, et al. (1992) Dynamic magnetic resonance imaging of human brain activity during primary sensory stimulation. *Proceedings of the National Academy of Sciences of the USA* **89:** 5675–9.

— Chesler DA, Weisskoff RM, et al. (1995) MR perfusion studies with T1-weighted echo planar imaging. *Magnetic Resonance in Medicine* **34:** 878–87.

Lou HC, Henriksen L, Bruhn P, et al. (1989) Striatal dysfunction in attention deficit and hyperkinetic disorder. *Archives of Neurology* **46:** 48–52.

— — — (1990) Focal cerebral dysfunction in developmental learning disabilities. *Lancet* **335:** 8–11.

Mountz JM, Tolbert LC, Lill DW, et al. (1995) Functional deficits in autistic disorder: characterization by technetium-99m-HMPAO and SPECT. *Journal of Nuclear Medicine* **36:** 1156–62.

Ogawa S, Lee TM, Kay AR, Tank DW. (1990) Brain magnetic resonance imaging with contrast dependent on blood oxygenation. *Proceedings of the National Academy of Sciences of the USA* **87:** 9868–72.

Paulesu E, Frith U, Snowling M, et al. (1996) Is developmental dyslexia a disconnection syndrome? Evidence from PET scanning. *Brain* **119:** 143–57.

Plante E. (1991) MRI findings in the parents and siblings of specifically language-impaired boys. *Brain and Language* **41:** 67–80.

— Swisher L, Vance R, Rapcsak S. (1991) MRI findings in boys with specific language impairment. *Brain and Language* **41:** 52–66.

Posner MI, Raichle ME. (1994) *Images of Mind.* New York: Scientific American Library.

Ramsey NF, Kirkby BS, Van Gelderen P, et al. (1996) Functional mapping of human sensorimotor cortex with 3D BOLD fMRI correlates highly with $H_2{}^{15}O$ PET rCBF. *Journal of Cerebral Blood Flow and Metabolism* **16:** 755–64.

Rumsey JM, Berman KF, Denckla MB, et al. (1987) Regional cerebral blood flow in severe developmental dyslexia. *Archives of Neurology* **44:** 1144–50.

— Andreason P, Zametkin AJ, et al. (1992) Failure to activate the left temporoparietal cortex in dyslexia. An oxygen 15 positron emission tomographic study. *Archives of Neurology* **49:** 527–34. Erratum published in *Archives of Neurology* (1994) **51:** 243.

Semrud Clikeman M, Filipek PA, Biederman J, et al. (1994) Attention-deficit hyperactivity disorder: magnetic resonance imaging morphometric analysis of the corpus callosum. *Journal of the American Academy of Child and Adolescent Psychiatry* **33:** 875–81.

Small SL, Noll DC, Perfetti CA, et al. (1996) Localizing the lexicon for reading aloud: replication of a PET study using fMRI. *Neuroreport* **7:** 961–5.

Sokoloff L, Reivich M, Kennedy C, et al. (1977) The [^{14}C]deoxyglucose method for the measurement of local cerebral glucose utilization: theory, procedure, and normal values in the conscious and anesthetized albino rat. *Journal of Neurochemistry* **28:** 897–916.

Tzourio N, Heim A, Zilbovicius M, et al. (1994) Abnormal regional CBF response in left hemisphere of dysphasic children during a language task. *Pediatric Neurology* **10:** 20–6.

13
PREVENTING AND MANAGING SPECIFIC LEARNING DIFFICULTIES IN THE CLASSROOM

Sonia Sharp

There are many ways in which teachers can prevent and manage learning difficulties. With the current emphasis on 'effective schooling' this has become a well-researched subject and this chapter aims to provide an overview of some of the established knowledge in this area. First, it may be worth considering the definition of learning difficulty and special educational need from an educational perspective. While a child or young person may have a specific impairment, this only creates a special educational need if it restricts access to the curriculum. A commonly cited example is visual impairment: many of us have a visual impairment that is corrected by wearing glasses or contact lenses, which is therefore not a disability and does not result in special educational need. Another example would be the student who uses a wheelchair. In a school with narrow doorways and many steps, access to the learning environment will be hampered and therefore the child will have a significant special educational need. In a school designed for wheelchair use, the child will have total access to learning opportunities and will have no special educational need. In educational terms, 'disability', 'special educational need', and 'learning difficulty' are defined by the match (or mismatch) between the needs of the individual student and what is being offered by the school. The educational perspective on learning difficulty is therefore ecological – a learning difficulty usually arises though a complex interaction between a number of factors, all of which have to be considered when designing an appropriate curriculum and learning environment for the individual student.

Attitude towards learning

Effective teaching is very much about what goes on in the classroom. Although this will largely depend on the approach of the teacher, his or her practice is likely to be shaped by the values and attitudes pervading the school. In 1996, the National Commission on Education reported a study of 11 schools in the UK that were successful despite significant disadvantages. The commission noted that these schools that were 'successful against the odds' had a clear philosophy about education shared by all staff. The philosophy was often an inclusive and optimistic one such as 'all children can succeed' (Maden and Hillman 1996). This kind of philosophy implies that success in learning is related to effort rather than ability and has been recognized as an important feature in positive motivation of students (Dweck 1986).

Promoting the relation between effort and successful learning is particularly important for students who experience specific learning difficulties. It is extremely likely that these students will have to invest more effort in learning and spend more time practising new skills than their peers. It is also likely that there will be other students in the class who have achieved competence in the very skill the student with learning difficulties is struggling with. It can sometimes seem as though the other students have acquired those skills with ease, although they too will have invested effort (perhaps not so much) in learning. The student who is finding the task or skill difficult to achieve can lose confidence, possibly becoming enmeshed in the 'failure cycle' (Westwood 1993). As the student loses confidence, they increasingly avoid tasks that involve the skill they are finding difficult. Consequently they minimize practice and therefore do not develop the skill. Their continued failure leads to further loss of confidence, self-esteem, and motivation. A similar failure cycle can be established when a student is encouraged to believe that they will not be able to learn a skill because of their specific difficulty. The student who experiences a specific literacy difficulty can begin to believe it is not worth investing effort in reading or writing. Of course, without practice there will be little improvement.

By explicitly linking success with effort and practice, teachers can encourage students who are experiencing difficulties to persist and to gain satisfaction from challenge. Prevention and management of learning difficulty needs to start with the expectation that every student will learn successfully if given the appropriate opportunities. Successful teaching is about discovering how this process can be facilitated.

Understanding learning

To be able to teach effectively, it is essential to understand how children learn. This relates not only to the learning process but also to the emotional state of the learner. There are four possible learning states that we progress through as we learn (Fig. 13.1). At first we are in a state of unconscious incompetence – we do not know that we do not know. Once we start learning, we become aware that we do not know something: we are 'consciously incompetent'. As we learn successfully, we still have to think about what we are doing and remind ourselves of how to do it successfully – in other words we are 'consciously competent'. Finally, as the skill or knowledge becomes automatic, we reach the state of 'unconscious competence'. If we spend too long in the state of conscious incompetence, our self-esteem falls. One key task of the teacher of a student experiencing learning difficulties is to minimize the amount of time spent in this state and to remind the student of the areas in which they have achieved unconscious competence.

Behavioural psychologists have described learning a new skill as a hierarchical process, in which the first stage is acquiring accuracy – this may be in recognizing letter shapes and linking them with sounds; learning the rules of addition; learning how to tie a shoelace. Once the student has become accurate in the skill, they can then practice and become fluent. Fluency helps learning to become more automatic and therefore less conscious. Automaticity is important in skills such as reading, as it enables the reader to concentrate on meaning. The skill is maintained through continued practice. Eventually the student is able to generalize the skill to novel situations, at first with direction and later independently. The theory underpinning this hierarchy is that until students have acquired accuracy and fluency they will not be able to retain the skill or apply or adapt it. Students who experience a specific

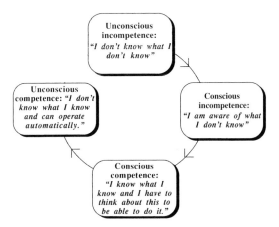

Fig. 13.1. States of learning.
(Source not known, but attributed to R Dubin.)

learning difficulty may need to work harder to acquire accuracy and fluency than their peers. Sometimes a student's failure to retain a skill over time is attributed to memory or learning problems when in fact accuracy and fluency were not established. To be able to generalize a new skill or knowledge the student needs to have developed good understanding. Marton and Saljo (1976) divided learning into 'surface' and 'deep' approaches. Surface approaches aim to increase knowledge, memorize information, or acquire facts or procedures. Deep approaches involve thinking about and questioning the information or skill and using it to change either pre-existing beliefs or ideas, or future action. The first three stages of the learning hierarchy (accuracy, fluency, and automaticity) require only surface approaches to learning, although learning at these stages will be more effective if deeper approaches are used. The final stages (generalization and adaptation) depend on the student's using deep approaches so that they are learning through understanding. Some educational researchers and cognitive psychologists would argue that real learning takes place only at this level. Edwards and Furlong (1978) analysed teacher–student talk about learning. They concluded that learning is not 'transmitted' from teacher to student. Learning occurs through a process of the student interpreting the teacher's meaning and making links between what the student already knows. We can help students to use deep approaches by structuring learning to include reflection, questioning, and adaptation of pre-existing knowledge. This can be achieved by encouraging the student to ask themselves at the outset questions such as, 'What do I know already about this subject?' and 'What do I want/need to know?' At the end of the task or activity, they can ask themselves, 'What have I learned about this subject?' or, 'Is anything I've learned surprising or unexpected?'

Learning is not a passive process. Watkins et al. (1996) noted that effective learners are active and strategic in the learning process. They can develop goals and understand their own learning. Self-management and self-regulation are both key features of successful learning. Self-management relates to the student's ability to work independently. It involves being able to organize materials and get ready to begin a task; knowing how to ask for help or to check work for errors; and being able to handle the usual school-day routines. Westwood

(1993), in a study comparing the progress of students with learning difficulties who were well integrated into the mainstream classroom with those who were not, found that well-integrated students were more skilled in self-management, were more aware of classroom routines, and spent more time 'on task'. Teachers can break down classroom routines into steps and teach these to students using mnemonics or provide picture prompt sheets for them to refer to. This is particularly important for students who experience specific learning difficulties, many of whom have a tendency to be disorganized.

Self-regulation relates to the student's ability to monitor and control his or her own thinking processes while engaged in a learning task. Successful learners are aware of a number of learning strategies and can select the most appropriate approach for the task. For example, if the task involves holding a piece of information in working memory, they will employ rehearsal strategies to assist them with this. If the information is too complex to do this through simple verbal or subverbal rehearsal, they may chunk or group the information, organize the information in some way, or make the information meaningful through linking it to existing knowledge. To be able to select the appropriate strategy they will have made a series of statements to themselves or asked themselves a series of questions relating to:

- problem identification (e.g. What do I have to do?)
- focusing attention (e.g. Which is the most important bit?)
- goal-setting and self-evaluation against the goal (e.g. I will work out what the first bit of this word says first . . . good, I've done that, what next?)
- error-correction strategies (e.g. I think I've made a mistake here . . . I will go back to the beginning and check.)

Paris et al. (1983) found that successful learners have three sorts of knowledge about thinking and learning strategies. They not only know which strategy to use, they also know how and when to use a strategy. Successful learners also often employ a more reflective approach to learning. Impulsive approaches are less effective (Walker 1985) and lead the student to make decisions too quickly, often increasing errors made. Teaching impulsive students strategies for self-management and self-regulation can help them to become more reflective and increase their success. Kluwe (1987) identified four metacognitive strategies essential for school-based learning:

- classification: identification of the nature of the learning activity;
- checking: determining progress while engaged in the learning activity;
- evaluation: making judgements about the quality of progress made;
- prediction: identifying alternative approaches for problem solving and their outcomes.

These four activities have been developed for specific areas of learning such as reading and mathematics. For example, Palinscar and Brown (1984) have identified four strategic approaches for improving reading comprehension: summarizing, questioning, clarifying, and predicting. The reader summarizes the content of the story or text and then asks questions about an important point in the text. The reader also clarifies any difficult parts of the text and then predicts what will happen next. This approach is particularly successful when introduced through an approach called 'reciprocal teaching'. The teacher and students read the passage to themselves initially. Then the teacher acts as an expert model, explaining and demonstrating the strategies first. The students then read another passage and this time they each demonstrate the strategies to their peers. Palinscar and Brown found that on average the students in their study made a 15-month gain in reading comprehension after only 3 months' teaching. A similar approach to improving reading comprehension is the 'PQRS' method: preview, question, read, and summarize. By 'previewing', the reader scans the passage to be read, attending to headings and diagrams to gain an overall impression of what the text is about. The reader can then ask himself or herself, 'What do I know about this already?' The reader then generates questions to help focus attention and guide the reading. While reading the passage the reader asks questions that check progress in relation to the reading goal, such as, 'Do I need to backtrack a bit here?' or, 'Is this answering my question?' Finally the reader summarizes what they have understood or learned through reading the text. Essentially, in all of these approaches the students are being taught to hold a dialogue with themselves that guides thinking and learning. Teachers can model 'thinking aloud' for students and can encourage them to think aloud for themselves.

Understanding teaching

There have been many well-documented studies on effective teaching, particularly in the USA, the UK, and the Netherlands (e.g. Brookover et al. 1979; Galton et al. 1980; Bennett et al. 1984; Hallinger and Murphy 1987; Mortimore et al. 1988; Levine and Lezotte 1990; Alexander 1991; Scheerens 1992). Collectively these studies support a model of successful teaching that include substantial time on task; intellectual challenge achieved through asking higher-order questions; good planning and clear structure; curriculum and teaching style matched to students' needs. It seems that there is not a particular teaching style that is more successful than others, but rather that successful teachers are those that achieve the above through applying a diverse range of approaches according to the situation.

Udvari-Solner and Thousand (1995) investigated effective practice in teaching students with learning disabilities in mainstream classrooms. As well as effective practice, they also identified barriers to effective practice. They found four common barriers: (1) reliance on familiar teaching approaches and limited adaptation of teaching style to accommodate the needs of the student; (2) overuse of parallel activities for the student that did not relate in any way to the activities the rest of the class were engaged in; (3) reliance on use of one-to-one support in the classroom to adapt the material or to assist the student; (4) dependence on one professional to meet the child's needs rather than a 'team' approach. Those authors found that effective teachers asked themselves a series of questions while planning how to deliver the curriculum. These included:

- What can the student do without any adaptation?
- Can the student's participation be increased by changing:
    the teaching arrangements?
    the lesson format?
    the teaching style?
    the classroom environment or lesson location?
    the instructional materials?

- Will the student need different goals?
- Will the student need personal assistance? If so, how can this be provided to maximize independent, active learning?
- Will the student need an alternative activity for him/herself and a small group of peers?

These questions aid successful differentiation and prevent some common problems such as low expectation of the student, lessening of the student's independence, and isolation of the student from peers. The case study on the next page illustrates an example of classroom practice taken from observation in a classroom of a secondary comprehensive school (that is, a school catering for children of all abilities), where the teacher was able to achieve successful learning outcomes for students with a range of difficulties as well as for their peers.

Teaching students with specific learning difficulties

The approaches we have considered so far are effective for students who experience a wide range of learning difficulties, including the specific learning difficulties discussed in this book. They provide a sound base upon which other more individually focused strategies can be introduced. The remainder of this chapter describes some teaching approaches that are helpful for students with specific learning difficulties.

FOCUSING ON THE INDIVIDUAL

Students who experience the specific learning difficulties discussed in this book may be able to engage in many of the more sophisticated and challenging aspects of the curriculum at a conceptual level but have great difficulty in independently recording their own thoughts, researching through reading, carrying out an activity involving fine motor skills, or focusing attention so as to complete a task successfully. This can be extremely frustrating for the student and can lead to additional behavioural problems in the classroom setting. When addressing individual need, the teacher not only has to design programmes to assist the individual students in developing those skill areas in which they experience difficulty but also find ways of engaging the individual students in activities that are sufficiently challenging while minimizing frustration. This is the artistry of teaching!

ADDRESSING THE DIFFICULTY

As mentioned earlier in this chapter, students develop skills only if they practice them regularly. Students who experience specific difficulties may unfortunately find that their opportunities to practice are reduced either if the teacher provides alternative approaches all or most of the time or if the student finds ways of avoiding tasks that involve the skill area in which they experience most difficulty. Opportunities to develop and practice regularly are essential to progress. Of course practice sessions must also be carefully structured for success so that the student is motivated to keep on practising. Lingard (1997) evaluated a programme to accelerate the development of literacy in students of secondary-school age who could read and write only poorly. The programme included intensive, daily involvement in meaningful reading and writing activities, individually and supported by an adult. This was supplemented by systematic teaching of phonology and spelling and by individual

Case study of successful secondary school classroom

- The room was prepared for the first activity to assist with organization.
- The students were welcomed into the room and settled down.
- Goals for the lesson were clearly stated.
- Activities were started and stopped clearly.
- Instructions were given in clear, short sentences and were repeated.
- Students were shown as well as told what to do.
- Additional individual instruction was provided for some students.
- Each task was carefully structured and sequenced.
- For some students tasks were broken down into the smallest steps – even down to how to hold a pencil appropriately.
- Some students were given guided practice either by the teacher or by a peer.
- The teacher asked questions that prompted correct responses.
- Students were given sufficient time to formulate a response.
- Activities were structured to require a high level of student involvement and discussion.
- Student performance was continually monitored and the teacher asked questions that encouraged the students to monitor their own performance in terms of learning and behaviour.
- Feedback was given on academic progress, including comments on thinking and learning.
- Throughout the lesson students were praised and encouraged.
- The teacher overtly linked progress with effort and practice.
- Sufficient time was given to clear materials away before the end of the lesson.
- The end of the lesson was marked by calm reflection on goals achieved.

help with written composition. The programme was delivered to groups of students during the timetabled lessons for English. The school deployed a combination of teachers, ancillary assistants, and older student volunteers to provide the individual support. The average reading age (yr.mo) of the students increased from 9.1 to 11.10 and spelling from 8.3 to 9.5 during the 9-month programme.

The area of learning in which students with specific learning difficulties most often experience difficulties is the development of literacy. Unfortunately much of the school curriculum is delivered through and dependent upon the use of reading and writing. Consequently if the curriculum is not managed appropriately, the student who experiences literacy difficulties is likely to be disabled for a significant proportion of the daily timetable. Learning to read and write are complex tasks for anyone. Literacy demands a combination of physiological, cognitive, and contextual processes such as visual and auditory perception, controlled eye and hand movement, memory, sequencing, comprehension, general knowledge, and specific knowledge about text and language. Students who experience specific learning difficulties often have some impairment hindering one or more of the processes necessary to facilitate literacy development. Literacy learning combines three central areas: meaning, phonics, and fluency (Reason and Boote 1994). Reason and Boote's model of literacy learning is presented in Figure 13.2. They emphasize that the three areas have a multiplying effect on each other as well as the potential for compensation from one area for limited knowledge or skill in another. Teachers need to address all three areas in a way that enables reading and writing activities to complement each other. Reason and Boote's (1994) practical

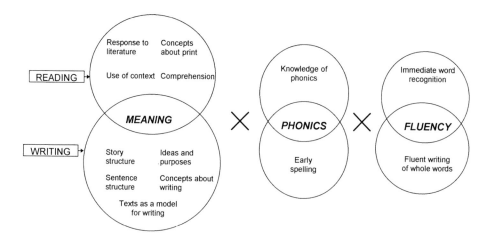

Fig. 13.2. A model of literacy learning. (Redrawn from Reason R, Boote R, 1994, *Helping Children with Reading and Spelling: A Special Needs Manual,* London, Routledge, with permisson.)

manual, *Helping Children with Reading and Spelling: A Special Needs Manual,* is a useful resource for concerned teachers and parents, including detailed strategies for each of the three areas.

Many approaches for teaching children and young people with specific learning difficulties are based upon use of the various sensory channels to assist learning – visual, auditory, and tactile. These approaches are usually called 'multisensory' (e.g. Fernald 1988) and typically involve the student looking at, tracing over, and saying out loud a word or letter to be learned. The student then writes the word or letter, checks it, and repeats the process until accuracy is achieved.

Building phonological skill and phonemic awareness is another important component of the development of literacy (Stanovich et al. 1984; Bryant and Bradley 1985). Phonological awareness is a cognitive component that governs sensitivity to segmentation of sounds and to the ordering, processing, and production of speech sounds. Lack of phonological awareness has now been identified as a significant factor in dyslexia (Frith 1995). Training in phonological awareness involves using phonemes, syllables, and particularly onset (initial sounds/sound clusters) and rime (final sound clusters) to develop an understanding of how words are constructed in speech and text. For example a student might be given the sound -all and asked to generate a list of five words with the same rime, such as *ball, fall, small, tall, wall.* Alternatively the child would be asked to generate a list of words with the same onset but different rimes, e.g. *shell, shawl, shocking.* Glass (1973) recognized that this kind of training enables youngsters to learn how letters cluster together within whole words and then to recognize clusters rather than individual letters.

DIFFERENTIATION

In addition to frequent direct teaching and plentiful practice to address specific areas of difficulty, differentiated approaches that enable the student to engage in classroom activities independently are needed. Lessons and tasks can be differentiated in a range of ways: by adapting instructional style, materials used, the nature of the task, the amount of time available, the goals set, etc. For example, a student who is very disorganized may need a checklist of equipment needed to enable them to organize themselves for a task. Another student who experiences difficulty writing fluently may benefit from being able to record their answers on a dictating machine, use a multiple-choice activity in which they select the appropriate answer, or draw pictures to illustrate their responses. A student who is slow in articulating verbal utterances could be allowed extra time to do so. A student who reads poorly could be introduced to technical vocabulary within the text prior to the lesson, so that during the lesson they can concentrate on meaning rather than on decoding. Differentiating tasks and lessons is essential for encouraging independent learning and for boosting student self-esteem.

SUPPORTING LEARNING

Adult and peer support for the student experiencing learning difficulties can be very beneficial but must be approached carefully. To provide a small amount of direct, individual teaching daily can be very effective if it is organized to demonstrate and instruct the student on specific objectives and is followed up by plentiful guided and independent practice. This can be provided by different people: the teacher, an ancillary assistant, a peer, a parent, a volunteer helper. If there is more than one adult working in the classroom, it will be necessary to define roles and tasks. Usually one person will be needed as 'general manager' to keep an overall view of classroom activity and to help regulate and organize student activity while the other spends time on specific activities or tasks with individual or small groups of students. The teacher and adult helper can take either role. Time spent on planning who will do what is essential if this support is to be used to maximum advantage. Situations in which the adult helper sits next to the student and 'translates' the curriculum for the student, or even completes work for them, can hinder learning and encourage dependence.

Tutoring by peers, either of the same age or older, can be beneficial for both parties (Cole and Chan 1990; Slavin 1991). The peer tutor can help the student to learn, practise, or review a skill. The peer can act as a model and guide for the target student, demonstrating appropriate learning behaviour and strategies as well as support in relation to the task or skill. Through this process the tutor also gains by consolidating his or her knowledge of the skill being taught or practised. Using students with specific learning difficulties as a peer tutor for younger students can help them to consolidate their own knowledge as well as boosting self-esteem.

DIRECT INSTRUCTION

Direct-instruction approaches (sometimes called structured teaching) have been found to be effective in enabling students to achieve accuracy and fluency (Scheerens 1992). Direct instruction involves setting clear goals and objectives that are phrased to specify what the student will be able to do in observable behaviours when she or he has acquired the skill. Lessons are then very carefully structured and rapidly paced so that the student achieves small manageable steps and overlearns so the skill becomes automatic. The teaching offers detailed explanation with many examples, along with plentiful active practice opportunities.

Students are given immediate feedback and correction, and student progress is continually monitored. The following step-by-step approach (often called 'task analysis') is applied in relation to each learning objective:

1 The learning objectives are stated in terms of student performance.
2 The skills to be learned are analysed in terms of specific tasks.
3 Each task is analysed to identify the actual steps and subskills involved. Prerequisite skills and knowledge are also identified.
4 All the component skills and knowledge are ordered in a logical teaching sequence.
5 The teacher determines which of the skills the student can already perform.
6 The teacher teaches, in a sequential order, the next step.
7 At each step student progress is evaluated in terms of the extent to which the student has learned the skill.

USING IT TO SUPPORT LEARNING

Computer-assisted learning provides opportunities for self-pacing, sequenced learning, and immediate feedback. It can be interactive and highly motivating for students, providing the right balance of challenge and success. Developments in hardware and software mean that the potential for teaching and supporting students through computerized packages is rich and varied, and there are now programmes targeted at students with specific learning difficulties (Day 1993). By the provision of a highly stimulating environment, students can be encouraged to practice and overlearn without becoming bored and demotivated. The quality of work produced can also be enhanced by allowing drafting and redrafting, and by introducing prompts and support strategies such as lists of key words, personalized dictionaries, and visual icons. Students with difficulties of motor coordination can have their work typed in for them, allowing them to concentrate on working on it rather than having to spend all their time on the mechanics of writing it down themselves. As schools adopt new technology such as voice-activated computers, students who experience specific difficulties are going to be more easily provided for within day-to-day teaching.

Summary

The teaching approaches that work for students who experience specific learning difficulties also work for many other students. The strategies used by successful students can be taught to less successful ones. Successful teaching and learning strategies are based upon a positive attitude towards learning and a belief that effort leads to success. They require lessons and tasks that are structured to enable the student to succeed, encourage the student's active involvement, and provide opportunities to model and practise new skills, and they require teaching about how to think and learn. In addition, students with specific learning difficulties need individual educational programmes that set explicit goals for addressing their educational needs. These are achieved by regular, focused teaching and plentiful opportunities for guided and independent practice. Lessons throughout the curriculum are appropriately differentiated so that the student can engage in the broad range of learning activities both independently and with support. Full use is made of information technology to support and extend learning.

REFERENCES

Alexander RJ. (1991) *Primary Education in Leeds: Twelfth and Final Report from the Primary Needs Independent Evaluation Project.* Leeds: University of Leeds.

Bennett SN, Deforges C, with Cockburn A, Wilkinson B. (1984) *The Quality of Pupils' Learning Experiences.* Hove: Lawrence Erlbaum.

Brookover W, Beady C, et al. (1979) *School Social Systems and Student Achievement: Schools Can Make a Difference.* New York: Praeger.

Bryant P, Bradley L. (1985) *Children's Reading Problems.* Oxford: Basil Blackwell.

Cole P, Chan L. (1990) *Methods and Strategies for Special Education.* New York: Prentice Hall.

Day J. (1993) *A Software Guide for Specific Learning Difficulties.* Coventry: National Council for Educational Technology.

Dweck C. (1986) Motivational processes affecting learning. *American Psychologist* **41:** 1040–8.

Edwards A, Furlong VJ. (1978) *The Language of Teaching.* London: Heinemann Educational.

Fernald G. (1988) *Remedial Techniques in Basic School Subjects.* Austin, TX: Pro-Ed. (Originally published in 1944).

Frith U. (1995) Dyslexia – can we have a shared theoretical framework? *Educational and Child Psychology* **12:** 6–17.

Galton M, Simon B, Croll P. (1980) *Inside the Primary Classroom.* London: Routledge.

Glass G. (1973) *Teaching Decoding as Separate from Reading.* Garden City, NY: Easier to Learn.

Hallinger P, Murphy J. (1987) The social context of effective schools. *American Journal of Education* **94:** 328–55.

Kluwe R. (1987) Executive decisions and regulation of problem solving behaviour. In: Weinert F, Kluwe R, editors. *Metacognition, Motivation and Understanding.* Hilldale, NJ: Lawrence Erlbaum.

Levine D, Lezotte L. (1990) *Unusually Effective Schools: A Review and Analysis of Research and Practice.* Madison [WI]: NCESRD Publications.

Lingard T. (1997) Literacy acceleration: an effective strategy for low-attaining secondary aged students. *Educational Psychology in Practice* **12:** 240–9.

Maden M, Hillman J. (1996) Lessons in success. In: National Commission on Education. *Success Against the Odds: Effective Schools in Disadvantaged Areas.* London: Routledge.

Marton F, Saljo R. (1976) On qualitative differences in learning: outcome and process. *British Journal of Educational Psychology* **46:** 4–11.

Mortimore P, Sammons P, Stoll L, et al. (1988) *School Matters: the Junior Years.* London: Open Books.

National Commission on Education. (1996) *Success Against the Odds: Effective Schools in Disadvantaged Areas.* London: Routledge.

Palinscar A, Brown A. (1984) Reciprocal teaching of comprehension-fostering and comprehension-monitoring activities. *Cognition and Instruction* **1:** 117–25.

Paris P, Lipson MY, Wixson KK. (1983) Becoming a strategic reader. *Contemporary Educational Psychology* **8:** 293–316.

Reason R, Boote R. (1994) *Helping Children with Reading and Spelling: A Special Needs Manual.* London: Routledge.

Scheerens J. (1992) *Effective Schooling: Theory, Research and Practice.* London: Cassell.

Slavin R. (1991) *Educational Psychology.* Englewood Cliffs, NJ: Prentice-Hall.

Stanovich KE, Cunningham AE, Feeman DJ. (1984) Intelligence, cognitive skills and early reading process. *Reading Research Quarterly* **14:** 278–303.

Udvari-Solner A, Thousand J. (1995) Effective organisational, instructional and curricular practices in inclusive schools and practices. In: Clark C, Dyson A, Millward A, editors. *Towards Inclusive Schools?* London: David Fulton.

Walker N. (1985) Impulsivity in learning disabled children: past research findings and methodological inconsistencies. *Learning Disabilities Quarterly* **8:** 85–94.

Watkins C, Carnell E, Lodge C, Whalley C. (1996) *Effective Learning.* Research Matters (5). London: Institute of Education.

Westwood P. (1993) *Common-Sense Methods for Children with Special Educational Needs.* London: Routledge.

14
MANAGEMENT OF BEHAVIOURAL PROBLEMS IN SPECIFIC LEARNING DISORDERS

Christopher Gillberg

The word *treatment* has a ring to it that invokes hope for a cure, or at least for major positive effects on the causative mechanisms or diseases underlying impairments. In the great majority of specific learning disorders, however, no treatment can be expected to produce such effects, either on the learning deficits as such or on the associated behavioural problems. It is therefore more appropriate to speak of 'intervention' when thinking about management or 'what to do' in the field of specific learning disorders.

Almost all the specific learning disorders are disabling chronic or subchronic conditions. At present, cure is possible only in exceptional cases, and most interventions should be undertaken to improve the situation of the individual and the family rather than to treat the underlying condition.

This chapter provides guidelines for dealing with behavioural problems in specific learning disorders. It emphasizes the role of a psychoeducational approach, driven by the conviction that usually the people with the problems, not the experts without the problems, are the ones most likely to be able to deal with them. In order to be able to do something about the problems, those afflicted – and relatives, friends, and teachers who regularly interact with them – need to have the best available knowledge and understanding of the nature of the problems. Diagnosticians (who need to be completely up to date in the field), support groups of various kinds (including parent and child groups), and teachers all need to work with the family, having the common goal of accepting that the child has a disorder and that adjustments of many different types will have to be made in order to minimize problems of psychosocial adaptation. Behaviour-modification programmes and pharmacotherapy may have to be used in certain instances but should not be accepted as the mainstay of intervention.

Diagnosis, work-up, and information

Making a diagnosis, taking a history, examining the child, performing an adequate work-up, and providing information about the disorder are essential elements of intervention in all disorders involving behavioural problems. This first step in the habilitation process is rarely acknowledged as perhaps the most important feature of intervention. Statements such as 'Why make a diagnosis when there is no specific treatment?' are testimony to the failure on occasion of even well-educated developmental paediatricians and child psychiatrists to appreciate the positive impact of skilful diagnosis and of information.

Information about the diagnosis and results of work-up should be as honest and detailed as possible, taking into account the specific needs of the individual and the family. The child needs information as well as the parents.

INFORMING THE CHILD

The child should be given specific information, depending on the child's age, about the diagnosis ('what is it called?'), usually with one or both parents present, though at times it may be necessary also to see the child alone. It is important to use the 'right' words, so that parents and children can use those words when communicating with each other about the nature of the disorder and about what needs to be done about it. It is too common for parents, even parents of a teenager, to feel uncertain about whether or not one should speak 'in front of the child' about such matters as dyslexia, attention-deficit/hyperactivity disorder (ADHD), and Asperger syndrome. Many parents and professionals appear to believe that one should wait for the child's 'coming of age' before one can begin to speak openly about matters to do with diagnosis. There is, instead, every reason to start speaking about the name and nature of the child's condition as early as possible – that is, when the diagnosis is made. There are of course exceptions to this general rule, but they are, and should be, rare. Most children do not experience the 'drama of diagnosis' that adults do, and having a name for your problems early in life is almost always helpful, not frightening or threatening. It is often much better to say to a child, 'You have Asperger syndrome and that means...' rather than trying to put it 'softly' by saying that 'You know you have some social interaction problems'. Things that have a name are usually much less frightening than those that do not.

There are now booklets specifically for children with various kinds of behavioural problems, in language and a format that make them accessible to the children themselves. These booklets are very often helpful in educating children about the nature of their condition. Support groups can usually provide such booklets, or information about them.

INFORMING THE PARENTS

Ideally both parents should be present when the information about the child's diagnosis is shared. Written information to supplement the oral communication is almost always helpful, and the diagnostic evaluation should usually be summarized in writing. Excellent leaflets, booklets, and books for parents are available in many languages on diverse topics, ranging from behaviourally defined syndromes such as attention disorders and Asperger syndrome on the one hand to genetic syndromes such as fragile X, Prader–Willi, and Williams syndromes on the other.

It is important to try to distinguish which aspects of the child's behavioural problems reflect the specific learning disorder as such and which are caused by a mismatch between the child's ability and demands from the environment. For instance, attention deficits, hyperactivity, and impulsivity are to a large extent biologically determined symptoms of ADHD or of deficits in attention, motor control, and perception (DAMP), whereas depression may well be a secondary reaction and signal the breakdown of coping mechanisms.

271

Parents usually want to know about outcome. The prognosis should never be treated either lightly or in terms of definitive statements. The outcome is always unknown, even in conditions for which we may have extensive information about the long-term outcome in studies of large groups of children: such studies do not reliably predict the outcome for the individual. In most disorders there is enormous variation of outcome, and this range should be acknowledged. It is essential to take a realistic view: very optimistic or very pessimistic attitudes are often inappropriate and may prolong the phase during which a family is trying to reorient after a period of shock and confusion.

Models for crisis development and intervention are usually hopelessly off key when it comes to children with specific learning disorders. 'Shock' almost never comes in a single blow when a child has a disorder such as dyslexia, ADHD, DAMP, or Asperger syndrome. Rather, a gradual process of learning and relearning is set in motion before, at, or after diagnosis. The family has to adjust to having an unusual child with a disorder rather than an ordinary child without major problems. It is often grossly inappropriate to speak of the need for crisis psychotherapy when what the family needs most is information, empathic support, advice about how to deal with behavioural problems in the home setting and the school, and practical help in arranging financial matters, day care, and sometimes respite care.

INFORMING THE TEACHERS

Once the child and the parents have been informed about the diagnosis and its consequences, it is usually helpful to inform one or more of the child's teachers – in collaboration with the family, of course. Changing the attitude of a teacher is often the one most important step in the management of behavioural problems in an individual with a learning disorder. An understanding teacher can make the difference between hopelessness and acceptance, so that behavioural problems may be considered in a new light and no longer be seen as extremely disabling either to the child or to others.

Support groups

Parent associations can be exceptionally helpful to families of individuals with learning disorders and behavioural problems. The tradition that parents and professionals work separately from each other is changing, and parents and professionals are finally coming together, whether in organizing conferences, in writing books, or in everyday clinical practice. In tailoring services for children with learning disorders it is essential to find out just what families need, and not to intervene in ways that are felt to be irrelevant by those closest to the patient.

Parent support groups need not always be anchored within parent associations, but may be formed in collaboration with a specialized clinic. Weekend conferences for groups of families whose children have a specific disorder are often felt to be the 'vitamin injection' needed when things get to be overwhelming or depressing. At such conferences, experts may contribute by surveying the latest developments in research and practice, while parents can support each other and develop support networks.

Parents of children with ADHD can be taught (by other parents or by professionals) to be better able to cope with behavioural problems in their children (Taylor 1986). This is also true of Asperger syndrome. Parents of children with this disorder very often need to learn how to deal with problems relating to eating, dressing, and hygiene (Beckman 1997, Gillberg 1997a). Learning how to create new routines and to avoid any vagueness in communication is essential if one is to reduce the secondary consequences (such as strange eating habits and refusal to brush teeth or wash hair) of the primary restriction of communication and imagination inherent in the syndrome (Bristol 1997).

Other support groups than those for parents can play an important role in dealing with behavioural problems in specific learning disorders. Groups for siblings of affected children and adolescents, and groups for the affected children and adolescents themselves can do a lot to alleviate problems of psychosocial stigma and may indirectly lead to amelioration of some behavioural problems. Also, particularly in the case of those who themselves have a specific disorder, support groups may be an excellent way of providing the social interaction that is often missing in their lives.

Changing attitudes in society

A most important aspect of intervention in specific learning disorders, and one that is closely linked with management of behavioural problems, is the effort by experts in the field to change societal attitudes to specific disorders. For instance, children and adolescents with dyslexia will always have behavioural and emotional problems if society continues to look upon individuals with dyslexia as being simply 'stupid' or fails to provide adequate training. Getting general acceptance for the notion that dyslexia is a kind of disability, different from yet conceptually similar to hearing problems, is possibly the single most important generalized intervention to be made in the field, and one that will prevent psychosocial problems in a substantial proportion of individuals who have dyslexia.

Educational measures

Almost all children who have behavioural problems associated with a specific learning disorder will need some adjustments in the school setting. The child with ADHD may need to be moved so as to always be close to the teacher and not be disturbed by seeing the movements of the other children (Barkley 1990). The child with dyslexia may need specific phonological training (Højen and Lundberg 1990), and the adolescent with Asperger syndrome may need a highly structured curriculum detailing the activities of each 15-minute period of the school day (Bristol 1997).

Most children with specific learning disorders need a lot of extra, individualized, one-on-one training to help overcome at least some aspects of the academic failure that is otherwise likely to ensue. Adapting the educational demands and the teaching strategy to the level of the individual child with a specific learning disorder will also help reduce behavioural problems (Beckman 1997).

Computer-aided training can be useful in improving academic skills in children with autism, and also in other neuropsychiatric disorders (Heimann et al. 1995).

Behaviour modification

Behaviour modification is the best-studied intervention for behavioural problems in people with developmental and learning disorders (Harris 1995). There are several different techniques. The application of the various methods and the choice of specific procedures must be decided by the clinician in charge of the individual patient, in collaboration with a psychologist specializing in behaviour modification. 'Rigorous' behaviour therapy is a complicated and costly form of treatment, which should be reserved for the most severely disabled individuals with behavioural problems (aggressive behaviour, self-injury, tantrums, rumination, etc.) associated with autism and severe global learning disability. However, elements of behaviour modification are usually present in most interventions directed at helping individuals with specific learning disorder also. Positive reinforcement, shaping behaviour, imitation, extinction, time-out, and gradual change are all part of good education. Sometimes such methods need to be used with more structure and a more explicit goal than usual in order to ameliorate aberrant behaviours. In such instances, it is always important to analyse behaviour in depth before suggesting specific measures. In behaviour analysis, the time and conditions present at the onset of a specific problematic behaviour are identified. Antecedents, consequences, frequency, duration, and intensity of the behaviour are listed, so as to provide a rational basis for the suggestion of a specific intervention.

Other psychotherapies
No studies have been published that support the use of psychoanalytically oriented psychotherapies in the management of behaviour problems associated with specific learning disorders. Nevertheless, in many countries such therapies are still suggested when parents apply for help because their child has a behaviour problem. Unless all children with behaviour problems that are deemed to be in need of intervention of some kind are examined by a team with expertise in specific learning disorders, there is a considerable risk that many individuals with such disorders will be subjected to ineffective treatments. Many children with specific learning disorders present with behaviour problems and may not be suspected of having an underlying learning disorder unless they are meticulously clinically examined by an expert in learning disorders.

There have been reports that supportive talks with young people with Asperger syndrome can improve their quality of life (Lögdahl 1994). Such talks initially focus on the individual's special interests and then go on to deal with the person's specific practical and social problems. One of the most important aspects of this kind of psychotherapy is that the therapist must thoroughly understand the basic dysfunctions in Asperger syndrome.

Group psychotherapy in which the group leader is unaware of the presence of DAMP, Tourette syndrome, and autism spectrum disorders can have disastrous effects. Symptoms, behavioural problems, and emotional lability that are specifically associated with the neuropsychiatric disorder may in such instances all be interpreted as resulting from traumatic experiences in childhood or later (Gerland 1996).

Psychopharmacological interventions
After decades of being considered second- or third-best interventions in child neuropsychiatry, psychopharmacological interventions have emerged as a legitimate option among a variety

of measures that should be considered in many children with major behavioural problems. This is not to say that the majority of children with behavioural problems need drugs: most such children should not be treated with drugs. However, children with ADHD and DAMP, Tourette syndrome and tics, obsessive–compulsive disorders, and depression sometimes need psychopharmacological treatment and should not be kept from good and safe medication simply because of a presumption that all behavioural problems should be dealt with in non-pharmacological ways.

Any developmental pediatrician or psychiatrist needs to be well informed mainly about three classes of drugs – namely central stimulants, neuroleptics, and antidepressants – and their effects, side effects, and possible indications.

CENTRAL STIMULANTS

It has been known since the 1930s that central stimulants can dramatically relieve symptoms of attention deficit, impulsivity, and hyperactivity (Jacobvitz et al. 1990). However, it is only recently that a long-term study demonstrated persisting benefits of amphetamine after 15 months in the treatment of children with severe attention deficit and hyperactivity problems (Gillberg et al. 1997).

Practice varies enormously across cultures in respect of stimulant treatment of childhood disorders. Millions of children and adolescents in the USA are likely to have been treated with methylphenidate or amphetamine because of attention-deficit syndromes (Ciaranello 1993), while only a few thousand are currently given such treatment in the Nordic countries. This discrepancy (treatment being given more than a thousand times more frequently in the USA) cannot be accounted for by the roughly tenfold difference in population between the two regions. School-age children in the USA with a clear diagnosis of ADHD would almost definitely be given a trial of stimulants. In the Nordic countries, such treatment would be considered only for the most severely disabled individuals with DAMP (Gillberg et al. 1997).

I suggest that the children who should be considered for a trial of central stimulants are those who are more than 5 years old; who fulfil the criteria either for severe DAMP (see Chapter 6) or for ADHD; who have been given comprehensive interventions as outlined in the foregoing (diagnosis, information, changes in the educational setting, etc.); who are severely psychosocially or academically disabled by their disorder; and who have not improved satisfactorily with regard to attention, activity level, academic functioning, and overall psychosocial adjustment. If one stimulant is not effective after 3 weeks at optimal dosage (which has to be individually titrated), another should be tried for another period of 3 weeks or so. It is reasonable to try amphetamine and methylphenidate before deciding that stimulant treatment is not effective. Sixty to eighty per cent of children with severe DAMP or ADHD respond favourably to stimulants, with markedly reduced overactivity and disruptive behaviour and improved academic functioning. Side effects, which are few, include mild nausea, decrease of appetite, some weight loss and – rarely – visual hallucinations (which appear early in treatment and disappear on reduction of dosage or on drug withdrawal).

NEUROLEPTICS

Neuroleptics are often prescribed, sometimes with good effect, for the treatment of tics (Green 1991). However, studies of their effects on tics and Tourette syndrome in children and adolescents are few, and there is usually no rationale for prescribing such drugs for mild or moderately severe tics (Gillberg 1997b).

Side effects of neuroleptics are common in children and include acute dystonia, tardive dyskinesias, drowsiness, mental blunting, and endocrinological impairments of various kinds (Campbell et al. 1988).

A recent review of publications about treating children and adolescents with neuroleptics concluded that such treatment should be reserved for individuals with extremely severe psychiatric disorders, particularly adolescent-onset psychosis and severe forms of Tourette syndrome in which there are major and severely disabling tics (Gillberg 1997b). In most other conditions these drugs should be used sparingly, if at all, and almost never for more than 6 months. Neuroleptics do have some positive effects in autism (Campbell 1989, Gadow 1992), but the chronic nature of the disorder, the relatively modest effect, and the high risk of side effects prevent their widespread use in this condition.

The atypical neuroleptics such as clozapine and risperidone may be useful in individuals with severe autism or schizophrenia combined with major behavioural problems such as aggression, hyperactivity, and self-injury (Siefen and Remschmidt 1996), but more studies regarding the efficacy and safety of these drugs are required before general recommendations can be issued. Clozapine in particular must be used with great caution, given the risk of agranulocytosis with this drug (Kane et al. 1988a,b).

It is already clear that neuroleptics should be prescribed to children and adolescents only by clinicians with expertise in neuropsychiatry.

ANTIDEPRESSANTS

There is little justification for prescribing the 'old' tricyclic drugs in most children with behavioural problems (Gillberg 1995). These drugs have side effects (dryness of mouth with deterioration of dental status, blurred vision, urine retention, fatigue, drowsiness, attention deficits and mental slowing, sensory–perceptual disturbance, mild tremor, and, albeit rarely, psychotic and confusional states) ranging from mild to very severe. Because these are usually difficult to explain to the child or youngster being treated, they can in themselves cause considerable psychological stress. Their clinical effectiveness has not been shown to outweigh the drawbacks in many cases. It is surprising that these drugs have been used in the treatment of nocturnal enuresis, for which they were for many years considered 'drugs of choice'. At least four case reports of sudden death in children being treated with imipramine or desipramine have appeared in the literature (Biederman 1991). Nevertheless, clinical experience suggests that in doses much lower than those recommended, amitriptyline, imipramine, and clomipramine (e.g. 5 to 10mg twice daily for 12- to 16-year-olds) may occasionally be effective in alleviating depression and irritability in ADHD/DAMP.

The new selective serotonin reuptake inhibitors (SSRIs) have fewer – and usually mild – side effects and appear to be at least as clinically effective as the old antidepressants. Too few studies have been published so far to permit generalized clinical recommendations, but it is already clear that drugs such as fluoxetine and paroxetine will have a place in the treatment of some behavioural and emotional disorders in childhood. SSRIs appear to ameliorate, in particular, obsessive–compulsive symptoms and social isolation (Riddle et al. 1992, Klein 1997).

OTHER DRUGS

Epilepsy carries a high risk of behavioural problems (Gillberg 1995), and distinguishing which are caused by the condition and which by the drugs is sometimes difficult or impossible (Deonna 1993). Antiepileptic drugs are commonly used in children and adolescents with disability, mostly for epilepsy, but sometimes in attempts to control explosive behaviours with or without associated epileptogenic discharge on the EEG. Sodium valproate and carbamazepine have relatively few behavioural side effects and are drugs of choice if children with epilepsy have major behavioural problems (Gillberg 1995). Lamotrigine may have specific psychotropic effects, but more studies are needed before it can be recommended as a first-line drug in the treatment of epilepsy (and possibly of some behavioural problems) in children and adolescents.

Sleep problems are common in children with disability (Harris 1995) and range from insomnia to hypersomnia. Sometimes pharmacological treatment is indicated. Unfortunately, no general guidelines can be provided, particularly since children with brain disorders very often react unexpectedly to drugs affecting brain functions. For instance, benzodiazepines very often lead to hyperactivity, aggression, and confusion rather than to relief of anxiety leading to drowsiness and sleep. Stimulants and other drugs may be needed in hypersomnia (including narcolepsy and the rare Kleine–Levin syndrome) but should be prescribed by specialists in sleep disorders with specific expertise in respect of treatment with stimulants.

Dyslexia is a frequent concomitant of attention-deficit syndromes, including DAMP (Hellgren 1994). There is some support for the use of piracetam (a so-called 'nootropic drug') in dyslexia (Wilsher and Taylor 1994), and it is unclear why this drug is used so rarely in the treatment of this sometimes socially and academically disabling condition.

Diets

Phenylketonuria is the classic example of a disease that can lead to severe disability with major behavioural problems and that can be treated with an appropriate diet. A few other identifiable metabolic disorders can be treated in the same fashion (Gillberg 1995, Harris 1995).

In recent years, claims have been made that other behavioural problems in children, including ADHD and autism, can be treated with diets. There is little empirical support for such notions. However, there is some evidence that children with attention deficits who also have allergies may benefit from diets excluding certain products (Egger et al. 1985). It is not known whether this is also true in populations of children with mental or physical disability. Further studies are needed before generalized conclusions can be drawn.

Alternative treatments

There are many 'alternative therapies' around for children with disabilities. Some of these are intended to be effective specifically for the underlying disease, whereas others attempt to cure the full range of signs and symptoms suffered by the individual, from major motor impairment to behavioural dysfunction. Holding therapy, pony therapy, organic brain dysfunction training, sensory integration training, auditory integration training, facilitated communication, and conductive education have all come and gone or have lingered without empirical support or in the face of negative outcome studies (Schopler 1989, Graves 1995). A common theme for these alternative treatments is the underlying refusal to accept the permanence of the disability. Very often there is a grain of truth in one or other aspect of the treatment. For instance, many children with physical disabilities and behavioural problems will have a good time while out pony riding, and it is possible that there may be at least temporary reduction of oversensitivity to sound in autism with auditory integration training (Bettison 1996). The major problems are that (i) proponents of these therapies usually make outlandish claims for cures or other extreme benefits of treatment and that (ii) children involved in such therapies may be withdrawn from other, more reasonable, interventions and from appropriate education.

Summary

Children who have learning disabilities that are complicated by behavioural and emotional problems often need interventions geared at alleviating the psychological problems. Providing help with regard to the learning problems is most important and will usually go some way towards ameliorating behavioural disorder also. A number of other interventions can be helpful, but only in exceptional cases can cures be achieved. Psychoeducational interventions, behaviour-modification programmes, individual talks, and medication may be required, singly or in various combinations. One of the most important aspects of intervention in this field is the dissemination of knowledge about the problems and the mechanisms involved in their pathogenesis. Changing the attitudes of parents, relatives, peers, and teachers should be the single most important feature of any intervention programme aimed at reducing behavioural problems associated with learning disorders in childhood and adolescence.

REFERENCES

Barkley RA. (1990) *Attention Deficit Hyperactivity Disorder.* New York: Guilford Press.
Beckman V. (1997) Projektet. Att leva med Aspergers syndrom, DAMP, dyslexi. Stockholm: Cura. In Swedish.
Bettison S. (1996) The long-term effects of auditory training on children with autism. *Journal of Autism and Developmental Disorders* 26: 361–74.
Biederman J. (1991) Sudden death in children treated with a tricyclic antidepressant. *Journal of the American Academy of Child and Adolescent Psychiatry* 30: 495–8.
Bristol M. (1997) Interventions in Asperger syndrome. Paper given at the Learning Disabilities Association International Conference, 19–22 February 1997, Chicago, IL, USA.
Campbell M. (1989) Pharmacotherapy in autism: an overview. In Gillberg C, editor. *Diagnosis and Treatment of Autism.* New York: Plenum.
— Adams P, Perry R, et al. (1988) Tardive and withdrawal dyskinesia in autistic children: a prospective study. *Psychopharmacology Bulletin* 24: 251–5.
Ciaranello RD. (1993) Attention deficit-hyperactivity disorder and resistance to thyroid hormone – a new idea? [editorial]. *New England Journal of Medicine* 328: 1038–9. [Comment on *New England Journal of Medicine* 1993 328: 997–1001; comment in *New England Journal of Medicine* 1993 329: 966–7.]
Deonna T. (1993) Annotation: cognitive and behavioural correlates of epileptic activity in children [review]. *Journal of Child Psychology and Psychiatry and Allied Disciplines* 34: 611–20. 46 references.

Egger J, Carter CM, Graham PJ, et al.. (1985) Controlled trial of oligoantigenic treatment in the hyperkinetic syndrome. *Lancet* **1:** 540–5.

Gadow KD. (1992) Pediatric psychopharmacotherapy: a review of recent research. *Journal of Child Pychology and Psychiatry* **33:** 153–195.

Gerland G. (1996) *En Riktig Människa.* Stockholm: Cura. In Swedish. 254 p.

Gillberg C. (1995) *Clinical Child Neuropsychiatry.* Cambridge and New York: Cambridge University Press. 366 p.

— (1997a) *Barn, Ungdomar och Vuxna med Aspergers Syndrom. Normala, Geniala, Nördar?* Stockholm: Cura. 192 p. In Swedish.

—. (1997b) Neuroleptikabehandling av barn och ungdomar. In: *SBU rapport - Behandling med Neuroleptika.* Volume 1, Chapter 10, p 193–208. Stockholm: Swedish Council on Technology Assessment in Health Care. In Swedish.

— Melander H, von Knorring A-L, et al. (1997) Long-term stimulant treatment of children with attention-deficit hyperactivity disorder. A randomized, double-blind, placebo-controlled trial. *Archives of General Psychiatry* **54:** 857–64.

Graves P. (1995) Therapy methods for cerebral palsy [review]. *Journal of Paediatrics and Child Health* **31:** 24–8. 34 references.

Green WH. (1991) *Child and Adolescent Clinical Psychopharmacology.* Baltimore: Williams and Wilkins.

Harris JC. (1995) *Developmental Neuropsychiatry. Volume 1, The Fundamentals.* New York and Oxford: Oxford University Press.

Heimann M, Nelson KE, Tjus T, Gillberg C. (1995) Increasing reading and communication skills in children with autism through an interactive multimedia computer program. *Journal of Autism and Developmental Disorders* **25:** 459–80.

Hellgren L. (1994) Psychiatric disorders in adolescence: longitudinal follow-up studies of adolescent onset psychoses and childhood onset deficits in attention motor control and perception [MD thesis]. Göteborg University, Göteborg, Sweden. 145 p. Available from Department of Child and Adolescent Psychiatry.

Højen T, Lundberg I. (1990) *Dysleksi.* Oslo: Gyldendals förlag. In Norwegian.

Jacobvitz D, Sroufe LA, Stewart M, Leffert N. (1990) Treatment of attentional and hyperactivity problems in children with sympathomimetic drugs: a comprehensive review. *Journal of the American Academy of Child and Adolescent Psychiatry* **29:** 677–88.

Kane JM, Honigfeld G, Singer J, Meltzer H. (1988a) Clozapine in treatment-resistant schizophrenics. *Psychopharmacology Bulletin* **24:** 62–7.

— Honigfield G, Singer J, Meltzer H. (1988b) Clozapine for the treatment-resistent schizophrenic: a double-blind comparison with chlorpromazine. *Archives of General Psychiatry* **45:** 789–96.

Klein RG. (1997) Treatment of ADHD. Paper read at conference on Treatment of ADHD and Treatment of Children and Adolescents with SSRIs, 7 April 1997, Uppsala, Sweden.

Lögdahl C. (1994) Autistiska tillstånd kräver nytänkande inom psykologisk behandling. *Psykologtidningen* **10:** 4–6. In Swedish.

Riddle MA, Scahill M, King RA, et al. (1992) Double-blind, crossover trial of fluoxetine and placebo in children and adolescents with obsessive–compulsive disorder. *Journal of the American Academy of Child and Adolescent Psychiatry* **31:** 1062–9.

Schopler E. (1989) Principles for directing both educational treatment and research. InL Gillberg C, editor. *Diagnosis and Treatment of Autism.* New York: Plenum. p 167–83.

Siefen G, Remschmidt H. (1986) Behandlungsergebnisse mit Clozapin bei schizophrenen Jugendlichen: Results of treatment with clozapine in schizophrenic adolescents. *Zeitschrift für Kinder- und Jugendpsychiatrie* **14:** 245–57.

Taylor EA. (1986) *The Overactive Child.* Oxford: Blackwell Scientific Publications.

Wilsher CR, Taylor EA. (1994) Piracetam in developmental reading disorders: a review. *European Child and Adolescent Psychiatry* **3:** 59–71.

15
PREVENTION AND MANAGEMENT OF SPECIFIC LEARNING DISORDERS

Martin Bax amd Kingsley Whitmore

This book had its origins in a meeting, sponsored by the Little Foundation, to consider the causes of specific learning disorders (SLDs) and to discuss the prevention of such neurodevelopmental disorders. The conclusion of that meeting was that if existing knowledge were applied the incidence of such disorders could be reduced. To what extent is that true? One can think of primary prevention, in which the disorder is actually prevented, and secondary prevention, in which, when the problem is known to be present, action is taken to obviate the disability.

Primary prevention

Primary prevention of the biological deficits is difficult. To reduce their incidence one needs to know the aetiology of the cases and, preferably, their nature – that is, whether they are due to dysfunction of normal CNS tissues or are a consequence of abnormal or damaged tissue.

In some specific learning disorders the problem is due to genetics (see Chapter 7). Theoretically, where there is a strong family history of specific reading difficulty, avoidance of pregnancy would be a method of prevention, but in practice this method would almost surely not be used. Genetic engineering to prevent such problems is still a long way off, but the process of understanding how genetic expression leads to morphological development of the brain is an area that is expanding tremendously. (Think, for example, of the field of behavioural phenotypes.) With growing understanding of the ways in which the expression of genes is translated to a functional outcome, sophisticated interventions, e.g. with neuropharmacology, may become possible.

Alternatively, the problem may lie in factors that may interfere with the process of brain development. Prominent among these are the perinatal adversities. However, as Hadders-Algra and Lindahl point out in Chapter 8, the prevalence of risk factors of very preterm birth, severe intrauterine growth retardation, and intrauterine exposure to substances such as alcohol or other environmental agents is low. Some three-quarters of learning problems – not all of which are specific learning problems – do not have a perinatal aetiology. Nevertheless if the problems of smoking and alcohol consumption were tackled more effectively the incidence of SLDs would undoubtedly be reduced. Equally, on the perinatal front there is the increased survival rate of the preterm infant, and many people are looking at the complex relations between early birth, neurological morbidity, and the organization of health-care delivery in perinatal medicine. Some sort of 'neuroprotection' of the small baby is seen as the most promising neurochemical way of avoiding brain lesions and long-term dysfunctions (Evrard, 1997). There is, therefore, some long-term hope of reducing some SLDs, but clearly it would be over-optimistic to count on substantial and imminent reduction in the incidence of SLDs by primary prevention – so what might be hoped for from secondary prevention?

Secondary prevention

Secondary (and tertiary) prevention are really aspects of the management of existing SLDs, of minimizing or, better still, of compensating for disability and preventing additional consequences. Secondary prevention begins with being aware of the risk of an SLD developing because of the child's family history of, for example, speech and language delay, because of the child's experience, or because of some physical or developmental anomaly.

For instance, many studies have now shown that some babies who have been in special-care units with one problem or another, though showing no obvious neurological signs, do get into difficulties in their school years. Children who have had head injury, epilepsy, or meningitis are unduly at risk of SLDs, and children who have, for example, a squint, an undescended testis, or congenital heart disease have all been shown to have higher rates of SLDs or other learning difficulties than children without these problems. More transient physical problems such as serous otitis media ('glue ear') have been said to carry a risk of SLD, but the long-term consequences are still under discussion (Maw 1995, Peters et al. 1997). And, most importantly, there are the children whose development in the preschool period seems to be delayed in one or more functions, such as motor function (clumsiness) and, especially, language: children with language and speech delay have been known since the pioneering work of Ingram (1959, 1971) to be particularly at risk of having an SLD.

We should not unduly stress these so-called markers or believe that by concentrating on them we would identify all the children with SLDs. In our own studies of children who had neurodevelopmental problems, for example, we found that the majority had not been in special-care baby units, and two-thirds or more of children with squint did not have significant learning difficulty. An SLD will probably not materialize in children with such markers, but the greater risk calls for a judicious watchfulness for early signs of its existence.

It is important to realize that the identification of a genetic or biological problem does not mean that the child cannot be helped. Throughout this book ways in which specific learning disorders can be dealt with have been mentioned. For example the application of remedial reading techniques (see Chapter 3 in this book, and Beitchman and Young [1997], Borström and Elbro [1997]) have been proven to be effective in children who are having specific reading problems. Some cases of developmental coordination disorder (DCD) may be helped by physiotherapy. Among behavioural issues, attention-deficit/hyperactivity disorder (ADHD) and deficits in attention, motor control, and perception (DAMP) can be tackled in the way suggested in Chapter 6, including in some instances the use of psychostimulant drugs, but it also requires a well organized programme of management of the child in school. Problems with academic learning can be helped by specific programmes in the classroom. The outcome may not necessarily be totally satisfactory, but at least some of the consequences of the SLD can be reduced.

Epidemiology

There is one problem with all these secondary interventions: how to prove that they are effective. To do that one would need to know the basic prevalence of an SLD before and after an intervention had been tried, with clearly defined criteria for the disorder and a rigorous methodology.

The epidemiology of SLDs has been bedevilled by the use of different criteria in different studies (such as the use of a cut-off point of 1 or 1.5 SD below the expected performance, or the measurement of delay in months or grades) and of different methodologies (such as tests used and ways of obtaining samples). Furthermore, as this book demonstrates, there are clearly different emphases and indeed different diagnoses between different experts in the field. Similarly, the same child seen by a variety of readers of this book might end up with a different primary diagnosis (in acronyms) of SLD – meaning 'specific learning disorder' or 'specific language disorder' – DCD, ADHD, or DAMP, depending on the preference of the author, particularly if the child has more than one specific learning disorder.

Under these circumstances our contributors have done no more than quote from published prevalence rates, aware that these may vary from country to country, place to place (e.g. urban or rural) and time to time. Gordon (Chapter 3) says it is estimated that about 3 to 10% of schoolchildren have dyslexia. O'Hare (Chapter 4) quotes the prevalence given by Gross-Tsur et al. (1996) for dyscalculia (6.5%) and that given by Benton (1975) for dysgraphia (3-4%). Polatajko (Chapter 5) gives the international estimate of 6% of school-aged children who have DCD (American Psychiatric Association 1994). Rassmussen and Gillberg (Chapter 6) give a clinical rate of 3.7% for the full DSM-IV criteria of ADHD among 7-year old children regardless of associations but 10.3% for a subclinical variant of individuals meeting most but not all of the DSM-IV criteria (Kadesjö and Gillberg 1998).

While researchers will of course argue about matters of labelling and prevalence, clinicians can take heart from the knowledge that nevertheless the actual management of the child should be broadly unaffected by these differences.

The association of SLDs

It is unusual for associations (comorbidities) to be mentioned in an epidemiological context. Many authors have concentrated on their own particular interests and it is often hard to discover from reported prevalences what the rate of associations was or whether it had been looked for and taken into account. It should have been: no one yet knows whether associated SLDs can exacerbate a disposition to a particular specific learning disorder, as, for instance, ADHD might.

There is repeated evidence of some associations:

- commonly of dyslexia and dysgraphia (spelling)
- of both dyslexia and (writing) dysgraphia with dyscalculia
- of reading and spelling difficulties with DCD

- of attention disorder with motor perception dysfunction (DAMP)
- of dyslexia and dyscalculia with ADHD

(Frith 1978, Share et al. 1987, Pennington 1991, Lewis et al. 1994, Shalev et al. 1995, Gross-Tsur et al. 1996, Landgren et al. 1996, Fletcher-Flinn et al. 1997). (For an example of an association, see the case history of CD in Chapter 3.)

Clearly the prevalence of 'SLDs' is not the sum of the prevalences of the individual LDs. Gaddes and Edgell (1993) estimated that 7 to 15% of the general school population have one or more such disorders. Perhaps neuroscientists should concentrate on the range of dysfunctions that might arise from morphological abnormalities rather than seek those morphological abnormalities associated with each specific dysfunction: are there strategic processes which may not be modality-specific (Henderson et al. 1994)?

Be that as it may, epidemiology is relevant only when problems have been identified and diagnosed. This has to be the responsibility of health and education services, ideally with the assistance of parents.

The early identification of specific learning difficulties

More than 30 years ago, in a paper describing an investigation into the early prediction of reading, writing, and spelling disabilities (i.e. 'the early identification of a specific pattern of dysfunction') in children referred to a clinic for paediatric langugage disorder, de Hirsch and Jansky (1966) wrote:

Twenty years' experience with intelligent and emotionally disabled children, whose learning drive was often severely damaged, has convinced us that [the] extraordinarily large proportion of them who developed reading, writing and spelling difficulties later, would not have needed remedial help then had their difficulties been recognised before first grade entrance.

and

The clinical impression of these youngsters was one of striking immaturity...their failure was characterised by the accumulation of deficits...that pointed to a profound and basic maturational deficit...so severe that it seemed rooted in the very biological matrix of the child.

Their original predictions had been based primarily on a clinical evaluation of the children's developmental level and only secondarily on their performance on a battery of tests assembled over the years (de Hirsch and Jansky 1966). Aware that whatever it was on which they had based their clinical judgement, it could not be handed on to someone else, they constructed a Predictive Index of ten single predictors that would most effectively identify children with a high risk of difficulty. In a heterogeneous group of children, this index identified 77% of those who failed to learn to read by the end of the second grade (age 8^1/$_2$ years) (Jansky and de Hirsch 1972). There were 19% false positives.

In 1990 Silver and Hagin summarized the technical aspects of 18 similar batteries, including the one (Search) that they had reported in 1972 which had given a correct prediction of reading achievement at 7 years in 87% of children tested at the age of 5^1/$_2$ years to 6^1/$_2$ years, with a false-positive rate of up to 9%. Shapiro et al. (1983) maintained that by shifting the focus from academic underachievement to deviant neurodevelopment (the identification of markers) it becomes possible to detect SLDs before school (at the age of 6 years). Later (1987), using an expanded neurological examination of 5-year-olds, they demonstrated impressive rates of correct classification of reading outcome at age 7 years, with a sensitivity of 0.8 and specificity of 0.79. Willems and his colleagues came up with a correct classification of 80%, with a sensitivity of 0.59 and a specificity of 0.79 (see Chapter 11).

These studies certainly show that before children go to school it is possible to forecast, reasonably accurately, the children who are likely to have serious difficulty in academic learning. Benasich and Spitz (see Chapter 9) have explained how even in 1-year-old infants it is possible to detect impairment in auditory temporal processing, a marker of specific language delay and dyslexia.

So why do so many educationalists and even some paediatricians seem to reject the concept of the early identification of SLDs? They argue that cognitive processes necessary for learning are not fully developed in early childhood (which is true enough, but irrelevant); that rates of learning are neither constant nor uniform enough to allow prediction of SLDs; that there is temporal instability in the development of children's behavioural characteristics and a greater modifiability in learning rates than has usually been assumed; that compensatory interactions occur between the abilities of children and their environment; that the basic skills of reading, writing, language, and mathematics can be taught to children regardless of their developmental readiness or their social background; that there are neither critical nor sensitive learning periods; and that it is doubtful whether remedial programmes based on a child's abilities and disabilities are any more successful than those based on sound instruction (see, for example, Lindsay [1979], Wedell and Lindsay [1980], and Leach [1981]). In other words, they will argue that it is preferable and certainly more expedient not to bother looking for precursors of SLDs; better wait until children show clear signs of having failed before dealing with their problems. So much for prevention!

METHODS OF EARLY IDENTIFICATION OF SLDs
Some influential paediatricians misconstrue all methods of early identification of 'learning and behavioural difficulties' as being developmental screening, which they then condemn as being inefficient and even as unethical because it fails to satisfy the traditional conditions laid down by Wilson and Junger (1968) and Holland (1974) for acceptable screening procedures for medical disorders; among these conditions are the requirement that the 'disease' should have a natural history, with a recognizable presymptomatic stage for which there should be an effective form of treatment, and that the screening techniques should be easy and quick for less specialized members of staff to administer. These paediatricians say that developmental screening, 'an invention of generations of developmental paediatricians since the sequence of normal development was described', has resulted in a system of poor predictive value with false positives and negatives, because of the difficulty of wide variation of 'normal' and the difficulty in showing it (Polnay 1989). This has certainly been clearly shown to be the case, for instance, in the use of the Denver Developmental Screening Test (see Cadman et al. [1988]), one of the best-known and most widely used. However, tests recording a child's age on reaching developmental milestones were not designed to *predict* either general or specific learning disorders. As we sought to explain (Whitmore and Bax

1988), in *clinical* practice, procedures for the early identification of all kinds of learning and behavioural problems in preschool entrants are *not* screening procedures, nor is their purpose per se to predict a child's success or failure in school. None of the above conditions of a screening test applies to SLDs; there is even a difference of opinion as to what an SLD is! Research workers, of course, are interested in predictions, because only by predicting correctly can they show that their tests are statistically valid, but clinicians are not primarily interested in predicting the educational outcome for a child; such tests are clinically relevant only as an additional element in an individual child's neurodevelopmental *assessment*.

The common-sense solution to the deficiencies of screening, according to Polnay (1989), is to rely on parents' observations, because 'there is an increasing body of evidence that parents are far more effective than professionals in the early diagnosis of a wide range of handicaps'. This is manifestly not so. We do not dispute that the observations of parents are sometimes instrumental in alerting paediatricians to their concern about the behaviour, both emotional and learning behaviour, and more often the physical health of their child; but *that is not making a diagnosis.* We are aware that a parental questionnaire may be useful in picking out children who have not already been identified as having learning difficulties or being in need of educational support in school (Sonnander 1987), but one has to remember that there is always an unknown proportion of parents, perhaps 1 in 6, who for a variety of social or biological reasons do not or cannot make use of the services that are available. The varied quality of preschool services to identify children with neurodevelopmental problems, which may be omens for SLDs, means that very often learning problems, and particularly SLDs, are likely to be identified later rather than sooner. Research that may follow the introduction of the testing of all 5-year-old entrants to schools in the UK in 1998 (in phonology, writing, speaking, mathematics, and social development) might show that such tests help in the early identification of SLDs, but at best this is educational screening and no substitute for an individual neurodevelopmental assessment that can detect strengths and weaknesses in a child's learning skills.

AN INTEGRATED HEALTH AND EDUCATION SERVICE IN SCHOOLS
We believe there are opportunities for the prevention and more effective treatment and management of SLDs. For these to be achieved there needs to more, not less, integration, both within the school health service and between the service and the schools, than there is at present.

There are two principal, related issues: who should carry out overall health and developmental assessments in school entrants and how can liaison with teachers be improved?

In the past, pupils in many European countries received routine periodic medical inspections, which were spread throughout a term so that school doctors attended weekly in most schools, but from our informal enquiries it appears that this is no longer the case except, we understand, in Switzerland and Belgium. In the Netherlands all children when they start school at 4 years of age and again at 5$\frac{1}{2}$ (before the formal teaching of academic skills) are examined by a doctor in the preventive paediatric service. In Germany there is an obligatory medical examination which pays a little attention to neurodevelopmental items; pupils receive further examinations during each of the kindergarten and elementary school years. In Sweden nurses in well-baby clinics provide health checks at the age of 5^1/$_2$ years, before the children start school at 6, and these checks include neurodevelopmental screening; children who fail such tests are referred to a school doctor of school psychologist (if there is one), but the school health system is almost non-existent in many schools because of financial problems.

In the UK the situation is very similar, except that the school health service, from being originally a school medical service, has become virtually a school-nurse service. Slack (1980), after seeing the work of school nurse practitioners in the US, questioned the need for both school doctors and school nurses. A recent working-party report (Polnay 1995) on the health needs of school-age children maintained that there was no additional benefit from a child's being seen by a school paediatrician on starting school if they had completed an adequate preschool surveillance programme uneventfully and where an interview with the school nurse, supported by a lack of parent and teacher concerns, indicated 'that the child is healthy'. The working party were evidently interested only in the physical health, and perhaps the emotional health, of school children, but not at all in their intellectual development and certainly not in the early identification of SLDs.

As in Sweden, there is very little consistency in what is actually provided in schools in the UK, and also school health services are currently being seen as 'soft targets' that would enable health authorities to deal with their overspending. Nurses are cheaper to employ than doctors. Similarly preschool health surveillance previously provided by health authorities' well-baby clinics is increasinly being done by health visitors attached to general practices or by the doctors themselves (enticed by a fee from the government), neither of whom also contribute to health services in the primary schools.

THE NEED FOR SCHOOLS TO HAVE APPOINTED SCHOOL DOCTORS AS WELL AS NURSES

We believe that in order for school health services to meet the needs of all children with learning difficulties, a doctor's regular presence is necessary in schools, as well as a nurse's. It is not satisfactory for a school nurse alone to undertake routinely a variety of screening tests largely of physical health to confirm the impressions of parents (and teachers) that all is well with the development of children at so important a point in their lives as when they start school. Children should be *assesssed* jointly by a school nurse and a school paediatrician who has the knowledge and skills to be far more sure the children do not have neurodevelopmental disabilities that might compromise their academic education. Of course the doctor cannot be certain: medicine is not an exact science, least of all neurodvelopmental paediatrics.

The parents of every school entrant should be offered an assessment by the school nurse and doctor, who should be free to use their discretion as to who does what. The parent may decline the offer, though in our experience this is rare. Even the parents of a child with an already identified educationally relevant problems are usually keen to discuss this with the paediatrician and the head teacher, who should be invited to attend the session. It may sometimes be the case that in a very stable community in which families and their children are well known to the school nurse and the teachers and there is close liaison with preschool health services, neither school nurse nor parent and teacher see the need for neurodevelopmental assessment by the doctor. However, in many parts of the developed world the majority of schoolchildren live in inner-city and suburban areas – in the UK in 1977 more than two-thirds (Office of Population Censuses and Surveys [1997]) – in which mobility and social disadvantage are high and the children do not receive satisfactory preschool surveillance. In our study of inner-city school entrants in London in the 1980s, at least one-third had no preschool health records, and of those with records 2 out of 5 had not been seen since the age of 2 years; half of these had health problems on entry, as did 40% of all the entrants (Whitmore and Bax 1986).

The type of approach to preschool children we would recommend was set out by Bax et al. (1990). The school nurse should rightly be responsible for initially contacting and even liaising with the preschool health services, but the size of the problem of all learning and behaviour disorders in 5- to 6-year-old children, and the fact that children with SLD may be found among the socially disadvantaged, points to the need for all school entrants with few exceptions to be assessed.

It is equally unsatisfactory that such assessments be made, before the child starts school, by doctors and nurses who are inexperienced in educational medicine and who do not also work in the schools. The interface between health and education is in the school. Effective educational medicine has to be practised not from clinics, surgeries, or hospitals, but within schools. Liaison is more than just communication; it means consulting with teachers and (educational) psychologists on the ground, in schools.

One might have thought that it was unnecessary to say this, but, sadly, it is not. Not so long ago a study based on interviews of teachers of pupils aged 7 to 11 years drew attention to the poor communication they had with school doctors about pupils with physical disabilities and chronic diseases who were in their classes: the consultancy role of the doctor was virtually nonexistent and the teachers' main source of information was the parents, though often this proved to be inadequate and inaccurate (Fitzherbert 1982). More recently, in a survey of children with asthma, it was found that many teachers did not know what to do for an acute attack: in only 57% of cases were the children allowed to keep inhalers at school, and half of these were locked away in cupboards (Pugh et al. 1995). Such reports are disappointing when it is remembered that traditionally school health services have been thought of as at least providing some input into the care of children with problems of physical health. Little wonder that the wisdom of integrating children with disabilities into ordinary schools has sometimes been questioned (Chazan 1980). In principle the policy of integration is sound for many, provided the schools are properly resourced, which they seldom have been. Will those children with learning and behaviour disorders fare any better without the resources customarily provided in special schools?

Being properly resourced includes having a school paediatrician and nurse not just visiting on an ad hoc basis but regularly accessible to class teachers. Of course there are practical difficulties for two parties to meet when each has fixed commitments. Liaison does not just happen; there has to be willingness on both sides to achieve it and maintain it. For the teachers such motivation is very much influenced by their past experience of a school health service. It takes time to change their attitudes and expectations, but once they are familiar with the kind of cooperation and service we have in mind (Whitmore 1985) 9 out of 10 teachers of infant classes (aged 5 to 7 years) cease to regard a doctor's appearance in the classroom as an interruption or in their common room as an intrusion, and instead appreciate it as a mission of support.

WHAT CAN SCHOOL DOCTORS AND NURSES OFFER TEACHERS?
So what can school paediatricians offer in the way of assistance and management of children who may have an SLD? Through a neurodevelopmental assessment on entry, with the parent present, they can elicit an uneven developmental profile that may be coupled with a family history of such a disorder. They can identify those particular functions that may be a cause for concern – for example a language delay that is in many cases a precursor of specific reading difficulties; the motor signs that may be suggestive of DCD; and the attentional problems or overactive behaviour characteristic of children with ADHD or DAMP. With the assistance of school nurses they can be satisfied that the child has no visual or auditory defect, and when in doubt can refer the child to specialists and inform the teacher of the result. They can gain a shrewd idea of the level of the child's intelligence and, if normal intellectual development is suspect, the extent to which any shortcoming might be related to adverse socioeconomic circumstances. They will be aware that in some countries the accepted definition of SLDs will, for both practical educational purposes and those of research and classification of SLDs, preclude the possibility of a diagnosis of SLD in a child whose visual, hearing, or intellectual capacity is impaired. However, at this stage in their assessment they will be interested, not in predicting, let along diagnosing, an SLD, but in ascertaining the reason for a child's uneven neurodevelopmental profile. This may or may not be associated with an SLD; only further observation and testing will settle the matter and this immediately involves collaboration with class teachers. This is the kernel of multidisciplinary assessment and care.

Paediatricians can personally explain to the class teacher their concerns and seek the class teacher's opinion based on observation of particular dysfunctions in the classroom and playground. The teacher's perceptions may be different and enlightening. From the child's response to early teaching, doctors and teacher can compare notes on the child's aptitudes. Equally it is important that the teacher is aware that the child's difficulties in learning may have a biological basis.

From the school nurse's parental interview when the child enters school, the paediatrician may first become aware that a child's living conditions at home are adverse – something the teacher may have suspected, or even known from having taught older siblings. There is little that paediatricians and teachers can personally do to modify social backgrounds, but if they suspect from their discussions that these are a factor in the child's difficulties, between them they can refer the family to social services, unless this has already been done. Even when biologically based SLDs are apparent, social factors may determine their severity (Hunt et al. 1988) and undermine the development of compensatory skills.

Paediatricians may also be the first to appreciate the emotional problems of young children, either from their history, their mother's concern, or their behaviour at an entrant

288

assessment. On the other hand the parents themselves may have mentioned their concern to the teacher about a child's worrying behaviour at home or the teacher may have soon noticed it. In either case teacher and paediatrician will need to confer. The paediatrician may be able to reassure the teacher when psychosomatic symptoms (e.g. headaches, abdominal pain) are prominent, and the teacher may soon be able to reassure both paediatrician and parent that the behaviour is not related to the child's introduction to school. However, it may take longer to establish that the child's behaviour is a reaction to neurodevelopmental difficulties, such as in reading and writing, or to relations between child and parents, or perhaps whether the learning difficulties and the behaviour problems have a common origin in a neurodevelopmental disorder, as in DAMP. In either case the paediatrician can advise the teacher not to assume too readily that the child is being naughty and is therefore eligible for chastisement.

Progress can be jointly reviewed each term or two. Signs and symptoms of SLD may vary with age, particularly between 5 and 7 years, being aspects of maturation and also of associations. Some children improve, but for those that do not the teacher may wish to seek the advice of the school's psychologist (if it has one), who then becomes another key member of the school's interdisciplinary team – and will need to be briefed by the paediatrician about the medical features before interpreting tests of intelligence and aptitudes or advising referral to a learning-disorder team. Equally the paediatrician may wish to refer the child to other specialists, e.g. a child neurologist, a physiotherapist, an occupational therapist, a speech and language specialist, a child psychiatrist, or a team for disabled children.

The point we are making is that the interrelation between educational, health, and social problems has to be borne in mind when the provision of services for children with SLD, no less than for children with general learning difficulties, is under discussion. First an action plan for any child who continues to show evidence of having an SLD requires input from paediatricians as well as class teachers and educational psychologists, because an anomaly in academic attainment is seldom the only anomaly. This means that school paediatricians, teachers, and psychologists must liaise so that each understands the opinions and intentions of the others and there is coordination between educational programs and health interventions. Nibbling at various facets of a problem, applying expertise in ignorant isolation, is illogical and likely to be inefficient. School doctors are the best catalyst for cooperation because of their role as neurodevelopmental paediatricians, bridging the disciplines of child neurology and education, and their firm commitment to prevention.

The outlook for children with SLDs
The natural history of many of the disorders discussed in this book – insofar as they are known – is not good. Young children with SLDs tend to go on having academic difficulties throughout childhood and adolescence (Tallal et al. 1997). Illiteracy hinders any person, quite apart from the possible experience of a secondary trauma arising from lack of self-confidence leading to school phobia and truancy or even more serious conduct disorders in adolescence – though evidently one should be cautious in attributing the latter to an SLD (Fergusson and Lynsky 1997). Gillberg et al. (1989), in following up 6- to 7-year-old children with DAMP into early adult life, have found convincing evidence that 4 out of 5

still have problems with school achievement or with behaviour at age 13 years (reviewed in Chapter 6), and poor outcomes in respect of psychiatric status at age 16 years (Hellgren et al. 1994) These results led them to recommend that all children in their late preschool years should be assessed for DAMP. That is what we think, too, provided the findings are discussed with the teachers. We are aware of evidence in support of the self-fulfilling prophecy, that teachers form inappropriately low expectations of children labelled as being of low ability (Rosenthal and Jacobson 1968). We do not believe, however, that teachers would make such naive assumptions if they had been briefed by a school paediatrician wise enough not to label a 5-year-old child as having an SLD but honest enough to explain that the child may have a neurodevelopmental disorder and to ask that the teacher monitor the child's progress in specific functions.

Nor do we believe that if clinicians are honest with parents it is unethical to seek evidence of SLDs by neurodevelopmental assessment at the age of 5 – as do those (Barlow et al. 1998) who regard such individual clinical assessments as a screening procedure with too many false-positive responses and no proven prospect of a cure. Most parents can understand and appreciate that the purpose of early identification of SLDs is to try to improve the quality of their children's lives. One cannot do this by turning a blind eye to a learning problem until it causes a crisis – such as the child truanting – because there is a chance it will resolve. It often does not. Equally, parents should be told that while there can be no guarantee yet that a biologically based SLD can be mitigated, because of the vagaries of development, there are teaching methods and therapies that have worked. Of course there is need for a great deal more research into early intervention, particularly an analysis of the specific effects of procedures and their experimental trial in school; but nothing ventured, nothing won!

Finally those whose responsibility it is to provide services need to know the size of the problem of SLDs in order to estimate the resources that are needed to deal with them. Authorities must be informed by practitioners of a realistic demand for services and respond with a budget that they will seek to implement as and when the finance and specialist staff can be made available. It is a defeatist attitude that sees no point in advising what is thought to be necessary because the services do not exist. In making recommendations medical and educational practitioners must work together, adamantly stating what help a child needs but when necessary giving more practicable advice about second-best alternatives.

There is a major challenge for health services to set up effective multidisciplinary services in schools. In many countries this is now the aim. Perhaps the necessary impetus to do so will come when all 3-year-old children are offered places in nursery school (as the UK government has recently promised). School health services could then be really integrated with the preschool services, and markers of SLDs could be identified and help offered at the age of 3 to 4 years instead of later, when help may have less chance of succeeding and secondary behavioural problems may have already developed, because of the child's basic learning difficulty. Thus early identification and planned management of the child who does have a problem can lead to effective secondary prevention of specific learning disorders, or, as we prefer, neurodevelopmental disorders.

REFERENCES

American Psychiatric Association. (1994) *Diagnostic and Statistical Manual of Mental Disorders.* 4th ed (DSM-IV). Washington, DC: American Psychiatric Association.

Barlow J, Stewart-Brown S, Fletcher J. (1998). Systematic review of the school entry examination. *Archives of Disease in Childhood* 78: 301–11.

Bax M, Hart H, Jenkins S. (1990) *Child Development and Child Health: The Preschool Years.* London: Blackwell Scientific Publications.

Beitchman JH, Young AR. (1997) Learning disorders with a special emphasis on reading disorders: a review of the past 10 years. *Journal of the American Academy of Child and Adolescent Psychiatry* 36: 1020–32.

Benton AL. (1975) Developmental dyslexia: neurological aspects. In: Freedlander WJ, editor. *Advances in Neurology* 17: 1–47. New York: Raven Press.

Borström I, Elbro C. (1997) Prevention of dyslexia in kindergarten: effects of phoneme awareness training of dyslexia with children of dyslexic parents. In: Hulme C, Snowling M, editors. *Dyslexia: Biology, Cognition and Intervention.* London: Whurr Publishers.

Cadman D, Walter SD, Chambers LW, et al. (1988) Predicting problems in school performance from preschool health, development and behavioural assessment. *Canadian Medical Association Journal* 139: 31–6.

Chazan M. (1980) *Some of Our Children: The Early Education of Children with Special Needs.* London: Open Books.

de Hirsch K, Jansky JJ. (1966) Early prediction of reading, writing and spelling ability. *British Journal of Disorders of Communication* 1: 99–108.

Evrard P. (1997) Neuroprotection. *Developmental Medicine and Child Neurology* 39: 717. (Editorial).

Fergusson DM, Lynsky MT. (1997) Early reading difficulties and later conduct problems. *Journal of Child Psychology and Psychiatry* 38: 899–907.

Fitzherbert K. (1982) Communication with teachers on the health surveillance of school children. *Maternal and Child Health,* March 1982, 100–3.

Fletcher-Flinn C, Elmes H, Strugnell D. (1997) Visual-perceptual and phonological factors in the acquisition of literacy among children with congenital developmental coordination disorder. *Developmental Medicine and Child Neurology* 39: 158–66.

Frith U. (1978) Spelling difficulties. *Journal of Child Psychology and Psychiatry* 19: 279–85. (Annotation).

Gaddes WH, Edgell D. (1993) *Learning Disabilities and Brain Function.* 3rd ed. New York: Springer-Verlag.

Gillberg IC, Gillberg C, Groth J. (1989) Children with preschool minor neurodevelopmental disorders. V: Neurodevelopmental profiles at age 13. *Developmental Medicine and Child Neurology* 31: 14–24.

Gross-Tsur V, Manor O, Shalev RS. (1996) Developmental dyscalculia: prevalence and demographic features. *Developmental Medicine and Child Neurology* 38: 25–33.

Hellgren L, Gillberg CI, Bagenholm A, Gillberg C. (1994) Children with deficits in attention, motor control and perception (DAMP) almost grown up: psychiatric and personality disorders at age 16 years. *Journal of Child Psychology and Psychiatry* 35: 1255–77.

Henderson ES, Barnett A, Henderson L. (1994) Visuospatial difficulties and clumsiness: on the interpretation of conjoined deficits. *Journal of Child Psychology and Psychiatry* 35: 961–9.

Holland WW. (1974) Screening for disease: taking stock. *Lancet* 2: 1494–7.

Hunt JV, Cooper BAB, Tooley WH. (1988) Very low birth weight infants at 8 and 11 years of age: role of neonatal illness and family status. *Pediatrics* 82: 596–603.

Ingram TTS. (1959) Specific developmental disorders of speech in childhood. *Brain* 82: 450–67.

— (1971) Specific learning difficulties in childhood. *British Journal of Educational Psychology* 41: Part 1.

Jansky J, de Hirsch K. (1972) *Preventing Reading Failure: Prediction, Diagnosis, Intervention.* New York: Harper and Row.

Kadesjö B, Gillberg C. (1998) Attention deficits and clumsiness in Swedish 7-year-old children. *Developmental Medicine and Child Neurology* 40: 796–804.

Landgren M, Petterson R, Kjellman B, Gillberg C. (1996) ADHD, DAMP and other neurodevelopmental/psychiatric disorders in 6-year-old children: epidemiology and co-morbidity. *Developmental Medicine and Child Neurology* 38: 891–906.

Leach DJ. (1981) Early screening for school learning difficulties: efficacy, problems, and alternatives. *British Psychological Society (Occasional Papers), Volume 5, No. 2.* p 46–60.

Lewis C, Hitch GJ, Walker P. (1994) The prevalence of specific arithmetic difficulties and specific reading difficulties in 9- to 10-year-old boys and girls. *Journal of Child Psychology and Psychiatry* **35**: 283–92.

Lindsay GA. (1979) Early identification of learning difficulties: a critique. Paper given to the British Psychological Society, Oxford, September 1979.

Maw AR. (1995) *Glue Ear in Childhood.* Clinics in Developmental Medicine No. 135. London: Mac Keith Press.

Office of Population Censuses and Surveys. (1977) *Demographic Review: A Report on Population in Great Britain.* Series DR No. 1. London: Her Majesty's Stationery Office.

Pennington B. (1991) *Diagnosing Learning Disorders.* New York: The Guilford Press.

Peters SAF, Grievink EH, van Bon WHJ, et al. (1997) The contribution of risk factors to the effect of early otitis media with effusion on later language, reading, and spelling. *Developmental Medicine and Child Neurology* **39**: 31–9.

Polnay L. (1989) Child health surveillance. *BMJ* **299**: 1351–2.

— (1995) *Health Needs of School Age Children.* London: British Paediatric Association.

Pugh E, Mansfield K, Clague H, Mattinson P. (1995) Children with asthma in schools: an opportunity for 'healthy alliances' between health and education authorities. *Health Trends* **27 (4)**: 127–9.

Rosenthal R, Jacobson L. (1968) *Pygmalion in the Classroom.* New York: Holt.

Shalev RS, Auerbach J, Gross-Tsur V. (1995) Developmental dyscalculia: behavioural and attentional aspects: a research note. *Journal of Child Psychology and Psychiatry* **36**: 1261–8.

Shapiro BK, Palmer FB, Antell S, et al. (1987) *Neurodevelopmental Precursors of Learning Disability: Final Report.* Springfield [VA]: National Technical Information Service, US Department of Commerce.

— — Wachtel RC, Capute AJ. (1983) Issues in the early identification of specific learning disability. *Journal of Developmental and Behavioral Pediatrics* **5 (1)**: 15–20.

Share DL, Silva PA, Adler CJ. (1987) Factors associated with reading-plus-spelling retardation and specific spelling retardation. *Developmental Medicine and Child Neurology* **29**: 72–84.

Silver AA, Hagin RA. (1990) *Disorders of Learning in Childhood.* New York: John Wiley and Sons.

Slack P. (1980) School nursing in the USA: lessons we can learn. *Nursing Times,* March 27, 557–8.

Sonnander K. (1987) Parental developmental assessment of 18-month-old children: reliability and predictive value. *Developmental Medicine and Child Neurology* **29**: 351–62.

Tallal P, Allard L, Miller S, Curtiss S. (1997) Academic outcomes of language-impaired children. In: Hulme C, Snowling M, editors. *Dyslexia: Biology, Cognition and Intervention.* London: Whurr Publishers.

Wedell K, Lindsay GA. (1980) Early identification procedures: what have we learned? *Journal of Remedial Education* **15**: 130–5.

Whitmore K. (1985) *Health Services in Schools: A New Look.* London: Spastics International Medical Publications.

— Bax M. (1986) The school entry medical examination. *Archives of Disease in Childhood* **61**: 807–17.

— — (1988) Screening or examining? *Developmental Medicine and Child Neurology* **30**: 673–6. (Annotation).

Wilson JMG, Junger G. (1968) *Principles and Practice of Screening for Disease.* WHO Public Health Papers No. 34. Geneva: World Health Organization.

INDEX

(Page numbers in *italics* refer to figures and tables.)

carbamazepine 277
cell-surface stimulation patterns, memory 46
central stimulants 275
cerebral blood flow
    funtional MRI 249
    regional 247
cerebral cortex
    damage 45, 48
    development 27, 28-29
    long-term memory storage 43, 46-49
    modules 36
    postnatal maturation 31-32
cerebral dysfunction, minimal 7, 8, 19, 228
cerebral dysfunction syndrome, minimal 7
cerebral hemispheres
    dominance 33-34, 37-42
    localization of function *36*
cerebral inhibition, reciprocal 39-40
cerebral morphogenesis 26-27
cerebral palsy 5, 20
child
    gifted and brain changes 18-19
    informing about diagnosis 271
    retarded 6
Children's Embedded Figures Test 108
choreiform dyskinesia 182
chromosomal aberrations, attention deficit 149
clomipramine 276
clozapine 276
clumsiness 121, 123-124
    dyslexia 88
    maturational delay 123, 125
    normal variance 123, 125
clumsy child syndrome *see* developmental coordi-
    nation disorder (DCD)
cocktail party syndrome 54, 55-56
Code of Practice of Department of Education
    (UK; 1994) 15-16
coeliac disease, overactivity 51
cognitive ability 14
cognitive development
    Groningen Perinatal Project 178-183, *184,* 185
    low-birthweight infants *170-173*
    social class 173
    visual–spatial 107
cognitive dysfunction, risk factors 169, 173
cognitive functioning, impulsivity 137-138
cognitive learning 59-61
coma 50
common environment 158
communication
    preverbal 57
    skills 16
comorbidity 282-283
comprehension 58, 59
    deficits and reading tests 237-238

computed tomography (CT) in autism 254
computer-aided training, autism 273
computer-assisted learning 268
conduct disorders
    ADHD distinction 138-140
    DAMP 147
consciousness 25, 49-50
consonant–vowel
    pair discrimination by infants 198-199, *201*
    transition stretching 206
corpus callosum
    absence 39
    dyslexia 83
cortical arousal loss 50
Crichton Active Vocabulary Scale 106
cross-cultural learning problem diagnosis 213
cultural factors, learning disorders 214

D
DAMP *135,* 140-148
    adolescence 146-147
    autism 143
    background factors 144
    case history 151
    central stimulants 275
    clinical course 144-147
    comorbid behavioural problems 147-148
    components 140, *141*
    conduct disorders 147
    definition 140-141
    diagnosis *141,* 142-143
    dyslexia 146
    early school years 146
    epidemiology 144
    infancy 145-146
    language problems 142-143
    motor function control 144
    motor–perceptual difficulties 145
    outcome 148
    outlook for children 289-290
    perceptual problems 142
    pre-school children 146
    preadolescence 146-147
    psychiatric problems 147
    severity 143
    sex ratio 144
    speech problems 142-143
DCD *see* developmental coordination disorder
deafness, central 62
deficits in attention, motor control, and perception
    see DAMP
déjà fait/déjà vu 44
Dejerine syndrome *104*
delinquency, reading difficulties 90-91
dendrites 29-30
dendritic spines 30

297

development 182-183, *184,* 185
genetic studies 162-163
global 62
identification at age of 5 years 227-229, 243
　　Brussels study 234-236, *237*
mental retardation differentiation 11
neurodevelopmental tests *238,* 239-240
professional approaches 4-5
psychosocial factors 221-224
risk factors 166
severe global 274
social environment 215
specific 1, 6, 9, 19-20
tests for schoolchildren 230-234
see also learning difficulties; SLD
learning-disabled, terminology 9
length judgement 232
lexical retrieval 233
lexicon 60-61
literacy 265
learning model 265-266
practice sessions 264-265
low-birthweight (LBW) infants 168-169, *170-172,*
173
neuropathological correlates of learning disor-
　　ders 169
socioeconomic status 216

M
MacArthur Communicative Development
　　Inventory 197, 203
magnetic resonance imaging (MRI) *see* imaging
magnetoencephalography (MEG) 251-252
magnocellular neuronal system abnormalities 193
magnocellular visual pathways 82, 83
male prevalence, reading disorders 214
male sex, cognitive dysfunction development 169
malnutrition, brain growth spurt 85
mamillary bodies 45
management of learning difficulties 259
mathematical disorder tests 238-239
meaning, literacy 265
memory 42-49
cell-surface stimulation patterns 46
conditioned sequence 54-55
declarative 42
deficits 240
explicit 42-43
false 44
implicit 42-43
localization 43-44
long-term 43-44
　　storage failure 48-49
molecular 47-48
motor 55
recall 42-43

reflex 42-43
saving 44-45
search 44
selective 43
sentence 240
short-term 43
attention 50
deficit 239
reading scores 233
tests for schoolchildren 233
storage 25, 44-45
synapses 46
time sequence 44
trace 24
verbal-sequential 240
meningitis, learning disability risk 281
mental age 6
mental disability 4
mental handicap 12
mental ratio 5
mental retardation 4, 11
causes 4-5
cultural/familial model 215
N-methyl D-aspartate *see* NMDA
methylphenidate 138, 253
microdomains 10
migraine, familial hemiplegic 113
mind 25
mirror interferences 39
mirror writing 110
motor coordination 96
DAMP 140, 141
motor development, impaired 88
motor learning 55
disorders 234-235
DCD 119
motor movements, writing 96
motor processes, DCD 128
motor skills 55
multisensory approaches 266
musical tone recognition/memory 35
mutism, akinetic 50
myelination 30-31
myelinogenesis, MRI 31, *32*

N
narcolepsy 277
National Commission on Education (UK; 1996)
259
National Joint Committee on Learning Disabilities
(USA) 9, 10
neurodevelopmental assessment 228
school-entrant health examinations 229-230
neurodevelopmental difficulties, language disor-
　　ders 235
neurodevelopmental dysfunction 20

301

right hemisphere syndrome, dyscalculia 112
risk factors
    learning disorders 166-168
    outcome measures *176*, 177
    peri-/pre-natal 168-169, *170-172*, 173-174
risperidone 276
Rolandic motor strip 56

S

Schonell Graded Word Spelling Test 99
school doctors/nurses 286-289
school-entrant health examinations 227-229
    abridged neurodevelopmental examination 240-242
    comprehensive 229-230
    diagnostic value for outcome 236, *237*
    neurodevelopmental assessment 229-230
    tests
        correlation with specific learning disorders 236, *238*
        learning disorders 230-234
        selection 237-240
schooling, effective 259-260
schools
    integrated health and education service 285-286
    multidisciplinary services 290
search, memories 44
second messengers 47, 48
selective serotonin reuptake inhibitors (SSRIs) 276-277
self-esteem
    lack 90
    low in DAMP 147
self-management, learning 261-262
semantic categorization deficit 237
semantics 56
sensory channels 266
sentence memory 240
sequential processing, dyslexia 83
serotonin, selective reuptake inhibitors 276-277
service administrator, views on SLDs 13-16
shoulder girdle movements in writing 96-97
simultanagnosia 237, 239-240
single photon emission computed tomography (SPECT) 247, 248
    ADHD *255*
    autism 253
    dyslexia 254-255
skill
    competence measurement 14
    learning hierarchy 260-261
SLD 1
    classifications 1, *2*, 3-4
    definitions 12
    professional approaches 4-5

researcher views 13-16
service administrator views 13-16
terminology 12-19
smoking 280
social class
    cognitive development 173
    perinatal risk factors 186
    protective effects 220-221
    reading environment 218
    risk factors for learning disorders 213
social conditions, cognitive dysfunction development 169, 173
social environment 215
social factors
    behavioural problem links 219-220
    cognitive development correlations 216-217
    comorbid problems 220
    interventions 221
    single disorders 220
social isolation, SSRIs 277
sociocultural disadvantage 15
sociocultural factors 214
socioeconomic status 213-214
    cognitive development 214
    factors for children at risk 221
    low-birthweight infants 216
    people with learning disorders 218
sodium valproate 277
soul 25
Southern California Sensory Integration Test 142
spatial reasoning weakness, dyscalculia 114-115
special educational treatment 15
specific developmental disorders 1, 3
specific learning disability/disorder 1, 6, 9, 19-20
    see also learning disability/disorder; SLD;
        learning difficulties
speech
    absence 55
    acquisition with brain damage 61
    centre 38
    DAMP 142-143
    delayed development and dysgraphia 102
    delayed learning 61-63
    development 57
    developmental delay 61-62
        with dyslexia 63-65
    expressive 35
    glue ear in slow development 61
    language absence 55
    left-ear dominance 38
    motor learning 55-58
    phonological system 56
    rate 58
    region localization 32
    sound formants 192
    without language 54

spelling
    assessment of competence 98
    auditory retrieval 99
    dyslexia 98-99
    see also dysgraphia
statoacoustic system 54
status epilepticus 49
stereotyped responses 53
Stott Test of Motor Performance 88
stratum, ADHD pathogenesis 252-253
strephosymbolia 65, 110
striatal cortex, dyslexia 84
stupidity 4, 5
Sturge–Weber syndrome, dyscalculia 113
support groups 272-273
symbol systems in language 60
synapses 46
syntax 56
    development 58

T
tactile stimuli, double 237
    discrimination of two points 239-240
Tallal Repetition Test 194, *197*
task analysis 268
teachers 13
    informing about diagnosis 272
    liaison with health services 287-288
    school health service contribution 288-289
teaching
    addressing difficulty 264-266
    barriers to effective practice 263
    differentiation 266-267
    direct instruction 267-268
    effective 259-260, 263-264
    focus on individual 264
    practice sessions 264-265, 267
    students with specific learning difficulties
        264-268
    supporting learning 267
temporal lobe 41
    ablation and memory loss 48
    language recognition 78
temporal processing
    language acquisition 200-201
    measures 197
temporoparietal dysfunction, bilateral 104
testosterone 80
thalamus 45
thinking strategies 262
thought 59-60
tics 276

Tourette syndrome 150, 255-256
    ADHD 150
    dyscalculia 113, 114, 115-116
    neuroleptics 276
toxic substances, fetal exposure 173-174
transitional cues in language 192
triple code model for dyscalculia 111
tuberous sclerosis 149
Turner syndrome 113

U
uncal lesions 45
underachievement, educational 6

V
verbal auditory agnosia *255*
verbal memory, writing 97
verbal reasoning 60
verbal-sequential memory 240
very-low-birthweight (VLBW) infants 168-169,
    170-172, 173
vision, reading 77
visual association area 34
    reading 35, 80-81
visual cortex 80
visual discrimination 232
visual function 88
visual input 81-82
visual pathway defects 82
visual perception 232
visual-habituation/recognition-memory task in in-
    fants 199-200
vocabulary, spatial 61

W
Wada test 33-34
Wechsler Intelligence Scale for Children 88
Wernicke's area 32
    damage 67
    dyslexia 83, 84
    position 38
word
    recognition in language area of temporal lobe
        78
    shape learning 78
word-blindness 4, 65, 78
writing
    normal development 96-97
    skills 69
    verbal memory 97
    see also dysgraphia

NOTES

NOTES

NOTES

NOTES

NOTES

NOTES